Pharmacotherapy of Depression

Pharmacotherapy of Depression

Applications for the Outpatient Practitioner

Edited by

JAY D. AMSTERDAM

Depression Research Unit
University of Pennsylvania
School of Medicine
Philadelphia, Pennsylvania

MARCEL DEKKER, INC. New York • Basel

Library of Congress Cataloging--in--Publication Data

Pharmacotherapy of depression: applications for the outpatient practitioner / edited by Jay D. Amsterdam.
p. cm.
Includes bibliographical references.
Includes index.
ISBN 0-8247-8209-7 (alk. paper)
1. Depression, Mental-- --Chemotherapy. 2. Antidepressants.
I. Amsterdam, Jay D.
[DNLM: 1. Antidepressive Agents-- --therapeutic use. 2. Depression-- --drug therapy. WM 171 P5365]
RC533.P43 1990
616.85'27061-- --dc20
DNLM/DLC
for Library of Congress 90-3834
CIP

MARCEL DEKKER, INC.
270 Madison Avenue, New York, New York 10016

Current printing (last digit):
10 9 8 7 6 5 4 3 2 1

PRINTED IN THE UNITED STATES OF AMERICA

Preface

In his timeless treatise, *The Anatomy of Melancholy*, Robert Burton described the affective disorders as a tapestry of symptoms which are different for each person and never constant within the same individual. "The tower of Babel, never yielded such confusion of tongues as the chaos of melancholy doth variety of symptoms. . . . There is in all melancholy *similitudo dissimilis*, . . . and as in a river we swim in the same place, though not in the same numerical waters . . . so the same disease yields diversity of symptoms."

In spite of exciting research advances in the field of neuroscience and an increasing clinical sophistication of "biologically oriented" neuropsychiatrists, in the broader scope it appears that not much has changed, since Burton's day, in our clinical approach to mood disorders. Depressive illness, in its tapestry of presentation, continues to confound clinicians and represents one of America's greatest silent epidemics. Despite the availability of effective antidepressant medications and specific psychotherapeutic interventions, depression continues to be one of the most misunderstood, underrecognized, and undertreated illnesses in the United States. Its incidence may be as high as 20% of the population, with about 5% experiencing a major depressive episode which necessitates medical intervention. Even when the illness is recognized, rarely does the sufferer receive adequate treatment. This is the case even by well-trained psychiatrists! Unfamiliarity with the clinical presentation of depressive illness, the persistence of a "psychopolitical cold war" between the psychodynamicists and psychobiologists, and a reluctance to apply psychopharmacologic treatment strategies in a consistent and aggressive fashion has now led to the emergence of a new syndrome called "refractory depression." As a consequence, millions of individuals seen in family practitioners' and psychiatrists' offices usually go undiagnosed or inadequately treated, and are condemned to live in the shadows of their chronic mood disturbance, exposed to an increased morbidity and greater risk of suicide. More than one study has demonstrated that the majority of completed suicides have occurred in patients with depressive illness, and more than 70% of these individuals had visited a physician within one month of their death! These are sobering statistics that mandate a wider recognition of affective illness by the medical community, and a clearer understanding of the current diagnostic and treatment approaches which are available. It is troubling that fewer than 20% of depressed patients under the care of a psychiatrist actually receive appropriate intervention with antidepressant medications. And these percentages are even lower for other medical specialties. The explanations for this difficult situation are complex and include factors like the paucity of psychopharmacologic training courses in medical and psychiatric residency programs, dependence on the *Physicians' Desk Reference* as the ultimate guide to medication selection and dosing regimens, a lack of familiarity with older antidepressants like monoamine oxidase inhibitors or the newer second generation antidepressants, fear of the legal profession which engenders a "defensive therapeutic posture" and a tendency to practice "overly" timid medicine, and a philosophical/historical orientation that all psychiatric illnesses (especially affective disorders) are of psychodynamic origin and primarily require psychotherapy (with medication used for adjunctive treatment).

Therefore, when the publishers approached me about the possibility of editing a book on antidepressant treatment strategies for use by the office-based physician, it was in this context that I agreed to assemble a comprehensive guidebook for general practitioners. It is not, however, meant to be a "cookbook" or "how-to" manual for treating depression, but rather a guidebook stressing clinically relevant concepts of a practical and utilitarian nature. As a consequence, the book has been divided into three broad areas of selected interest. The first presents chapters on differential diagnosis, the usefulness of biochemical and neuroendocrine tests in depressed patients, and the most recent concepts of psychopharmacology and how antidepressant drug therapies may be working. The second area attempts to focus on the use of specific pharmacologic treatment modalities, including general guidelines for the use of tricyclic antidepressants, monoamine oxidase inhibitors, lithium carbonate, anticonvulsant medications, psychostimulants, and combination drug therapies. The final chapters deal with treatment approaches to specific patient groups that are often seen in a general practitioner's office and, as a result of concurrent problems, require special attention towards antidepressant treatment. For example, these chapters include guidelines for treating depressed medically ill patients, elderly, pregnant, and adolescent patients, and patients with treatment-resistant depression.

Although the present scenario of inadequate recognition of affective disorders, and a failure to apply systematic treatment approaches to patients with these illnesses is troubling, there is a brighter side to the picture, and the future seems to hold promise. In this regard, there is an increasing awareness among physicians of recent diagnostic and treatment advances in the field, and the lay community is finally beginning to view affective illness as "disease state" rather than the consequence of a "weak mind."

It is my hope, therefore, and the hope of each contributor, that our effort will assist our clinical colleagues—those practitioners in "the trenches" who constantly confront the enemy—in advancing their understanding, recognition, and treatment approaches to patients' affective disorders.

Jay D. Amsterdam

Contents

Contributors

Jay D. Amsterdam, M.D. Depression Research Unit, University of Pennsylvania School of Medicine, Philadelphia, Pennsylvania

Thomas A. Ban, M.D. Department of Psychiatry, Vanderbilt University, Nashville, Tennessee

Neil J. Berwish, M.D. Depression Research Unit, University of Pennsylvania School of Medicine, Philadelphia, Pennsylvania

Donald W. Black, M.D. Department of Psychiatry, University of Iowa College of Medicine, Iowa City, Iowa

Jerry L. Carter, M.D. Department of Psychiatry, University of Iowa Hospitals, Iowa City, Iowa

Dennis S. Charney, M.D. Psychiatry Service, West Haven VA Medical Center, West Haven; Clinical Neuroscience Research Unit, Connecticut Mental Health Center; Department of Psychiatry, Yale University School of Medicine, New Haven, Connecticut

C. Edward Coffey, M.D. Associate Professor of Psychiatry and Medicine (Neurology), Duke University Medical Center, Durham, North Carolina

Brian Cook, D.O. Assistant Professor, Department of Psychiatry, University of Iowa College of Medicine and VA Medical Center, Iowa City, Iowa

Sharon M. Curlik, D.O. Assistant Professor, Department of Psychiatry, Medical College of Pennsylvania, Philadelphia Geriatric Center, Philadelphia, Pennsylvania

Pedro L. Delgado, M.D. Psychiatry Service, West Haven VA Medical Center, West Haven; Clinical Neuroscience Research Unit, Connecticut Mental Health Center; Department of Psychiatry, Yale University School of Medicine, New Haven, Connecticut

Josephine Elia, M.D. Department of Psychiatry, Medical College of Pennsylvania/Eastern Pennsylvania Psychiatric Institute, Philadelphia, Pennsylvania

James C. Garbutt, M.D. Department of Psychiatry, University of North Carolina School of Medicine, Chapel Hill, North Carolina

Michael Garvey, M.D. Associate Professor, Department of Psychiatry, University of Iowa College of Medicine and VA Medical Center, Iowa City, Iowa

Robert H. Gerner, M.D. Associate Research Professor, Department of Psychiatry, University of California, Los Angeles; West Los Angeles VA Medical Center; Center for Mood Disorders, Los Angeles, California

Alexander H. Glassman, M.D. Professor of Clinical Psychiatry, College of Physicians and Surgeons of Columbia University, Chief, Clinical Psychopharmacology, New York State Psychiatric Institute, New York, New York

John H. Griest, M.D. Professor of Psychiatry, Co-Director, Lithium Information Center, University of Wisconsin Center for Health Sciences, Madison, Wisconsin

Carroll W. Hughes, Ph.D. Psychiatric Research Institute, St. Francis Regional Medical Center; Department of Psychiatry, University of Kansas School of Medicine; Psychiatry Service, Wichita Veterans Administration Medical Center, Wichita, Kansas

Steven P. James, M.D. Laboratory of Human Chronobiology, Depression Research Unit, University of Pennsylvania School of Medicine, Philadelphia, Pennsylvania

James W. Jefferson, M.D. Professor of Psychiatry, Director, Center for Affective Disorders, Co-Director, Lithium Information Center, University of Wisconsin Center for Health Sciences, Madison, Wisconsin

Roger G. Kathol, M.D. Department of Psychiatry, University of Iowa Hospitals, Iowa City, Iowa

Ira Katz, M.D., Ph.D. Associate Professor, Director, Geriatric Psychiatry, Medical College of Pennsylvania, Philadelphia Geriatric Center, Philadelphia, Pennsylvania

John H. Krystal, M.D. Psychiatric Service, West Haven VA Medical Center, West Haven; Clinical Neuroscience Research Unit, Connecticut Mental Health Center; Department of Psychiatry, Yale University School of Medicine, New Haven, Connecticut

Neil M. Kurtz, M.D. Medical Director, CNS Clinical Research, Miles, Inc., Pharmaceutical Division, West Haven, Connecticut

Mark Kutcher, M.D. Department of Psychiatry, Vanderbilt University, Nashville, Tennessee

Alfred J. Lewy, M.D., Ph.D. Departments of Psychiatry, Ophthalmology and Pharmacology, Oregon Health Sciences University, Portland, Oregon

Peter T. Loosen, M.D. Departments of Psychiatry and Medicine, Vanderbilt University Medical Center and Veterans Administration Medical Center, Nashville, Tennessee

George A. Mason, Ph.D. Department of Psychiatry, University of North Carolina School of Medicine, Chapel Hill, North Carolina

Russell Noyes, Jr., M.D. Professor, Department of Psychiatry, University of Iowa College of Medicine and VA Medical Center, Iowa City, Iowa

Patricia Parmelee, Ph.D. Senior Research Psychologist, Philadelphia Geriatric Center, Philadelphia, Pennsylvania

Marcella Pascualy, M.D. Geriatric Psychiatry Fellow, Seattle Veterans Administration Medical Center, Department of Psychiatry, University of Washington School of Medicine, Seattle, Washington

Robert M. Post, M.D. Chief, Biological Psychiatry Branch, National Institute of Mental Health, Bethesda, Maryland

Arthur J. Prange, Jr., M.D. Department of Psychiatry, University of North Carolina School of Medicine, Chapel Hill, North Carolina

Sheldon H. Preskorn, M.D. Psychiatric Research Institute, St. Francis Regional Medical Center; Department of Psychiatry, University of Kansas School of Medicine; Psychiatry Service, Wichita Veterans Administration Medical Center, Wichita, Kansas

Steven P. Roose, M.D. Associate Professor of Clinical Psychiatry, College of Physicians and Surgeons of Columbia University, Research Psychiatrist, New York State Psychiatric Institute, New York, New York

Nicholas Rosenlicht, M.D. University of California, Davis, VA Medical Center, Martinez, and Center for Mood Disorders, Los Angeles, California

Janusz K. Rybakowski, M.D. Department of Psychiatry, Medical Academy of Bydgoszcz, Bydgoszcz, Poland

Robert L. Sack, M.D. Departments of Psychiatry, Ophthalmology, and Pharmacology, Oregon Health Sciences University, Portland, Oregon

Richard S. Shelton, M.D. Departments of Psychiatry and Medicine, Vanderbilt University Medical Center and Veterans Administration Medical Center, Nashville, Tennessee

George M. Simpson, M.D. Professor and Director, Clinical Psychopharmacology, Medical College of Pennsylvania/Eastern Pennsylvania Psychiatric Institute, Philadelphia, Pennsylvania

Hardeep Singh, M.D. Department of Psychiatry, Medical College of Pennsylvania/Eastern Pennsylvania Psychiatric Institute, Philadelphia, Pennsylvania

Steven M. Southwick, M.D. Psychiatric Service, West Haven VA Medical Center, West Haven; Clinical Neuroscience Research Unit, Connecticut Mental Health Center; Department of Psychiatry, Yale University School of Medicine, New Haven, Connecticut

Richard C. Veith, M.D. Director, Geriatric Research, Education and Clinical Center; American Lake Veterans Administration Medical Center; Associate Professor, Department of Psychiatry and Behavioral Sciences, University of Washington School of Medicine, Seattle, Washington

Thomas A. Wehr, M.D. Clinical Psychobiology Branch, National Institute of Mental Health, Bethesda, Maryland

Richard D. Weiner, M.D., Ph.D. Associate Professor of Psychiatry, Duke University Medical Center, Durham, North Carolina

1

Clinical Characteristics of Depressive Disorders

NEIL J. BERWISH and JAY D. AMSTERDAM

University of Pennsylvania School of Medicine
Philadelphia, Pennsylvania

INTRODUCTION

Many psychiatrists believe that depression has a physical basis, reflecting defects in the actions of neurotransmitters and their receptors, alterations in biorhythms, and dysfunction of the neuroendocrine system. The success of tricyclic and other antidepressants in a large percentage of patients tends to support this hypothesis.

At present, the diagnosis of depression is based upon clinical symptoms. Depressive episodes may begin after a stressful event, although more commonly they begin insidiously. Unfortunately, these disorders often go undiagnosed, and when they are recognized, they are rarely treated adequately, despite the availability of effective medications. The symptoms of depressive illness (Table 1) are not always easy to recognize, and some patients may lack the most obvious symptom—that of a depressed mood. Some may also have concurrent medical or psychiatric disorders that might initially appear to account for the patient's symptoms, and many depressed patients will present clinically with a bewildering array of somatic complaints. Therefore, a high index of clinical suspicions must be maintained to more fully appreciate the myriad of presentations of depressive illness.

Table 1 Summary of DSM-III-R Criteria for Major Depressive Episode

A. At least five of the following symptoms have been present during the same 2-week period and represent a change from previous functioning; at least one of the symptoms is either (1) depressed mood, or (2) loss of interest or pleasure.
   1. Depressed mood most of the day, nearly every day, by subjective or objective report.
   2. Markedly diminished interest or pleasure in all, or almost all, activities most of the day, nearly every day.
   3. Significant weight loss or gain when not dieting, or decrease or increase in appetite nearly every day.
   4. Insomnia or hypersomnia nearly every day.
   5. Psychomotor agitation or retardation nearly every day (observable by others).
   6. Fatigue or loss of energy nearly every day.
   7. Feelings of worthlessness or excessive or inappropriate guilt (which may be delusional) nearly every day.
   8. Diminished ability to think or concentrate, or indecisiveness nearly every day.
   9. Recurrent thoughts of death (not just fear of dying), suicidal ideation with or without a specific plan, or suicide attempt.

B. 1. It cannot be established that an organic factor initiated and maintained the disturbance.
   2. The disturbance is not a normal reaction to the death of a loved one.

EPIDEMIOLOGY

It is estimated that 20-26% of women and 8-12% of men will suffer from a major depression during their lifetime. Almost one-fourth of sufferers will experience at least one severe episode. Although current prevalence rates average 5.3% for unipolar illness and less than 0.5% for bipolar illness, lifetime risk rates average 12% and 0.6%, respectively. Women suffer unipolar depression twice as often as men, whereas bipolar disorder has a 1:1 gender ratio.

Several lines of evidence suggest a genetic contribution to the disease. Twin studies have demonstrated as much as 70% concordance in identical (monozygotic) twins with bipolar disorder and a 20% concordance rate in fraternal (dizygotic) twins, compared with the 5% risk in the general population. Recent studies among the Pennsylvania Amish have demonstrated a high rate of bipolar illness, which is thought to be associated with a dominant gene located on the short arm of chromosome 11. Other studies have suggested a linkage of bipolar disorder with certain markers (e.g., Xg blood type and color blindness) on the X chromosome. However, these studies have been difficult to reproduce and remain controversial.

SYMPTOMS OF MAJOR DEPRESSION

Symptoms (see Table 1) most often develop insidiously over weeks to months. Classically there is no apparent reason for the patient's symptoms, but it is common for an episode to begin after a psychosocial stressor. The most frequently reported symptom is an altered mood (dysphoria), usually, although not invariably, reported as feeling sad, "down," or "blue." This may also manifest as feelings of hopelessness, worthlessness, or poor self-esteem. A nearly universal symptom is anergy, or loss of energy, frequently accompanied by fatigue, loss of motivation, loss of interest, difficulty in initiating activities, and difficulty in completing activities once started. These are often the presenting complaints. Feelings of worthlessness and lowered self-esteem are intensified by the impairment in daily function, and self-reproach and guilt are common. In severe depressions, ruminations of guilt may become delusional.

Apathy may be accompanied by anhedonia, or the inability to feel pleasure or enjoyment in previously pleasurable activities; libido is frequently impaired as well. Patients must be asked specifically about this symptom; it is volunteered infrequently, particularly if sexual performance is affected along with desire.

Changes in cognitive function are commonplace, with complaints of slowed or unclear thinking, lapses in memory, and impaired concentration. Patients may fear they are "getting senile" or "going crazy." The severely depressed patient may be slowed motorically as well as psychically, exhibiting decreased motor activity, stilled facial expressions, and monotonic speech, which is slowed and barely audible. Word content may be sparse, and answers to questions delayed or absent.

In contrast, patients may report nervousness and anxiety, increased worry, irritability, panicky feelings, or subjective agitation. Objective signs of agitation may include jitteriness, nail-biting, increased smoking, handwringing, pacing, or full-fledged panic attacks. Physical complaints are common, and may include changes in gastrointestinal function, tachycardia, dyspnea, diaphoresis, paresthesias, headaches, and "shakiness." These somatic symptoms may become continuous or incapacitating and are frequently the original complaints made to the primary care physician.

There may be a diurnal variation in mood or energy. Classically, the morning is worse, with some improvement as the day progresses, but this order may be reversed, with deterioration as the day goes on. This symptom is thought to result from alterations in the diencephalic "biological clock."

Disturbances in sleep are prominent symptoms of unipolar depression. Disruptions in sleep patterns include difficulties falling asleep (early insomnia), waking intermittently during the night (middle insomnia), or waking in the early hours of the morning (late insomnia; early-morning awakening). Hypersomnia, or oversleeping, may exist alone or following difficulties in initiating or maintaining sleep. Both insomnia and hypersomnia may be accompanied by daytime fatigue or sleepiness, for which naps may not provide relief.

Patterns of appetite disturbances may encompass increased or decreased desire for food. In either event, patients may actually eat more or less than usual, and tend to gain or lose weight accordingly. They frequently complain that food lacks taste, and that they eat only because they have to. Some patients will crave certain types of food, such as "sweets" and foods high in carbohydrate or fat content (cookies, crackers, pastas, ice creams, and chocolate). Depressed patients with the symptom cluster of hyperphagia and hypersomnia are sometimes described as having "atypical" depression, and these patients may respond better to treatment with monoamine oxidase inhibitors.

Thoughts of death are common, from death wishes without suicidal ideation to suicidal ideation or plans. Actions taken in furtherance of suicidal ideas or plans, such as purchasing a supply of pills or a gun, setting affairs in order, or giving away possessions, indicate a patient at extreme risk for attempting suicide. The patient at this point may feel that suicide has become the only alternative for relief from pain. Prompt hospitalization may be lifesaving and ensure more aggressive treatment. Another high-risk period may occur after initiating antidepressant therapy, if the patient's dysphoria and suicidal ideation remain active while energy increases to the point at which self-destructive plans can be implemented.

Psychotic symptoms may sometimes occur in severe depression and lead to an erroneous diagnosis of schizophrenia or "schizoaffective" disorder. Delusional symptoms in schizophrenia seem bizarre and devoid of affective content, and tend to involve themes of persecution, or thought or body control by outside agents. In depression, the delusional focus tends to be on personal inadequacy, death, disease, nihilism, or deserved punishment.

The subjective feeling of an endogenous depression is different from the "normal" depressive feelings experienced after the loss of a loved one (i.e., grief or bereavement) and these are not considered biochemical disorders. The reaction to loss may not be immediate, but onset rarely occurs after the first 2-3 months. Although symptoms such as anorexia, weight loss, and insomnia are frequent in bereavement, it is uncommon to encounter morbid preoccupation with worthlessness, prolonged and marked functional impairment, and marked psychomotor retardation. If these symptoms are present, or if bereavement lasts longer than 6-12 months, it suggests the superimposition of a major depression, often called a prolonged grief reaction.

OTHER PRESENTATIONS OF DEPRESSIVE DISORDER

Dysthymic depressions are similar to major depression, although less severe (Table 2). They appear to be more heterogenous in etiology than major depression, and the evidence for a clear-cut biological cause is less certain. Some dysthymic disorders occur in the setting of preexisting psychiatric disorders, whereas others may represent sequelae to, or incomplete remissions from, a previous major depressive episode. These conditions more frequently begin in the late 30s or 40s, and do not usually have a premorbid pattern of depressive symptoms. In contrast, other dysthymic disorders begin insidiously before the age of 25, and follow a protracted course. The occurrence of superimposed major depressive episodes in these individuals represents a so-called "double depression," and recovery from these episodes is often characterized by return to the premorbid dysthymic level. These illnesses may be the most common affective disorders seen in the primary care physician's office.

The depressive syndrome frequently appears in less typical forms, particularly in the very young and the elderly. The patient with "masked" depression may present with ruminations about perceived somatic symptoms, including fatigue, headache, myalgias, gastrointestinal complaints, sleep disturbances, or nearly any symptom affecting any organ system. In the face of poor symptom localization and lack of clear organic etiology, primary depressive illness should be suspected and investigated. "Secondary depressions" occasionally are associated with a host of other medical illnesses (Table 3), particularly viral infections, stroke, severe pulmonary or cardiac diseases,

Table 2 Summary of SMS-III-R Criteria for Dysthymic Disorder

A. Depressed mood (by subjective or objective report) for most of the day, more days than not, for at least 2 years; never without the symptoms in A and B for more than 2 months at a time
B. At least two of the following while depressed:
   1. Poor appetite, or overeating
   2. Insomnia or hypersomnia
   3. Low energy or fatigue
   4. Low self-esteem
   5. Poor concentration, or difficulty making decisions
   6. Feelings of hopelessness
C. No evidence of an unequivocal major depressive disorder during the first 2 years of the disturbance
D. Has never had a manic or hypomanic episode

Table 3 Illnesses Associated with Depression

Cardiac disease	Neurological disorders
Congestive heart failure	Dementias
Myocardial infarction	Multiple sclerosis
Open-heart surgery	Normal pressure hydrocephalus
Endocrine disease	Parkinson's disease
Addison's disease	Subarachnoid hemorrhage
Cushing's disease	Subdural hemorrhage
Diabetes	Stroke (CVA, TIA)
Hypoglycemia	Tumor
Hypoparathyroidism	Pulmonary disease
Hypo- or hyperthyroidism	Chronic obstructive pulmonary disease
Sheehan's syndrome	Emphysema
Gastrointestinal disease	Pneumonia
Colitis	Rheumatological disease
Irritable bowel syndrome	Rheumatoid arthritis
Hematological disease	Systemic lupus
Anemias	Viral infections
Incapacitating disorders	AIDS
All (e.g., postsurgical, traumatic)	Hepatitis
Intoxications	Influenza
Heavy metals (mercury, thallium)	Mononucleosis
Malignancy	Other
Pancreatic carcinoma	Tertiary syphilis
Uterine carcinoma	

or incapacitating illnesses. In these instances, symptoms such as anorexia, weight loss, insomnia, fatigue, motor retardation, and agitation may be caused by the primary medical illness, and as such, they may not be helpful diagnostically. The best indicators of depression are likely to be feelings of dysphoria, loss of interest and pleasure, feelings of worthlessness and guilt, and loss of libido.

Depressive symptoms are also known to follow the use of many medications (Table 4), most notably steroids, α-methyldopa, cimetidine, guanethidine, β-blocking agents, and reserpine. Drug-induced depression is the most common form of iatrogenic psychiatric disorder. In the elderly, the "pseudodementia" of depression must be differentiated from the dementias associated with the organic changes in infarction and Alzheimer's disease. Deficits of attention and memory are seen in both types of dementia, but the patient

Table 4 Commonly Used Drugs Associated with Depression

Amphetamines (withdrawal)
Anticancer drugs
Antidepressants (toxicity)
Antihypertensives
α-Methyldopa
β-Blocking agents
Clonidine
Guanethidine
Hydralazine
Reserpine
Barbiturates
Benzodiazepines
Cimetidine
Digitalis
Ethanol
L-Dopa
Phenothiazines
Steroids
Sulfonamides

with pseudodementia demonstrates an apologetic and self-reproachful awareness of his cognitive deficits, whereas the demented patient is likely to confabulate (make up) answers. Pseudodementia is characterized by a relatively rapid onset, mood changes that precede cognitive changes, and a relative stability of mood thereafter. In dementia, the onset is usually slow and insidious, mood changes follow the cognitive changes, and mood may remain labile.

BIPOLAR DISORDER

The diagnosis of bipolar disorder rests on the identification of a manic or hypomanic episode in the patient's history—only one is required, even if in the distant past. These episodes may be relatively brief and mild, or they may last many months. Such episodes usually present as periods of abnormal elation or euphoria, although they may manifest as irritability. Associated symptoms may be grandiosity or inflated self-esteem, with the feeling that one "can do anything." There may be a tremendous availability of energy, sometimes described as feeling "supercharged," often accompanied by a decreased or absent need for sleep, despite the increase in ability to accomplish physical tasks. Thoughts may seem to be racing, often jumping from one subject to another, with a distractible inability to focus concentration, and the patient may be more talkative than usual or feel pressure to keep talking. Impulsivity is common, and patients may indulge in unrestrained spending sprees, give away money, make foolish business investments, absent themselves from work, or take impulsive trips, all with disregard for potential negative consequences. Hypersexual feelings are frequent, along with increased goal-directed activity in sexual, social, or vocational spheres. Marked difficulty in occupational functioning or usual social activities or relationships, or the need for hospitalization, is the hallmark of a truly manic episode. Hypomanic episodes do not exhibit a similar level of impairment and may be far less severe, or even quite subtle. The ability to function may continue unabated, or even be enhanced by effective use of the increased energy and decreased need for sleep.

A patient with one or more episodes of major depression whose history includes at least one manic episode is usually classified as *bipolar I* subtype. A patient whose elated mood has been only hypomanic is considered *bipolar II*. With advancing age, depressive episodes are more frequent, more severe, and longer lasting than are manic or hypomanic episodes.

In contrast, *cyclothymia* represents a much milder form of bipolar disorder, characterized by numerous periods of mild hypomania and depression that usually present for more than 2 months at a time over several years. In these cases, the depressive episodes are not severe enough to be considered "major depression," and this disorder may bear the same relationship to bipolar illness as dysthymic disorder does to major depression.

A more controversial category is that of *atypical bipolar disorder*. This syndrome is essentially a subtype of the bipolar II disorder in which the hypomanic episode is extremely mild. The major depression initially may appear to exist in isolation (i.e., the diagnosis may seem to be one of unipolar major depression). Antidepressants may repeatedly "lose their effectiveness" after good therapeutic response, or there may be a series of partial responses to a variety of agents. A careful review of history may reveal vague or transient mood variations that do not reach the proportions of a hypomanic episode in number or intensity of symptoms. In addition, these patients will often have a family history of some type of bipolar disorder, postpartum depression (usually commencing several weeks to months after parturition) or thyroid disease. Another clue to atypical bipolar disease is a history of "switch" phenomenon, in which depressed patients given antidepressants may suddenly become hypomanic.

Manic and hypomanic episodes often feel very good subjectively, and patients are frequently loathe to embark on a course of treatment that promises to obliterate the elated mood or facilitated function. Nonetheless, what goes up *will* come down; the danger from uncontrolled manic or hypomanic episodes is the certainty of an abrupt plummet to the depressed state, rather than a gentle relaxation of the altered mood back to a "normal," undepressed state. Such a "crash" can occur even with antidepressant therapy in place.

CONCLUSION

In conclusion, depressive illness is extremely common, and is frequently underrecognized, underdiagnosed, and undertreated. It carries a high morbidity in terms of shattered relationships, disrupted child-rearing, alcoholism, substance abuse, unemployment, and financial loss. The most serious consequence of an unrecognized (or undertreated) depression is that of suicide: 10-15% of all deaths of patients with affective disorder are attributable to suicide, a rate 30 times higher than for the general populace. Furthermore, approximately half of completed suicides (over 28,000 people in the United States alone in 1985) suffered from major depression. It is clearly of paramount interest and importance to recognize these disorders accurately, and to institute adequate treatment promptly.

SUGGESTED READING

Akiskal, H. S. (1984). The interface of chronic depression with personality and anxiety disorders. *Psychopharm. Bull. 20*:393-398.

Akiskal, H. S. (1983). Diagnosis and classification of affective disorders: New insights from clinical and laboratory approaches. *Psychiatr. Dev. 2*:123-160.

Akiskal, H. S. (1983). Dysthymic disorder: Psychopathology of proposed chronic depressive subtypes. *Am. J. Psychiatry 140*:11-20.

Akiskal, H.S. (1981). Subaffective disorder: Dysthymic, cyclothymic and bipolar II disorders on the "borderline" realm. *Psychiatr. Clin. North Am. 4*:25-46.

Akiskal, H. S., Rosenthal, R. H., Rosenthal, T. L., et al. (1979). Differentiation of primary affective illness from situational, symptomatic, and secondary depressions. *Arch. Gen. Psychiatry 36*:635-643.

American Psychiatric Association (1987). *Diagnostic and Statistical Manual of Mental Disorders.* 3rd ed., revised. Washington, D.C., American Psychiatric Association.

Berwish, N. J., and Amsterdam, J. D. (1986). Differentiating the types of depression. *Diagnosis 8*:92-103.

Boyd, J. H., and Weissman, M. M. (1981). Epidemiology of affective disorders: A re-examination and future directions. *Arch. Gen. Psychiatry 38*:1039-1046.

Clark, D. C., Cavanaugh, S. V., and Gibbons, R. G. (1983). The core symptoms of depression in medical and psychiatric patients. *J. Nerv. Ment. Dis. 171*:705-713.

Coryell, W. (1987). Outcome and family studies of bipolar II depression. *Psychiatr. Ann. 17*:28-31.

Coryell, W., Andreasen, N. C., Endicott, J., et al. (1987). The significance of past mania or hypomania in the course and outcome of major depression. *Am. J. Psychiatry 144*:309-315.

Coryell, W., Zimmerman, M., and Pfohl, B. (1985). Short-term prognosis in primary and secondary major depression. *J. Affect Disord. 9*:265-270.

Clayton, P. J. (1986). Bipolar illness. In *Medical Basis of Psychiatry*. Edited by G. Winokur. Philadelphia, W.B. Saunders.

Dunner, D. L. (1987). Stability of bipolar II affective disorder as a diagnostic entity. *Psychiatr. Ann. 17*:18-20.

England, J. A., Gerhard, D. S., Pauls, D. L., et al. (1987). Bipolar affective disorders linked to DNA markers on chromosome 11. *Nature 325*:783-787.

Gershon, E. S., Weissman, M. M., Guroff, J. J., et al. (1986). Validation of criteria for major depression through controlled family study. *J. Affect. Disord. 11*:125-131.

Gullege, A. D., and Calabrese, J. R. (1988). Diagnosis of anxiety and depression. *Med. Clin. North Am. 72*:753-763.

Guze, S. B., and Robins, E. (1970). Suicide and primary affective disorders. *Br. J. Psychiatry 117*:437-438.

Kamerow, D. B. (1988). Anxiety and depression in the medical setting: An overview. *Med. Clin. North Am. 72*:745-751.

Keeler, L. L., and Othmer, E. (1987). Atypical bipolar disorder: Is it a distinct entity? *Psychiatr. Ann. 17*:21-27.

Keller, M. B., Klerman, G. L., Lavori, P. W., et al. (1984). Long-term outcome of major depression. *JAMA 252*:788-792.

Kidd, K. K., Egeland, J. A., Molthan, L., et al. (1984). Amish study, IV: Genetic linkage study of pedigrees of bipolar probands. *Am. J. Psychiatry 141*:1042-1048.

Klerman, G. L. (1987). The classification of bipolar disorders. *Psychiatr. Ann. 17*: 13-17.

Risch, N., Baron, M., and Mendlewicz, J. (1986). Assessing the role of X-linked inheritance in bipolar-related major affective disorder. *J. Psychiatr. Res. 20*:275-288.

Roose, S. P., Glassman, A. H., and Walsh, B. T. (1983). Depression, delusions, and suicide. *Am. J. Psychiatry 140*:1159-1162.

Roy, A., Breier, A., Doran, A. R., et al. (1985). Life events in depression: Relationships to subtypes. *J. Affect. Disord. 9*:143-148.

Schlesser, M. A., and Altschuler, M. Z. (1983). The genetics of affective disorder: Data, theory, and clinical applications. *Hosp. Commun. Psychiatry 34*:415-421.

Weissman, M. M., Gershon, E. S., Kidd, K. K., et al. (1984). Psychiatric disorders in the relatives of probands with affective disorders. *Arch. Gen. Psychiatry 41*: 13-21.

Winokur, G. (1986). Unipolar depression. In *Medical Basis of Psychiatry*. Edited by G. Winokur. Philadelphia, W.B. Saunders.

Young, M. A., and Grabler, P. (1985). Rapidity of symptom onset in depression. *Psychiatry Res. 16*:309-315.

2

Current Status of the Receptor Sensitivity Hypothesis of Antidepressant Action:

Implications for the Treatment of Severe Depression

DENNIS S. CHARNEY, STEVEN M. SOUTHWICK,
PEDRO L. DELGADO, and JOHN H. KRYSTAL

West Haven VA Medical Center
West Haven, Connecticut
Connecticut Mental Health Center
and Yale University School of Medicine
New Haven, Connecticut

INTRODUCTION

The original catecholamine hypothesis postulated that a deficit in central nervous system (CNS) norepinephrine (NE) was responsible for depression and that the therapeutic action of antidepressants was related to an ability to increase brain NE by interfering with NE reuptake (tricyclic antidepressants) or by inhibition of monoamine oxidase (MAO) (1,2). However, this theory has recently been challenged on the basis of several observations. Some drugs that are potent NE-reuptake blockers (such as cocaine and amphetamine) are not effective antidepressants. Conversely, effective antidepressants, such as iprindole and mianserin, do not block uptake of NE or inhibit MAO. Furthermore, studies of drug metabolism or pharmacokinetics have failed to find a "dose-response" relationship between clinical improvement and NE blockade. Instead, effective antidepressants have varied markedly in their ability to effect NE reuptake. The catecholamine hypothesis has also failed to account for the temporal discrepancy between the rapid onset of NE-reuptake inhibition and delayed clinical improvement. The former occurs within hours, whereas the latter can take at least 7-14 days after the initiation of drug treatment (3,4).

A second, competing pharmacologic hypothesis of depression, the indolamine hypothesis, stated that a functional deficit in the neurotransmitter, serotonin (5-HT), produced depressive symptoms and that antidepressants worked by increasing 5-HT activity through inhibition of 5-HT reuptake or MAO (5,6). This theory has also been challenged on the same grounds as the NE hypothesis.

In recent years, with the development of more sophisticated neurobiological methodologies, investigators have increased their understanding of the multiple effects of antidepressants on neurotransmitter systems. This has resulted in a number of "receptor sensitivity" hypotheses that suggest the ability of long-term antidepressant treatment to reduce certain neurotransmitter (β- or α_2-adrenergic) receptor sensitivity or to enhance (serotonergic or α_1-adrenergic) receptor sensitivity may be related to the mechanism of action of antidepressant treatments (3,4). The goal of this chapter theses and to explore the applicability of these findings to the treatment of major depression. To develop a foundation from which to consider these hypotheses, the chapter begins with a review of the basic elements of neurotransmission.

FUNDAMENTALS OF SYNAPTIC NEUROTRANSMISSION

Information in the brain is transmitted by electrical impulses within neurons. These impulses travel through the cell's axon and cause the release of neurotransmitters from the axon terminal into the synaptic cleft. More than 36 putative neurotransmitters have now been identified. Although the general belief has been that individual neurons produce only one neurotransmitter, recent studies have shown the presence of two or more neurotransmitters within the same neuron. Of the numerous neurotransmitters now identified, norepinephrine, serotonin, dopamine, and acetylcholine have received the most attention in the study of antidepressant mechanisms.

Once neurotransmitters have been released into the synaptic cleft, they can bind to either pre- or postsynaptic receptors on the neuronal membrane. Some receptors are directly linked to channels that regulate the influx of sodium, potassium and calcium ions, and others are part of a protein complex within the cell membrane. These complexes relay information through the cell membrane that ultimately leads to activation of intracellular enzymes. The receptor complex has at least three components: The receptor recognition site, to which neurotransmitters attach, is on the outer membrane surface. Attachment of neurotransmitters to this receptor causes a conformational change that promotes complexing to the transmembrane G-protein that, when stimulated, links to the intracellular enzyme, adenylate cyclase, which then converts ATP to cyclic AMP (cAMP; also referred to as a second messenger). A cascade of biochemical events follows, ending with the phosphorylation and activation of target enzymes. Another second-messenger system, linked to the breakdown of phospholipids, is the phosphatidylinositol system, by which stimulation of G-protein activates phospholipase C, rather than adenylate cyclase. Both the cAMP and phosphatidylinositol second-messenger systems involve transmembrane activation of enzymes and are important mediators of signal transduction.

Of the numerous receptor types now identified, our primary focus will be the adrenergic and serotonergic receptors. There are at least four adrenergic receptor subtypes: β_1-, β_2- and α_1-adrenergic postsynaptic receptors, and α_2-adrenergic pre- and postsynaptic receptors. Presynaptic α_2-receptors are called autoreceptors because they mediate negative-feedback through NE in the synaptic cleft. As autoreceptors, they inhibit the firing of NE neurons.

The 5-HT receptor subtypes relevant to antidepressant action appear to be the 5-HT_1 and 5-HT_2. The 5-HT_1 is further subdivided into 5-HT_{1A}, 5-HT_{1B}, 5-HT_{1C} and 5-HT_{1D} subtypes. The 5-HT_{1A} receptor functions as an autoreceptor when located presynaptically, analogous to the α_2-adrenergic receptor. The 5-HT_2 receptor is located postsynaptically.

Neurotransmitters are removed from the synaptic cleft, once they have served their function, by reuptake into the presynaptic terminal or through metabolic degradation by MAO. Neurotransmitters that have been taken up by presynaptic mechanisms may be repackaged and released again (see Ref. 7 for review).

RECEPTOR SENSITIVITY HYPOTHESES OF ANTIDEPRESSANT ACTION

Each of the major receptor sensitivity hypotheses are discussed in light of current preclinical and clinical investigations. Clinical studies of the neurobiological effects of antidepressant drugs and therapeutic approaches based upon receptor sensitivity hypotheses of antidepressant efficacy will also be reviewed to assess the validity of the different hypotheses.

β-Adrenergic Receptor Downregulation Hypothesis

The β-adrenergic receptor downregulation hypothesis postulates that the net effect of chronic antidepressant administration is a reduction of neurotransmission through β-adrenergic receptors. The hypothesis was developed on the basis of preclinical observations that long-term, but not brief, administration of antidepressants reduce the density of brain β-adrenergic receptors and the cAMP response mediated by these receptors. Because postsynaptic β-adrenergic receptors were functionally reduced, this hypothesis appeared to be a reversal of the original low NE catecholamine hypothesis, since these new observations indicate that antidepressants decrease, rather than increase, noradrenergic function (8).

Several antidepressants, including maprotiline, nomifensine, bupropion, mianserin, citalopram, and fluoxetine, have either no effect or weak effects in reducing the β-adrenergic receptor cAMP response.

Few clinical paradigms have been developed to assess the effect of antidepressant treatments on β-receptor function in depressed patients. One method has been to measure the effect of antidepressant treatment on melatonin secretion, a pineal gland hormone under β-adrenergic control. Some, but not all, antidepressants increase the secretion of melatonin, suggesting a net increased rather than decreased effect on noradrenergic transmission (9), contrary to that predicted by the β-receptor downregulation hypothesis of antidepressant action.

Therapeutic Studies

The role of β-adrenergic receptor downregulation in the therapeutic actions of antidepressants has been evaluated indirectly by determining if a combination of the tricyclic antidepressant, desipramine, and the α_2-receptor blocker, yohimbine, would result in a more rapid antidepressant effect. This study was based on the observation that the combined antidepressant-yohimbine treatment in laboratory rats resulted in a reduction in β-adrenergic receptor function and density within 4 days of drug administration, compared with the 2-3 weeks usually required by antidepressants alone. However, the desipramine-yohimbine combination was not effective in depressed patients who, subsequently, had therapeutic responses to lithium-antidepressant combinations (10).

Another evaluation approach for clinical validity of the β-adrenergic receptor hypothesis was to determine the effects of centrally acting drugs with specific actions on β-adrenergic receptors in depressed patients. From this hypothesis, the β-receptor antagonist propranolol would be expected to improve depressive symptoms. Instead, propranolol has been implicated as a cause of depression in vulnerable individuals (11).

The β-adrenergic downregulation hypothesis also predicts that treatments that antagonize a decrease in β-receptor density should prevent antidepressant responses. High doses of triiodothyronine (T_3) increase β-adrenergic receptor density in certain brain areas and block the decrease in β-adrenergic receptor downregulation produced by imipramine and desipramine (12). However, clinical investigations indicate that T_3 augments, rather than inhibits, antidepressant effects (13).

Summary

Although not all antidepressants reduce β-adrenergic receptor function and density, the β-receptor downregulation hypothesis of antidepressant action continues to be viable and requires further testing (Table 1). However, the relative paucity of preclinical behavioral models and clinical paradigms that

Table 1 Preclinical Studies of the β-Receptor Downregulation Hypotheses of Antidepressant Action

Antidepressant category	NE-isoproterenol-mediated cAMP	β-Receptor binding	β-Receptor neurophysiological sensitivity	β-Receptor behavioral sensitivity
NE-reuptake inhibitors	↓	↓	↓0	↓
Mixed NE- and 5-HT-reuptake inhibitors	↓	↓	↓0	↓
5-HT-reuptake inhibitors	↓0	↓0	0	–
MAOI	↓	↓	↓	–
Atypical antidepressants				
Trazodone	–	↓	–	–
Bupropion	0↓	0↓	–	–
Mianserin	0↓	0↓	–	–
Nomifensine	0	0	–	–
Maprotiline	0	0↓	↓	–
ECT	↓	↓	0	↓

Symbols used: ↓ decrease; 0 no change; – not tested; averaged over different brain regions and different drugs; mixed results are indicated by more than one symbol.

are capable of assessing β-receptor function and are relevant to antidepressant actions has limited the conclusions about the therapeutic relevance of β-receptor downregulation (Table 2). To date, those clinical studies that have been conducted do not support the β-receptor downregulation hypothesis. Figure 1 illustrates schematically the hypothesized effects of antidepressant treatments on α- and β-adrenergic receptors.

α_2-Receptor Downregulation Hypothesis

Because the presynaptic α_2-adrenergic receptor inhibits NE neuronal activity, this hypothesis proposes that net NE function is increased by chronic antidepressant administration. In preclinical studies, the effect of antidepressants on α_2-adrenergic receptor function has been investigated by measurement of receptor binding and determination of receptor-mediated second-messenger function, NE neuronal activity, and behavior (14,15).

Studies on the effect of α_2 adrenergic receptor-mediated cAMP accumulation suggest that antidepressants may reduce responses to α_2-adrenergic receptor agonists by shifting the receptor to an "antagonist-preferring" state.

Table 2 Therapeutic Studies Relevant to β-Adrenergic Receptor Downregulation Hypothesis of Antidepressant Action

Study	Results
Desipramine-yohimbine combination treatment of depression	Because this combination produced a rapid downregulation of β-adrenergic receptors in laboratory rats, it was predicted it would have rapid antidepressant effects. However, the combination was not effective in depressed patients who subsequently responded to other antidepressant combinations.
T_3 augmentation of antidepressant action	Clinical investigations have demonstrated that T_3 administration augments antidepressant effects. However, contrary to the β-adrenergic downregulation hypothesis of antidepressant action, in laboratory rats T_3 blocks the decrease in β-adrenergic receptor down regulation produced by antidepressants.
Propranolol use in cardiovascular disease	Contrary to the β-adrenergic downregulation hypothesis of antidepressant action, propranolol, when used for cardiovascular disease, produces depression in vulnerable individuals.

A review of the available studies indicates that α_2-receptor binding is not systematically altered by antidepressant treatment, with increases, decreases, and no change reported. Similarly, neurophysiological and behavioral studies suggest that the ability to reduce α_2-adrenergic autoreceptor sensitivity is not shared by all antidepressants.

Clinical investigations have assessed the effect of antidepressant drugs on α_2-adrenergic autoreceptor sensitivity by determining the effects of the α_2-receptor agonist, clonidine, on plasma 3-methoxy-4-hydroxyphenylglycol (MHPG), blood pressure, and sedation. Desipramine, amitriptyline, and the MAO inhibitor clorgyline reduce these effects of clonidine, suggesting development of α_2 presynaptic autoreceptor subsensitivity. However, similar actions were not observed with long-term treatment with trazodone or mianserin.

The growth hormone response to clonidine, which probably reflects *postsynaptic* α_2-adrenergic receptor function is not changed by extended antide-

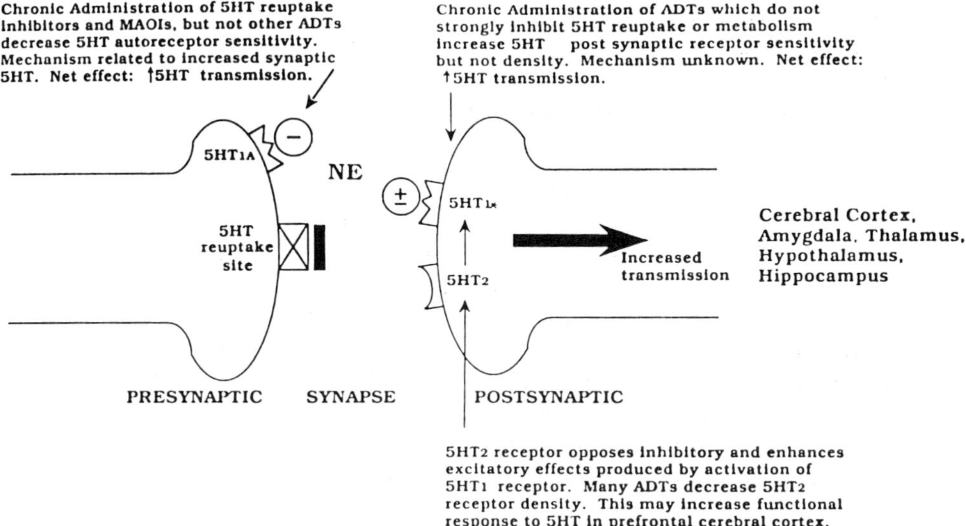

Figure 1 Schematic representation of the effects of prolonged antidepressant treatments (ADTs) on norepinephrine (NE) neuronal function relected by neurophysiological responses, receptor binding, and second-messenger activity. Most consistent ADT effects are a reduction in β-adrenergic receptor-mediated transmission. There is data suggesting enhancement of α_1-receptor-mediated transmission and inconsistent actions on α_2-receptor functions by ADTs. Brain regions with high densities of the specific adrenergic receptors are indicated. – NE has inhibitory effect on neuronal activity; + NE has excitatory effect on neuronal activity; * blocks frequency accommodation and enhances efficiency of sensory inputs.

pressant treatment; whereas, treatment with imipramine, amitriptyline, and lithium has decreased platelet [–H]clonidine binding (16).

Summary

Preclinical and clinical investigations have demonstrated that an ability to reduce α_2-receptor sensitivity is a property shared by only select antidepressants with strong NE-uptake inhibition or MAO inhibition properties. These data indicate that α_2-receptor downregulation probably does not represent a common therapeutic mechanism of action of antidepressant treatments. Studies designed to differentiate the functional properties of pre- and postsynaptic α_2-receptors and the relative effects of antidepressants on these receptors will be valuable. In addition, certain depressive subtypes (e.g., bipolar disorder) may have therapeutic responses to α_2-receptor antagonists. Such studies are in progress with the α_2-receptor antagonist, idazoxan.

α_1-Receptor Upregulation Hypothesis

The α_1-receptor upregulation hypothesis suggests that the mechanism of antidepressants' action may be related to an ability of these agents to increase the function of postsynaptic α_1-adrenergic receptors (17,18).

Receptor-binding investigations have not identified consistent effects of antidepressants on α_1-receptor binding (19,20). α_1-Receptor-mediated activation of inositol phospholipid turnover is not altered by antidepressant treatment. In contrast, single-unit electrophysiological investigations have identified enhanced α_1-adrenergic responsiveness in various postsynaptic brain regions after long-term antidepressant administration (17).

Several behavioral paradigms have been developed to assess the function of α_1-receptors in the brain; however, these studies do not reveal consistent effects of antidepressants on α_1-receptor-mediated behaviors (21).

In clinical investigations, α_1-adrenergic receptor function has been examined by measuring the phenylephrine-induced dilation of iris. This response is increased after long-term administration of MAO inhibitors, unchanged by mianserin, and decreased by desipramine. There is some evidence that α_1-receptors are stimulatory to corticosteroid release. The corticosteroid response to amphetamine is decreased in depressed patients, but this is not affected by tricyclic drug administration or electroconvulsive therapy (ECT) (3,4).

Summary

Improved clinical methods are required to appropriately evaluate α_1-receptor function in human subjects, and tests for the validity of the α_1-receptor hypothesis of antidepressant action are also indicated.

Enhancement of Serotonin Neurotransmission Hypothesis

It has also been hypothesized that the mechanism of antidepressants' action is related to changes in serotonin neuronal function (22). This was originally thought to occur by inhibition of serotonin neuronal reuptake. The work of deMontigny and colleagues, and other groups, has led to the development of a serotonin hypothesis which suggests that during long-term antidepressant administration, antidepressant efficacy involves alterations in serotonin receptor sensitivity, thereby producing enhanced serotonin neurotransmission (3,4,6,23).

Prolonged antidepressant treatment has inconsistent effects on [^{3}H]5-HT binding. Recent investigations with radioactive-labeled receptor-binding

Table 3 Preclinical Studies of the Serotonin Neurotransmission Potentiation Hypothesis of Antidepressant Action

Antidepressant category	Receptor binding			Neurophysiological sensitivity			Behavioral sensitivity	
	$5\text{-}HT_1$	$5\text{-}HT_2$	IMI	5-HT autoreceptor	5-HT postsynaptic	$5\text{-}HT_1$	$5\text{-}HT_{1A}$ autoreceptor	$5\text{-}HT_2$
NE-reuptake inhibitors	0↓	↓	↓0	0	↑	↓	↓	↑0
Mixed NE-and 5-HT-reuptake inhibitors	0	↓	↓0	0	↑	↓	↓	↑↓0
5-HT-reuptake inhibitors	0	↑0	↑	↓	0	↓	↓	↓0
MAO1	↓	↓	↑0	↓	0	↓	↓	↓
Atypical anti-depressants								
Trazodone	0	↓	–	–	–	–	–	0↑
Bupropion	–	0	0	–	–	–	–	–
Mianserin	0	↓	0	–	↑	–	↓	0↓
Nomifensine	–	–	–	–	–	–	–	–
Maprotiline	–	0	–	–	–	–	–	–
ECT	0	↑	↓0	–	↑	↓↑	↓	↓

Symbols used: ↑ increase; ↓ decrease; 0 no change; – not tested; averaged over different brain regions and different drugs; mixed results are indicated by more than one symbol.

ligands such as spiperone and ritanserin, which label 5-HT_2 receptors, have observed that these receptors are decreased in density by some antidepressant drugs (Table 3). For many of these drugs, the reduction in 5-HT_2 density appears to require long-term administration. However, an important exception is mianserin, which has this effect after a few doses. However, mianserin requires extended administration for therapeutic activity; therefore, there is a dissociation between mianserin's ability to reduce 5-HT_2 receptors and its clinical efficacy. Electroconvulsive therapy increases 5-HT_2 receptor density, opposite the effects of antidepressant drugs (24).

Single-unit electrophysiological investigations have consistently shown that long-term antidepressant administration enhances serotonergic neurotransmission in various brain regions, either by autoreceptor desensitization or postsynaptic receptor supersensitivity (3,4,6,23). Extended treatment with specific serotonin-reuptake inhibitors and MAO inhibitors increases serotonergic transmission by inducing a desensitization of the serotonin autoreceptor, without altering postsynaptic serotonin sensitivity (25,26). In contrast, tricyclic antidepressant drugs and iprindol induce postsynaptic serotonin receptor supersensitivity, but do not change autoreceptor function (23). The explanation for this observation may be that tricyclic antidepressants are rapidly demethylated into their secondary metabolite forms, which are weak serotonin uptake inhibitors. These results suggest that sustained blockade of serotonin reuptake is probably required for desensitization of the 5-HT autoreceptor.

Behavioral investigations of the effects of antidepressant treatments on serotonin function do not reveal uniform effects of these treatments on serotonin function. The inability of these studies to assess brain regions involved in antidepressant action is a major limitation. For example, the serotonin-induced head twitch response in rats, although associated with 5-HT_2 receptors, does not involve receptors located in the frontal cortex (27).

Many clinical studies designed to evaluate monoamine receptor function with pharmacologic probes have evaluated serotonergic function. A series of studies have determined the effect of a variety of antidepressant drugs on the ability of intravenous tryptophan to increase prolactin. Extensive evidence (reviewed elsewhere) indicates that the prolactin response to tryptophan can be used as a reflection of serotonergic function, perhaps involving the 5-HT_1 receptor. Many antidepressants, including fluvoxamine, amitriptyline, tranylcypromine, and desipramine, increase the prolactin response to tryptophan in depressed patients (28-30). However, potentiation of this response is not universal among the antidepressants because, trazodone, mianserin, and bupropion do not enhance the tryptophan-induced increase in prolactin in these patients (31). The inability of trazodone and mianserin to increase the prolactin-tryptophan response probably relates to the postsynaptic serotonin antagonist properties of these drugs.

Another paradigm used to evaluate serotonin function is the cortisol increase following 5-hyroxytryptophan (5-HTP) administration. Depressed patients who received imipramine, desipramine, or nortriptyline exhibited a decreased cortisol response to 5-HTP, compared with the drug-free condition. These findings contrast with the enhancement of serotonin function identified by the tryptophan infusion test. This may be because 5-HTP-induced increases in cortisol are related to effects on the 5-HT_2 receptors, whereas the neuroendocrine actions of tryptophan appear to result from 5-HT_1 receptor stimulation. Additionally, 5-HTP may have peripheral effects at the adrenal gland level as well as actions on catecholamine and indoleamine function (32).

Therapeutic Studies

The addition of lithium (which increases 5-HT synaptic release) to ongoing antidepressant treatment, in patients either refractory or partially responsive to treatment, was based on the hypothesis that an enhancement of serotonin function was critical to therapeutic efficacy. The original open study (33) and the double-blind placebo-controlled study (34), have now been replicated by numerous investigations and have established lithium augmentation as a routine clinical treatment (35-47).

The initial studies demonstrating that parachlorophenylalanine (PCPA), which decreases 5-HT synthesis, induces a recurrence of depressive symptoms in recovered depressed patients, who are receiving antidepressant treatment, provided important support of a critical role for 5-HT in antidepressant action (48,49). Our research group has recently replicated these findings by a novel method for quickly depleting plasma tryptophan (TRP) with a 24-hr, 160-mg/day, low TRP diet, followed the next morning by a TRP-free amino acid drink (TFD). This paradigm results in a reduction in plasma TRP of over 90% 5 hr after the TFD. Ongoing investigations indicate that over 60% of remitted patients maintained on antidepressant medication experience depressive symptoms 2-7 hr after the TFD, with a gradual return over 24 hr to the remitted state with normal TRP intake (50). Preliminary observations suggest that patients who respond to 5-HT-enhancing drugs are more vulnerable to the effects of the TFD than patients who responded to NE-reuptake inhibitors.

Summary

Neurophysiological studies have consistently indicated that a spectrum of antidepressant drugs increase serotonergic neurotransmission (Fig. 2). The increase in serotonin neurotransmission observed in neurophysiological studies has not been associated with an increase in the density of serotonin receptors. In contrast, 5-HT_2 receptor density is reduced by most antidepressant treatments; ECT is a major exception. The apparent contradictory findings

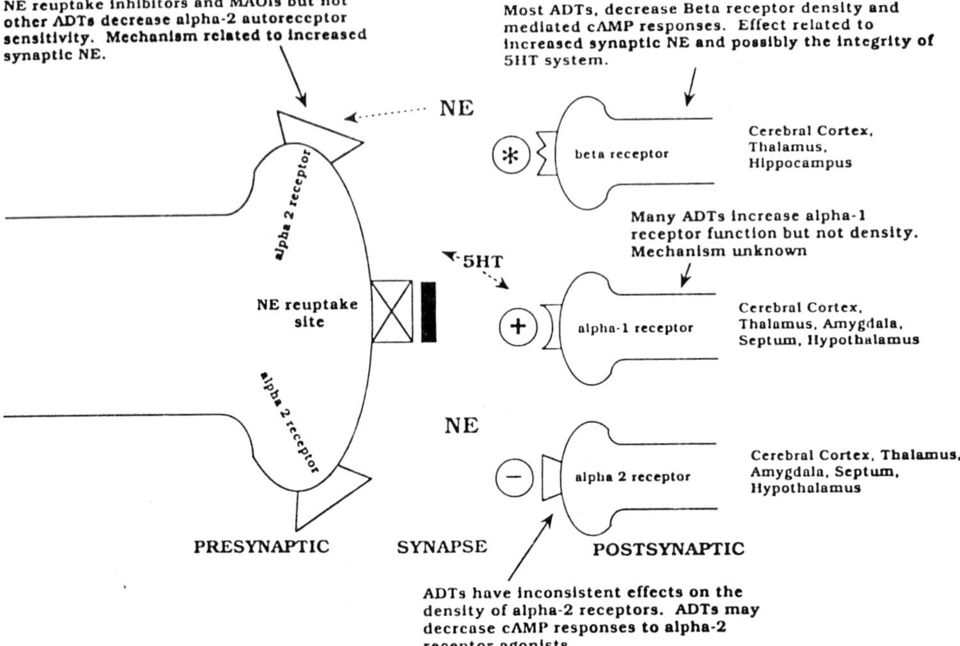

Figure 2 Schematic representation of the effects of chronic antidepressant treatments (ADTs) on serotonin (5-HT) neuronal function reflected by neurophysiological responses and receptor binding. Neurophysiological studies indicate most ADTs increase serotonin neurotransmission either by 5-HT autoreceptor desensitization or 5-HT postsynaptic supersensitivity. Many ADTs decrease 5-HT_2 receptor binding (an exception is ECT which increases 5-HT_2 binding). Brain regions with high densities of serotonin receptors are indicated: − 5-HT has inhibitory effect on presynaptic neuronal activity; ± 5-HT has excitatory (e.g., facial motor nucleus) or inhibitory (e.g., prefrontal cortex) effects on postsynaptic neuronal activity depending upon the brain region; * The 5-HT receptor mediating the neurophysiological responses of postsynaptic neurons (e.g., hippocampus) to 5-HT may be distinct from radioligand techniques (see text).

of the neurophysiological and binding studies probably result from assessment of different 5-HT receptor subtypes by the two methods and from reciprocal functional interactions between 5-HT_1 and 5-HT_2 receptors (see Table 3).

Clinical investigations have shown that most, but not all, antidepressants enhance serotonin neurotransmission. Important exceptions are bupropion, trazodone, and mianserin. From a clinical perspective, a major difficulty with the serotonin hypothesis as currently proposed (i.e., enhancement of 5-HT function) is that it may be overly simplistic. It is clear from infusion studies of serotonin precursors (tryptophan) and receptor agonists M-chlorophenylpiperazine (MCPP) and from therapeutic augmentation of antidepressants with serotonin-enhancing agents that there is no linear relationship between increased serotonin neurotransmission and improvement in depressed mood. The relationship between antidepressant-induced changes in serotonin function and therapeutic response is probably more complex.

However, the ability of lithium to potentiate antidepressant efficacy in treatment-refractory patients, the rapid reversal of antidepressant responses when serotonin function is rapidly reduced by PCPA, or the 90% reduction in plasma tryptophan by a TFD are supportive of an important role for antidepressant-induced alterations in serotonin function as an antidepressant action mechanism (Table 4).

Other Neurotransmitter Receptor Hypotheses of Antidepressant Action

α-Aminobutyric Acid Receptor Upregulation

A series of investigations suggest that long-term, but not brief administration of many antidepressants may increase tritiated α-aminobutyric acid (GABA) binding to $GABA_B$-receptors in frontal cortex (51). An upregulation of $GABA_B$ recognition sites possibly results in enhancement of monoaminergic neurotransmission. The $GABA_B$ sites occur on NE terminals in the rat

Table 4 Therapeutic Studies Relevant to Serotonin Neurotransmission Potentiation Hypothesis of Antidepressant Action

Hypothesis and therapeutic approach	Results and implications
Serotonin depletion reverses antidepressant action	Consistent with the serotonin neurotransmission potentiation hypothesis of antidepressant action, PCPA, a tryptophan hydroxylase inhibitor that reduces serotonin synthesis and rapid depletion of plasma tryptophan by a tryptophan-free amino acid drink, reverses the therapeutic effects of antidepressants.
Lithium augmentation of antidepressant action	In numerous investigations, lithium has been demonstrated to augment the therapeutic effects of several antidepressant drugs in treatment-refractory depressed patients. This treatment was developed and based upon the serotonin neurotransmission potentiation hypothesis of antidepressant action.

cerebral cortex. Baclofen, a $GABA_B$ agonist, enhances NE-stimulated cAMP production, which is potentiated by long-term imipramine treatment. Five days of combined baclofen-imipramine adminstration results in significant decreases in β-adrenergic receptor density and NE-stimulated cAMP accumulation, effects not induced by either drug alone. The findings suggest that $GABA_B$ agonists, either alone or in combination with antidepressants, may be useful antidepressant treatments (52).

Enhancement of Dopamine Neurotransmission

Antidepressant drugs do not have consistent effects on dopamine D_2 receptor density in the limbic system (53). However, there is evidence that brief administration of several antidepressants decreases dopamine D_1 receptor binding, as reflected by changes in [^{3}H]Sch 23390 binding in the striatum and limbic forebrain (54). Biochemical and behavioral studies indicate that long-term antidepressant administration does not consistently alter dopamine autoreceptor function (53,55-57).

Clinical studies indicate apomorphine-stimulated growth hormone release is not consistently altered by repeated ECT and is decreased by long-term amitriptyline treatment. However, the validity of this model of dopamine function has been questioned. Apomorphine-induced prolactin inhibition has been increased by repeated ECT in two of three investigations, and bromocriptine-induced prolactin inhibition has been increased by long-term amitriptyline treatment (53).

Clinical efficacy studies that used dopamine precursors or drugs that increased dopamine release, indicated that simply increasing the availability of synaptic dopamine is not an effective antidepressant treatment for many depressed patients. However, the dopamine agonist, piribedil, may have antidepressant properties, particularly in patients whose pretreatment cerebral spinal fluid (CSF) level of homovanillic acid (HVA) is low (58). Nomifensine, which is a potent antagonist of neuronal dopamine reuptake, has robust antidepressant properties (59). Anecdotal data indicate that nomifensine is effective for some depressed patients refractory to conventional treatments. Unfortunately, it is no longer generally available because of hematological side effects. Therefore, an effort should be made to develop and evaluate the effects of other potent dopamine-reuptake inhibitors in depressed patients.

Downregulation of Cholinergic Function

At clinical doses some tricyclic antidepressants are potent cholinergic receptor blockers; however, the rank order of their anticholinergic and antidepressant activities differ (60). Despite the evidence for a role of cholinergic mechanisms in the development of depressed mood, an evaluation of the anticholinergic effects of antidepressants, demonstrates that if anticholinergic action is important, at best, it is an enhancing, rather than an underlying, primary therapeutic action. Placebo-controlled investigations of the antidepressant efficacy of centrally acting selective anticholinergic drugs could more definitively address this.

A COMMON MECHANISM FOR ANTIDEPRESSANT ACTION?

One of the purposes of this chapter was to determine if, during long-term antidepressant treatment, a specific alteration in receptor sensitivity has been identified that can account for the therapeutic mechanism of action of all, or even most, antidepressant treatments. Preclinical paradigms of receptor function have not yet revealed an alteration of receptor function that is consistent across the spectrum of therapeutic agents, and clinical studies have also failed to determine the neurobiological actions of antidepressant treatment.

However, the ability of long-term antidepressant treatment to enhance serotonin function appears relevant to therapeutic activity. For example, methods that reduce serotonin availability (such as PCPA and TFD) produce depressive symptomatology in patients remitted from their depression, which suggests that the integrity of the serotonin neuronal system may be necessary for the maintenance of the remission induced by at least some antidepressant drugs.

The serotonin neuronal enhancement hypothesis has led to a new, effective treatment approach. The original studies of lithium augmentation were based upon a clearly defined preclinical hypothesis of a psychotropic drug mechanism (i.e., potentiation of serotonin function). Although the demonstrated efficacy of lithium augmentation was consistent with the preclinical prediction, there is no direct clinical demonstration of this action mechanism. The recent observations of Price et al. (47) indicate that the rapid antidepressant effect of lithium augmentation (fewer than 7 days) is less common than originally suggested and that up to 3 weeks of lithium administration may be required to obtain therapeutic responses. This suggests that lithium's immediate effect of increasing presynaptic serotonin release may not be the primary therapeutic mechanism, and that the actions of lithium on the regulation of serotonin neurotransmission must be considered. Lithium may work by stabilizing (61) homeostatic systems that may be dysregulated in patients with affective disorders (61-63). This may explain why the addition of the serotonin precursors, tryptophan and 5-HTP, and fenfluramine to antidepressant regimens in treatment-refractory patients has been therapeutically disappointing.

BIOLOGICAL HETEROGENEITY OF DEPRESSIVE ILLNESS AND THE TREATMENT OF DEPRESSION

It is widely accepted that the available antidepressants are broad-spectrum agents with actions on numerous neurotransmitter systems and possess actions far beyond those required to reverse the pathology related to depressive illness.

A major advance in the treatment of depression would be the development of methods that are capable of biologically subtyping the different forms of depressive illness and, thereby, could guide treatment choice. For example, patients whose depression is related to reduced serotonin function may respond preferentially to serotonin-reuptake inhibitors, such as fluoxetine and fluvoxamine alone, or in combination with lithium (64). Recently, it has been speculated that MAOIs may be a better alternative to tricyclic antidepressants for treating depressed patients with decreased serotonin activity (65). There is clinical support for the effectiveness of MAOI-tryptophan and MAOI-lithium combinations in treatment of refractory depressed patients (66).

A subgroup of patients may be depressed because of a reduction in noradrenergic neuronal activity. Some evidence suggested that bipolar depression is characterized by decreased NE function; therefore it would be interesting to determine if α_2-receptor antagonists, such as yohimbine and idazoxan, which cause large increases in noradrenergic neuronal activity, are effective in this biologically defined subgroup.

Similarly, it is probable that some depressed patients will benefit from an enhancement of dopamine function. This is supported by the observations that the dopamine-reuptake inhibitor, nomifensine, was particularly effective in selected patients. The beneficial effects of antidepressant-stimulant combinations in some refractory depressed patients may relate to an augmentation of dopamine function (67).

There are also effective treatments for refractory depression that do not indicate specific neurotransmitter mechanisms. For example, the addition of T_3 to tricyclic antidepressants and MAOIs has been clinically useful (13, 68), perhaps by T_3 augmentation of NE function by increasing NE synthesis and β- and α_1-noradrenergic receptor sensitivity. It has been argued that certain depressed patients may suffer from a subclinical hypothyroid state accompanied by normal routine thyroid indices.

An extensive body of evidence supports an important role for ECT in the treatment of refractory depression, particularly for patients with psychotic symptoms. However, the mechanism of ECT's superior antidepressant efficacy remains obscure because, although preclinical studies identify numerous effects of ECT on brain neurotransmitter function, very few clinical neurobiological investigations of ECT have been conducted.

THE DEVELOPMENT OF NOVEL THERAPEUTIC APPROACHES FOR REFRACTORY DEPRESSION

Logical avenues exist for the development and investigation of novel therapeutic approaches to depressive illness. The study of drugs with actions beyond inhibition of neurotransmitter uptake, metabolisms, or receptor stimulation or antagonism will be important. A new pathway for antidepressant action may involve changes in second- and third-messenger (intracellular) function, including G-proteins, protein kinases, phosphoproteins, and phospholipids. The putative antidepressant, rolipram, which inhibits calmodulin-independent cAMP phosphodiesterase, may represent a new and novel class of antidepressant compounds (69).

An area, which may be therapeutically useful, is determination of the antidepressant effects of drugs with specific actions on serotonin receptor subtypes. Preliminary evidence indicates that the 5-HT_{1A} receptor agonist, gepirone, and the 5-HT_2 receptor antagonist, ritanserin, may be useful for depression (70,71).

It has been suggested that GABA function may relate to antidepressant action. Fengabine is a putative antidepressant that may represent a new class of antidepressant compounds with primary actions on GABA. Fengabine increases $GABA_B$ binding on frontal cortex, similar to other antidepressants. The antidepressant potential of fengabine is supported by open clinical studies in severely depressed patients of whom 65% demonstrated good to excellent responses to the drug (72).

The development of drugs that affect brain peptide function may result in new antidepressant compounds. The most promising lead here is drugs with corticotropin-releasing factor (CRF) antagonist properties because preclinical studies have related CRF to behavior associated with animal models of depression.

Technological advances in basic neuroscience are identifying new peptides, neurotransmitters, and receptor systems, thereby contributing to an increased understanding of signal transmission from the receptor recognition site through second- and third-messenger systems. This knowledge provides reason for optimism that in the near future a new generation of centrally active compounds will be identified that will have a potential of benefit for the many treatment-refractory depressed patients.

REFERENCES

1. Bunney, W. E. and Davis, J. M. (1965). Norepinephrine in depressive reactions. *Arch. Gen. Psychiatry 13*:483-493.
2. Schildkraut, J. J. (1965). The catecholamine hypothesis of affective disorders. *Am. J. Psychiatry 122*:502-522.

3. Charney, D. S., Menkes, D. B., and Heninger, G. R. (1981). Receptor sensitivity and the mechanism of action of antidepressant treatment. *Arch. Gen. Psychiatry 38*:1160-1180.
4. Heninger, G. R. and Charney, D. S. (1987). Mechanism of action of antidepressant treatments: Implications for the etiology and treatment of depressive disorders. In *Psychopharmacology: The Third Generation of Progress.* Edited by H. Y. Meltzer. New York, Raven Press, pp. 535-544.
5. Coppen, A., Shaw, D. M., and Malleson, A. (1965). Tryptamine metabolism in depression. *Br. J. Psychiatry 111*:993-998.
6. Meltzer, H. Y. and Lowy, M. T. (1987). The serotonin hypothesis of depression. In *Psychopharmacology: The Third Generation of Progress.* Edited by H. Y. Meltzer. New York, Raven Press, pp. 513-526.
7. Cooper, J. R., Bloom, F. E., and Roth, R. H. (1986). *The Biochemical Basis of Neuropharmacology.* New York, Oxford University Press.
8. Sulser, F., Vetulani, J., and Mobley, P. L. (1978). Mode of action of antidepressant drugs. *Biochem. Pharmacol. 27*:257-261.
9. Murphy, D. L., Aulakh, C. S., and Garrick, N. A. (1986). How antidepressants work: Cautionary conclusions based on clinical and laboratory studies of the longer-term consequences of antidepressant drug treatment. In *Antidepressants and Receptor Function.* Edited by R. Porter, G. Bock, and S. Clark. Chichester, John Wiley & Sons, pp. 106-120.
10. Charney, D. S., Price, L. H., and Heninger, G. R. (1986). Desipramine-yohimbine combination treatment of refractory depression: Implications for the β-adrenergic receptor hypothesis of antidepressant action. *Arch. Gen. Psychiatry 43*:1155-1161.
11. Avorn, J., Everitt, D. E., and Weiss, S. (1986). Increased antidepressant use in patients prescribed β-blockers. *JAMA 255*:357-360.
12. Mason, G. A., Bondy, S. C., Nemeroff, C. B., Walker, C. H., and Prange, A. J., Jr. (1987). The effects of thyroid state on beta-adrenergic and serotonergic receptors in rat brain. *Psychoneuroendocrinology 12*:261-270.
13. Goodwin, F. K., Prange, A. J., Post, R. M., Muscettola, G., and Lipton, M. A. (1982). Potentiation of antidepressant effect by triiodothyronine in tricyclic nonresponders. *Am. J. Psychiatry 139*:34-38.
14. Crews, F. T. and Smith, C. B. (1978). Presynaptic alpha-receptor subsensitivity after long term antidepressant treatment. *Science 202*:322-324.
15. Finberg, J. P. (1987). Antidepressant drugs and downregulation of presynaptic receptors. *Biochem. Pharmacol. 36*:3557-3562.
16. Siever, L. (1987). Role of noradrenergic mechanisms in the etiology of the affective disorders. In *Psychopharmacology: The Third Generation of Progress*, Edited by H. Y. Meltzer. New York, Raven Press, pp. 493-504.
17. Menkes, D. B., Kehne, J. H., Gallager, D. W., Aghajanian, G. K., and Davis, M. (1983). Functional supersensitivity of CNS α_1-adrenoceptors following chronic antidepressant treatment. *Life Sci. 33*:181-188.
18. Lipinski, J. F., Cohen, B. M., Zubenko, G. S., and Waternaux, C. M. (1987). Adrenoceptors and the pharmacology of affective illness: A unifying theory. *Life Sci. 40*:1947-1963.

19. Mogilnicka, E., Zazula, M., and Wedzony, K. (1987). Functional supersensitivity to the α_1 adrenoceptor agonist after repeated treatment with antidepressant drugs is not conditioned by β-down-regulation. *Neuropharmacology 26*:1457-1461.
20. Stockmeier, C. A., McLeskey, S. W., Blendy, J. A., Armstrong, N. R., and Kellar, K. J. (1987). Electroconvulsive shock but not antidepressant drugs increases α_1-adrenoceptor binding sites in rat brain. *Eur. J. Pharmacol. 139*:259-266.
21. Maj, J. (1984). Central effects following repeated treatment with antidepressant drugs. *Pol. J. Pharmacol. Pharm. 36*:87-99.
22. Lapin, I. P. and Oxenkrug, G. F. (1969). Intensification of the central serotonergic processes as a possible determinant of the thymoleptic effect. *Lancet 1*: 132-136.
23. deMontigny, C., Blier, P., and Chaput, Y. (1984). Electrophysiologically-identified serotonin receptors in the rat CNS: Effect of antidepressant treatment. *Neuropharmacology 23*:1511-1520.
24. Green, A. R., Heal, O. J., and Goodwin, G. M. (1986). The effects of electroconvulsive therapy and antidepressant drugs on monoamine receptors in rodent brain. In *Antidepressant and Receptor Function*. Edited by R. Porter, G. Bock, and S. Clark. New York, John Wiley & Sons, pp. 246-259.
25. Blier, P., deMontigny, C., and Azzaro, A. J. (1986). Modification of serotonergic and noradrenergic neurotransmissions by repeated administration of monoamine oxidase inhibitors: Electrophysiological studies in the rat central nervous system. *J. Pharmacol. Exp. Ther. 237*:987-994.
26. Chaput, Y., deMontigny, C., and Blier, P. (1986). Effects of a selective 5-HT reuptake blocker, citalopram, on the sensitivity of 5-HT autoreceptors: Electrophysiological study in the rat brain. *Naunyn-Schmiedebergs Arch. Pharmakol. 333*:342-348.
27. Willner, P. (1985). Antidepressants and serotonergic neurotransmission: An integrative review. *Psychopharmacology 85*:387-404.
28. Charney, D. S., Heninger, G. R., and Sternberg, D. E. (1984). Serotonin function and mechanism of action of antidepressant treatment: Effects of amitriptyline and desipramine. *Arch. Gen. Psychiatry 41*:359-365.
29. Price, L. H., Charney, D. S., and Heninger, G. R. (1985). Effects of tranylcypromine treatment on neuroendocrine, behavioral, and autonomic responses to tryptophan in depressed patients. *Life Sci. 37*:809-818.
30. Price, L. H., Charney, D. S., Delgado, P. L., and Heninger, G. R. (in press). Effects of desipramine and fluvoxamine treatment on the prolactin response to L-tryptophan: A test of the serotonergic function enhancement hypothesis of antidepressant action. *Arch. Gen. Psychiatry.*
31. Price, L. H., Charney, D. S., and Heninger, G. R. (1988). Effects of trazodone treatment of serotonergic function in depressed patients. *Psychiatry Res. 24*: 165-175.
32. Meltzer, H. Y., Lowy, M., Robertson, A., Goodnick, P., and Perline, R. (1984). Effect of 5-hydroxytryptophan on serum cortisol levels in major affective disorders. *Arch. Gen. Psychiatry 41*:391-397.

33. deMontigny, C., Grunberg, F., Mayer, A., and Deschenes, J. P. (1981). Lithium induces rapid relief of depression in tricyclic antidepressant drug nonresponders. *Br. J. Psychiatry 138*:252-256.
34. Heninger, G. R., Charney, D. S., and Sternberg, D. E. (1983). Lithium carbonate augmentation of antidepressant treatment: An effective prescription for treatment-refractory depression. *Arch. Gen. Psychiatry 40*:1335-1342.
35. deMontigny, C., Cournoyer, G., Morissette, R., Langlois, R., and Caille, G. (1983). Lithium carbonate addition in tricyclic antidepressant-resistant depression: Correlations with the neurobiologic actions of tricyclic antidepressant drugs and lithium ion on the serotonin system. *Arch. Gen. Psychiatry 40*:1327-1334.
36. Nelson, J. C. and Byck, R. (1982). Rapid response to lithium in phenelzine nonresponders. *Am. J. Psychiatry 141*:85-86.
37. Price, L. H., Conwell, Y., and Nelson, J. C. (1983). Lithium augmentation of combined neuroleptic-tricyclic treatment in delusional depression. *Am. J. Psychiatry 140*:318-322.
38. Birkhimer, L. J., Alderman, A. A., Schmitt, C. E., and Ednie, K. J. (1983). Combined trazodone-lithium therapy for refractory depression. *Am. J. Psychiatry 140*:1382-1383.
39. Joyce, P. R., Hewland, H. R., and Jones, A. V. (1983). Rapid response to lithium in treatment-resistant depression. *Br. J. Psychiatry 142*:204-205.
40. Louie, A. K. and Meltzer, H. Y. (1984). Lithium potentiation of antidepressant treatment. *J. Clin. Psychopharmacol. 4*:316-321.
41. deMontigny, C., Elie, R., and Caillé, G. (1985). Rapid response to the addition of lithium in iprindole-resistant unipolar depression: A pilot study. *Am. J. Psychiatry 142*:220-223.
42. Joyce, P. R. (1985). Mood response to methylphenidate and the dexamethasone suppression test as predictors of treatment response to zimelidine and lithium in major depression. *Biol. Psychiatry 20*:598-604.
43. Schrader, G. D. and Levien, H. E. M. (1985). Response to sequential administration of clomipramine and lithium carbonate in treatment-resistant depression. *Br. J. Psychiatry 147*:573-575.
44. Roy, A. and Pickar, D. (1985). Lithium potentiation of imipramine in treatment resistant depression. *Br. J. Psychiatry 147*:582-583.
45. Nelson, J. C. and Mazure, C. M. (1986). Lithium augmentation in psychotic depression refractory to combined drug treatment. *Am. J. Psychiatry 143*:363-366.
46. Kushnir, S. L. (1986). Lithium-antidepressant combinations in the treatment of depressed, physically ill geriatric patients. *Am. J. Psychiatry 143*:378-379.
47. Price, L. H., Charney, D. S., and Heninger, G. R. (1986). Variability of response to lithium augmentation in refractory depression. *Am. J. Psychiatry 143*:1387-1392.
48. Shopsin, B., Friedman, E., and Gershon, S. (1976). Parachlorophenylalanine reversal of tranylcypromine effects in depressed patients. *Arch. Gen. Psychiatry 33*:811-819.

49. Shopsin, B., Friedman, E., Goldstein, M., and Gershon, S. (1975). The uses of synthesis inhibitors in determining a role for biogenic amines during imipramine treatment in depressed patients. *Psychopharmacol. Commun. 1*:239-249.
50. Delgado, P. L., Charney, D. S., Price, L. H., Goodman, W. K., Aghajanian, G. K., Landis, H., and Heninger, G. R. (1988). Behavioral effects of acute tryptophan depletion in depressed and obsessive compulsive disorder (OCD) patients. *Soc. Neurosci. Abstr. 14*:970.
51. Lloyd, K. G., Thuret, F., and Pilc, A. (1985). Upregulation of γ-aminobutyric acid $GABA_B$ binding sites in rat frontal cortex: A common action of repeated administration of different classes of antidepressants and electroshock. *J. Pharmacol. Exp. Ther. 235*:191-199.
52. Enna, S. J., Karbon, E. W., and Duman, R. S. (1986). $GABA_B$ agonists and imipramine induced modifications in rat brain β-adrenergic receptor binding and function. In *GABA and Mood Disorders.* Edited by G. Bartholini, K. G. Lloyd, and P. L. Morselli. New York, Raven Press, pp. 23-31.
53. Willner, P. (1983). Dopamine and depression: A review of recent evidence. III. The effects of antidepressant treatments. *Brain Res. Rev. 6*:237-246.
54. Klimek, V. and Nielsen, M. (1987). Chronic treatment with antidepressants decreases the number of [^{3}H]SCH 23390 binding sites in the rat striatum and limbic system. *Eur. J. Pharmacol. 139*:163-169.
55. Chiodo, L. A. and Antelman, S. M. (1980). Repeated tricyclics induce a progressive dopamine autoreceptor subsensitivity independent of daily drug treatment. *Nature 287*:451-454.
56. Mac Neill, D. A., and Gower, M. (1982). Do antidepressants induce dopamine autoreceptor subsensitivity? *Nature 298*:302-303.
57. Diggory, G. L. and Buckett, W. R. (1984). Chronic antidepressant administration fails to attenuate apomorphine-induced decreases in rat striatal dopamine metabolites. *Eur. J. Pharmacol. 105*:257-263.
58. Post, R. M., Gerner, R. H., Carman, J. S., Gillin, J. C., Jimerson, D. C., Goodwin, F. K., and Bunney, W. E. Jr. (1978). Effects of dopamine agonist piribedil in depressed patients. *Arch. Gen. Psychiatry 35*:609-615.
59. Brogden, R. N., Heel, R. C., Speight, T. M., and Avery, G. S. (1979). Nomifensine: A review of its pharmacological properties and therapeutic efficacy in depressive illness. *Drugs 18*:1-24.
60. Richelson, E. (1984). The newer antidepressants: Structures, pharmacodynamics, and proposed mechanisms of action. *Psychopharmacol. Bull. 20*:213-223.
61. Rudorfer, M. V., Karoum, F., Ross, R. J., Potter, W. Z., and Linnoila, M. (1985). Differences in lithium effects in depressed and healthy subjects. *Clin. Pharmacol. Ther. 37*:66-71.
62. Siever, L. J. and Davis, K. L. (1985). Overview: Toward a dysregulation hypothesis of depression. *Am. J. Psychiatry 142*:1017-1031.
63. Price, L. H., Charney, D. S., Delgado, P. L., and Heninger, G. R. (1989). Lithium treatment and serotoninergic function: Neuroendocrine and behavioral responses to intravenous tryptophan in affective disorder. *Arch. Gen. Psychiatry 46*:13-19.

64. Delgado, P. L., Price, L. H., Charney, D. S., and Heninger, G. R. (1988). Efficacy of fluvoxamine in treatment-refractory depression. *J. Affect. Dis. 15*:55-60.
65. Aulakh, C. S., Cohen, R. M., Dauphin, M. M., McLellan, C. A., and Murphy, D. L. (1988). Role of serotonergic input in the down-regulation of β-adrenoceptors following long-term clorgyline treatment. *Eur. J. Pharmacol. 156*:63-70.
66. Price, L. H., Charney, D. S., and Heninger, G. R. (1985). Efficacy of lithium-tranylcypromine treatment in refractory depression. *Am. J. Psychiatry 142*: 619-623.
67. Wharton, R. N., Perel, J. M., and Dayton, P. G. (1971). A potential clinical use for methylphenidate (Ritalin) with tricyclic antidepressants. *Am. J. Psychiatry 127*:619-1625.
68. Joffe, R. T. (1988). Triiodothyronine potentiation of the antidepressant effect of phenelzine. *J. Clin. Psychiatry 49*:409-410.
69. Bobon, D., Breulet, M., Gerard-Vandenhove, M.-A., Guiot-Goffioul, F., Plomteux, G., Sastre-y-Hernandez, M., Schratzer, M., Troisfontaines, B., von Frenckell, R., and Wachtel, H. (1988). Is phosphodiesterase inhibition a new mechanism of antidepressant action? *Eur. Arch. Psychiatr. Neurol. Sci. 238*:2-6.
70. Robinson, D. S. (1988). Clinical effects of 5-HT_{1A} partial agonists in the treatment of depression. Presented at the 27th Annual Meeting of American College of Neuropsychopharmacology, San Juan, Puerto Rico.
71. Data on file, Janssen Pharmaceutica, N.V. B-2340 Beerse, Belgium.
72. Lloyd, K. G., Zivkovic, B., Sanger, D., Depoortere, H., and Bartholini, G. (1987). Fengabine, a novel antidepressant GABAergic agent. I. Activity in models for antidepressant drugs and psychopharmacological profile. *J. Pharmacol. Exp. Ther. 241*:245-241.

3

Thyroid Axis Syndromes in Depression
Definitions and Interpretations

ARTHUR J. PRANGE, JR., GEORGE A. MASON, and JAMES C. GARBUTT

University of North Carolina School of Medicine, Chapel Hill, North Carolina

The purpose of this chapter is to acquaint the practitioner with the hypothalamic-pituitary-thyroid (HPT) axis findings that often occur in depressed patients. To do this, some preliminary paragraphs are necessary to outline HPT axis physiology and the tests that are available to measure the hormones involved or to measure some parameters (e.g., binding space on proteins) that influence them. We then will describe the HPT axis syndromes often seen in depression and comment on their significance. From this exercise we hope the practitioner will be better able to choose appropriate tests of HPT axis function and to interpret their results. Touching on several areas, we will not treat any of them in depth. To offset this fault we will provide references to their fuller treatment. In any event, it is not thyroidology or its relevant laboratory science or depression that is the focus of this chapter; it is their conjunction.

PHYSIOLOGY OF THE HYPOTHALAMIC-PITUITARY-THYROID AXIS: AN OVERVIEW

From the many accounts of HPT axis physiology (1-4) we have taken the treatise by Ingbar (5) as our main reference point. Although Ingbar uses the word *thyrotoxicosis* to denote the metabolic converse of hypothyroidism (HO), our purposes are best served if we use *hyperthyroidism* (HR) as the metabolic converse of HO.

The HPT axis is a homeostatically controlled neuroendocrine system that comprises both central (hypothalamus) and peripheral (pituitary gland and thyroid gland) tissues (Fig. 1) and their various secretions (Table 1). Thyroid hormones affect many metabolic processes, among them the activity of many enzymes, the metabolism of many other hormones, and the response of many tissues to certain neurotransmitters. Probably no single mechanism of action can account for this plethora of effects with thyroid hormones acting at multiple sites within the cell. Recently, a thyroid hormone receptor has been identified at a specific DNA locus (6).

Thyrotropin-releasing hormone (TRH), a tripeptide, is secreted from nerve terminals in the median eminence of the hypothalamus into the hypothalamic-pituitary-portal venous system. In this system, it is then carried to the anterior pituitary gland, where it binds to specific membrane receptors on thyrotroph cells, which respond by releasing thyroid-stimulating hormone (TSH) into the general circulation. The TSH binds to receptors on thyroid cells to induce the synthesis and release of tetraiodothyronine (thyroxine, T_4) and 3,5,5′-triiodothyronine (T_3). Evidence that T_4 must first be deiodinated to

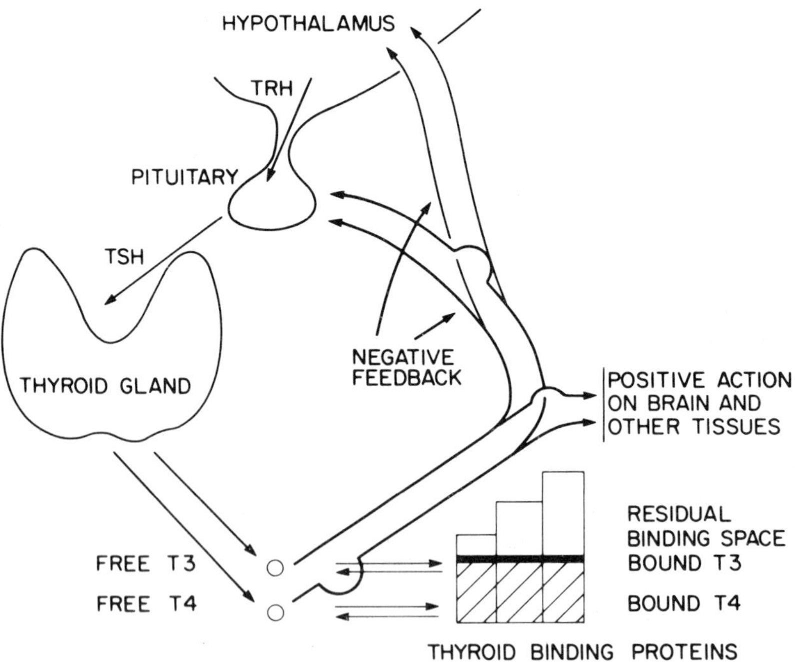

Figure 1 Control of the HPT system.

Table 1 Hormones of the Thyroid Axis

Hormone	Abbreviation	Main origin	Function
Thyrotropin-releasing hormone	TRH	Brain	Stimulates release of TSH; neuromodulator
Thyroid-stimulating hormone	TSH	Anterior pituitary	Stimulates synthesis and release of thyroid hormones
Thyroxine	T_4	Thyroid gland	Acts as precursor of T_3; shares functions with T_3
Triiodothyronine	T_3	Thyroid gland; deiodination of T_4 by peripheral tissues	Stimulates growth, development, and metabolism; maintains central and sympathetic nervous system function
Reverse triiodothyronine	rT_3	Deiodination of T_4 by peripheral tissues	Inhibits conversion of T_4 to T_3

T_3 to produce a metabolic effect suggests that T_4 functions primarily as a prohormone, or precursor, for the more active hormone T_3. About 80% of serum T_3 arises from deiodination of T_4 by peripheral tissues, rather than from direct thyroidal secretion. More than 99% of circulating T_4 and T_3 is bound to three serum proteins: thyroxine-binding globulin (TBG), thyroxine-binding prealbumin, and albumin. It is the remaining unbound, or free, fraction that is active and, by negative-feedback, tends to damp TSH (and TRH) secretion.

Circulating thyroid hormone levels (especially free thyroid hormone levels) are regulated to maintain metabolic homeostasis. Departure from normal ranges almost always indicates thyroid axis dysfunction or more generalized systemic illness. Hormone synthesis and secretion by the thyroid gland is controlled largely by the serum level of TSH. Furthermore, TSH secretion is stimulated by TRH and inhibited by free thyroid hormone levels. Because TSH secretion is tightly regulated by the sum of these influences, TSH is usually the best single indicator of peripheral thyroid status. However, in some conditions, such as starvation and certain forms of illness, the usual controls of thyroid function are relaxed in an apparent effort to conserve energy by lowering peripheral metabolism. Although the mechanisms underlying this process are not well understood, it is under such conditions that the thyroid economy of the central nervous system (CNS) and its regulation may become dissociated from that of the peripheral organs. In part, because of the brain's great ability to convert T_4 to T_3, the thyroid status of the CNS is maintained, even in the presence of decreasing levels of circulating thyroid hormones. This suggests that euthyroidism (EU), if only local EU, is important to brain function.

LABORATORY TESTS OF THE HYPOTHALAMIC-PITUITARY-THYROID AXIS: AN OVERVIEW

The paragraphs that follow are based, to some extent, on primary sources, but largely on fuller reviews of the subject (7,8).

For reasons that we will later clarify, we think that the practitioner should be interested in the thyroid state of patients with depression. The satisfaction of this interest should not be limited to laboratory investigations, but a medical history of thyroid-related symptoms, such as skin changes and temperature insensitivities, should be obtained. One should do a physical examination, because a patient may have a goiter that will be revealed only by palpation. Inventories for the systematic historical assessment of both HO (9) and HR (10) are available.

However, laboratory examination will often reveal faults in the HPT axis when history is equivocal and physical examination is negative. The various tests available for examination of the HPT axis have increased in step with the description of the chemical identity of the hormones. The technique of radioimmunoassay (RIA) has been a main contributor to this development, and the relationship between these events was implicit in the Nobel Prize for Physiology or Medicine in 1978, which was awarded to Guillemin (11) and to Schally (12) for the description of TRH and to Yalow (13) for the innovation of RIA.

Ingbar (5) has classified "commonly employed laboratory tests of thyroid hormone economy" as follows: (1) direct tests of thyroid function (e.g., thyroid radioiodine uptake); (2) tests related to concentrations and binding of thyroid hormones in blood (e.g., serum total T_4); (3) tests that assess metabolic impact of thyroid hormones (e.g., basal metabolic rate); (4) tests that assess mechanisms for regulating thyroid function (e.g., serum TSH); (5) miscellaneous tests (e.g., measurement of antithyroid antibodies). For the psychiatrist, we have selected tests from categories 2, 4, and 5 and classified them as standard (Table 2), that is, readily available through most laboratories, or as specialized test (Table 3), that is, often less available and used mainly to follow-up some diagnostic lead. With one exception, the tests we

Table 2 Some Standard Laboratory Tests of Thyroid Axis Function

Test	Method of measurement	Approximate normal range[a]	Interpretation of abnormal result
T_4 (total)	RIA	4-12 μg/dL	↓ HO and/or decreased TBG binding ↑ HR and/or increased TBG binding
T_3 (total)	RIA	70-190 ng/dL	↓ HO and/or decreased TBG binding ↑ HR and/or increased TBG binding
T_3 uptake	Resin or antibody uptake of radiolabeled T_3	40-60% saturation	↓ Increased TBG binding ↑ Decreased TBG binding
Free thyroxine index (FTI)	Calculated from T_4 and T_3U	Usually about same as total T_4 (4-12)	↓ HO ↑ HR
TSH (basal)	Immunoradiometric assay of serum	<3.5 μIU/mL	↑ Primary HO or pituitary tumor

[a]Normal ranges vary among laboratories.

Table 3 Some Specialized Tests of Thyroid Axis Function

Test	Method of measurement	Normal result	Interpretation of abnormal result
TSH (stimulated by TRH)	Immunoradiometric assay of serum 0,15,30,45 min after TRH	TSH >5 μIU/mL	↓ In hyperthyroidism or secondary hypothyroidism (pituitary disease) ↑ In primary hypothyroidism
Free T_4	Equilibrium dialysis or RIA	0.5-1.8 ng/mL	↓ HO ↑ HR
Free T_3	Equilibrium dialysis or RIA	3-7 pg/ml	↓ In hypothyroidism ↑ In hyperthyroidism
Reverse T_3 (RT_3; total)	RIA	70-300 pg/mL	↓ In hypothyroidism ↑ In hyperthyroidism—caloric deprivation
Thyroid antibodies Antithyroglobulin Antimicrosomal	Hemagglutination tests	Negative	Positive in Hashimoto goiter, most primary hypothyroidism, and variants of Graves' disease

will discuss depend only on taking a blood sample. However, the TRH stimulation test requires the administration of TRH under controlled conditions. Remember that this chapter does not pretend to exhaust the laboratory means of assessing thyroid function, and the psychiatrist must sometimes consult an endocrinologist for a more detailed examination.

Serum Thyroxine

The serum T_4 level, usually expressed in micrograms per deciliter (μg/dL), is now routinely measured by RIA in most hospital laboratories. A measure of total (bound plus free) T_4 is elevated by HR, an abnormally high TBG concentration, or by decreased peripheral conversion of T_4 to T_3. Elevated TBG may be a genetic condition, or it may be a consequence of high estrogen levels resulting from pregnancy or use of oral contraceptives. Reduction of peripheral conversion of T_4 occurs in caloric deprivation or acute illness.

Serum T_4 levels are low when thyroidal secretion is reduced in HO or when TBG levels are low. Levels of TBG are decreased in nephrosis, cirrhosis, several disorders involving elevated serum androgens and, rarely, in inherited TBG deficiency.

From the foregoing, it must be apparent that an abnormal total T_4 value by itself tells the practitioner that something is amiss and needs investigation, but it is not pathognomonic of either HR or HO. Similarly, a normal value does not prove EU.

Serum Triiodothyronine

The measurement of the serum T_3 level (bound plus free) is available in most hospital laboratories, but may not be a part of a routine thyroid workup. Although serum T_3 varies with serum T_4 in most conditions, the two may diverge in starvation, in acutely ill EU patients, in patients with impaired T_4 to T_3 conversion or, rarely, in patients with "T_3 thyrotoxicosis," in which T_3 is elevated and T_4 is normal. The usefulness of a serum T_3 value as an only measurement is subject to the same limitations that apply to a solitary T_4 value.

Triiodothyronine Uptake and Free Thyroxine Index

Because the concentration of *free* T_4 is not affected appreciably by variations in TBG levels or by the presence in serum of foreign substances (e.g., salicylates) that interfere with protein binding of T_4, it is a valuable determination. Its measurement by equilibrium dialysis is rather laborious; it has been supplanted by RIA or by two other tests. Calculations from the results of these tests yield, over a wide range of values, one that is proportional to free T_4. The results from the (total) T_4 test and the T_3 uptake (T_3U) test are used in conjunction to calculate a free thyroxine index (FTI).

The T_3U test, contrary to what its name suggests, is not a measure of T_3, but rather, of the TBG-binding capacity of a serum sample; the name comes from the use of radiolabeled T_3 as a reagent. The test is performed by adding labeled T_3 to a serum sample. The labeled T_3 binds to sites on TBG—the major binding protein in the sample—that are not occupied by endogenous thyroid hormones. More labeled T_3 is used than TBG can bind; thus, after incubation, some labeled T_3 is leftover. This leftover reagent is taken up by a resin or an antibody and its radioactivity counted. This radioactivity is compared with that of a reference serum and expressed as a percentage retention, or ratio. Because there is no single reference serum, the units for the T_3U test are arbitrary; furthermore, T_3U results from different assay systems have different normal ranges.

More useful to the clinician than the total T_4 and the T_3U is the value of the FTI, which is calculated from them. Each laboratory establishes a normal range for the FTI, which is expressed as a number without units. The FTI is elevated in HR, low in HO, and normal in EU. Conveniently for the practitioner, a normal FTI result is obtained both in a patient whose total T_4 level is elevated because of high TBG and in a patient whose total T_4 level is diminished because of low TBG binding. In the former EU patient, the high total T_4 level would be "corrected" downward by a low T_3U value resulting from an abundance of unsaturated TBG-binding sites; in the latter EU patient, the low total T_4 level would be "corrected" upward by a high T_3U caused by a paucity of T_3 TBG-binding sites for the T_3 reagent.

Thyroid-Stimulating Hormone

The employment of immunoradiometric assay (IRMA) technology in conjunction with monoclonal antibodies in commercially available reagent kits has greatly improved the sensitivity and specificity of TSH measurements available to clinicians from hospital clinical laboratories or from commercial service laboratories. These assays can detect TSH levels as low as 0.03 μIU/mL, which are usually found only in HR patients. Because of their greater specificity, the newer IRMA assays yield normal TSH values somewhat lower than those of older RIA procedures. The older procedures sometimes produced values that were falsely elevated because of cross-reactions with molecules similar to TSH or with TSH fragments that are nonfunctional.

Basal TSH levels are markedly elevated in primary (thyroidal) HO. Levels are low or normal in HO when it arises from a dysfunction in the pituitary or in the hypothalamus, both of which are uncommon conditions.

The Thyrotropin-Releasing Hormone Stimulation Test

The measurement of TSH after stimulation of the pituitary gland with intravenous TRH is often used in diagnosing HR in patients with borderline elevations of serum T_4. The expected rise in TSH (> 5 μIU/mL) in response to 0.5 mg TRH is blocked by the excessive negative-feedback exerted on the pituitary by the elevated levels of free thyroid hormones present in the serum of these patients. In primary HO, the TSH response to TRH administration is exaggerated, often grossly, even when diminutions of circulating thyroid hormones are slight. The test is also useful in identifying the origin site of a disturbance within the HPT axis (i.e., hypothalamus, anterior pituitary gland, or thyroid gland).

The TRH stimulation test has been employed extensively as a research tool in the study of psychiatric patients. A blunted response is observed in about 25% of patients in certain psychiatric populations. An exaggerated TSH response to TRH stimulation may indicate a subclinical form of HO, in which levels of free thyroid hormones, although within the "normal" range, are insufficient to render a normal inhibitory effect on the pituitary.

Free Serum Thyroxine

Free T_4 concentration usually is determined by RIA after overnight equilibrium dialysis of serum, which does not disturb the bound/free hormone ratio, although a recently developed method employing direct RIA (without dialysis) of serum is available. Elevations of free T_4 are indicative of HR, whereas free T_4 levels are generally reduced in HO.

Free Serum Triiodothyronine

Methods for measuring free T_3 are analogous to those for measuring free T_4. A determination of free T_3 may be useful, especially when clinical findings are not congruent with values for total serum T_3 and when T_4 measures are not informative. Levels of free T_3 are elevated in HR and low in HO.

Reverse Triiodothyronine

Reverse T_3 (3,3′,5′-triiodothyronine; rT_3), similarly to T_4 and T_3, is a normal component of human serum, although it is seldom measured in routine clinical assessments. Most rT_3 arises from peripheral monodeiodination of the inner tyrosyl ring of T_4. Levels of rT_3 are elevated in many conditions, such as starvation or acute systemic illness, in which T_3 levels are usually low. Although rT_3 itself is metabolically inert, it inhibits the conversion of T_4 to its metabolically active metabolite T_3. Therefore, the presence of higher concentrations of rT_3 may be adaptive during conditions for which energy conservation is critical. Elevations of rT_3 are also found in HR; low levels are found in HO.

Antithyroid Antibodies

In recent years, greater attention has been paid to the role of autoantibodies in the development and progression of thyroid disease. Complete reagent kits are now commercially available for the detection and quantification of antithyroglobulin and antimicrosomal antibodies in human serum. In these hemagglutination procedures, serum samples of 10-12 different dilutions are incubated in the presence of animal erythrocytes to which are attached either microsomal antigen from human thyrotoxic gland (antimicrosomal antibody test) or thyroglobulin extracted from human thyroid gland (antithyroglobulin antibody test). These "sensitized" red cells will agglutinate in the presence of specific autoantibodies. A positive result is reported by citing the highest dilution at which at least 50% of the sensitized red cells agglutinate.

In most clinical evaluations, a reason to test for one antibody is a reason to test for the other. This procedure will detect practically all autoimmune thyroiditis (Hashimoto's disease) and about 90% of primary HO. Moreover, HR also often occurs on an autoimmune basis, and many patients with HR will show the presence of one or the other antibody.

Positive thyroid antibody tests may predict future thyroid disease in patients with some other existing autoimmune disorder or in members of families predisposed to organ-specific autoimmunity.

HYPO- AND HYPERTHYROIDISM: AN OVERVIEW

Some disorders of the HPT axis (e.g., nontoxic goiter) cause neither HO nor HR. We will not consider them in this precis. We will consider only those conditions that produce either some degree of HO or HR or, in HO, some basis for suspecting it (e.g., a slightly elevated TSH level). The thyroid gland communicates with the brain through its secretions; thus, we are concerned only with those disorders that cause changes in the thyroid hormone economy. We will set aside HO arising either in the anterior pituitary gland (secondary HO) or in the hypothalamus (tertiary HO). They are uncommon disorders, and they can usually be distinguished from thyroidal (primary) HO by the hormonal patterns and, especially, by the TSH response to a TRH stimulation test. We will give special attention to the syndrome of subclinical HO: it may have special importance in psychiatry.

The most common cause of primary HO is total or partial ablation of the thyroid gland, either from surgical operation or from radioactive iodine treatment, usually for Graves' disease, which is a cause of HR. A number of other conditions, with goiter as a finding common to all of them, can cause HO. They include Hashimoto's thyroiditis, endemic iodine deficiency, ingestion of antithyroid agents (especially iodides), heritable defects in thyroid hormone synthesis, and peripheral resistance to thyroid hormone action. Ingbar (5) has provided a description of all these disorders and outlined their relationships. However, primary (thyroidal) idiopathic HO is the main interest of the psychiatrist.

To characterize primary idiopathic HO, we can do no better than to quote Ingbar (5):

> Primary HO . . . is more common in women than in men and occurs most often between the ages of 40 and 60. The cause is unknown. The presence of circulating thyroid antibodies in up to 80% of the patients and the clinical and immunological overlap with autoimmune diseases suggest, however, that it represents the end stage of an autoimmune thyroiditis in which goiter either was absent or had gone unnoticed.

Hashimoto's thyroiditis can be viewed as a related disorder because its autoimmune basis is even clearer. However, it differs from idiopathic HO in several respects: there is gross lymphocytic infiltration of the thyroid gland; there is usually goiter; the patient, at least early in the course of the illness, can be EU.

Both idiopathic HO and Hashimoto's thyroiditis may lead to severe HO; during progression to this end point, either disease may cause a syndrome known as diminished thyroid reserve or subclinical HO. In recent years, increased capacity to test the dynamics of the thyroid axis has given rise to definitions of degrees of this syndrome and of their relationship to overt HO. These relationships, as proposed by Evered et al. (14) and Wenzel et al. (15) are shown in Table 4. Our group (16) and others (17) have proposed the recognition of what is shown as grade 4, a condition in which the only abnormality is the presence of thyroid antibodies.

Grade 1 HO is synonymous with overt HO, defined by the usual criteria for this disorder. In *grade 2*, levels of thyroid hormones are within the normal

Table 4 Grades of Primary (Thyroidal) Hypothyroidism

Grade	FTI	Basal TSH	Stimulated TSH	Antibodies
1 HO (overt)	↓	↑	↑	Usually +
2 HO (subclinical)	N[a]	↑	↑	Usually +
3 HO (subclinical)	N	N	↑	Usually +
4 HO (subclinical)	N	N	N	+

[a]Normal

range, but there is other evidence of disturbance. In *grades 3* and *4* there is a stepwise retreat in the laboratory findings. It is within these categories that the isolated finding of thyroid antibodies may have clinical significance in depressed patients.

As noted earlier, HO sometimes arises in the pituitary or the hypothalamus. In contrast, HR is not now considered to arise at these levels. It arises in the thyroid gland itself as an autoimmune process (or from such cause as ectopic thyroid tissue or ingesting excessive amounts of thyroid hormone). However, the older literature is replete with accounts of Graves' disease following a severe life crisis and with accounts of a personality profile and life history that may predispose to the illness (18). Of course, an autoimmune basis for an illness does not preclude a contribution from the nervous system. However this may be, the HR state usually proceeds from Graves' disease (80%), toxic multinodular goiter (10%), or toxic adenoma (5%) (19).

"Graves' disease is characterized by diffuse goiter, thyrotoxicosis, infiltrative ophthalmopathy, and occasionally infiltrative dermopathy" (5). The serum of these patients usually contains thyroid-stimulating antibodies, which attach themselves to receptors on cells in the thyroid gland that are normally the targets for TSH. This usually leads to the synthesis and release of excessive amounts of thyroid hormones, although some patients with Graves' disease remain EU. Because of its apparent autoimmune basis, Graves' disease bears a pathophysiological relationship to both idiopathic HO and Hashimoto's thyroiditis. Over a period of years, Graves' disease may "burn out" leaving the patient HO. Thus, this disorder, a prime cause of HR, may eventually become a cause of HO.

HYPOTHALAMIC-PITUITARY-THYROID AXIS SYNDROMES IN DEPRESSION

Systematic data are sparse concerning the prevalence of disorders of the HPT axis in patients with any mental illness, including depression. Nevertheless, we think that changes in the thyroid economy are relevant to mental illness, especially depression. The few pertinent studies, along with informal observation, suggest that several HPT axis diseases or syndromes may be more common in depressed patients than in the general population, although there seem to be no HPT axis diseases or syndromes that are specific to depressed patients.

We have adopted a theoretical scheme that lends order to certain data concerning onset of affective illness, and propose that many factors can alter the threshold for the development of depressive illness. Factors, such as the thyroid economy, need not be regarded as necessary for the occurrence or remission of the illness, they merely contribute to its presence. Thus, changes in the thyroid economy may play no role at all in some patients, whereas in others, such changes may be of critical importance to the development of depressive illness.

There are five HPT axis syndromes that, when considered together, form a nexus that suggests a continuous dynamic role of the HPT axis in depression.

Overt Hypothyroidism

We postulate that overt or subclinical HO may contribute to depression. For these disorders, Table 5 shows the typical results from the ten HPT axis tests. The most important findings for each disorder are underlined. Overt HO is easily recognized if one takes a relevant history, is mindful of the usual physical findings, and obtains two standard HPT axis measures—the FTI and the basal TSH. The prevalence of overt HO in a population of hospitalized psychiatric patients has been found to be 0.5% (20). What one may occasionally encounter is a patient who has responded poorly to antidepressant treatment and is then discovered to suffer from HO. In this connection the clinician should recall that lithium treatment is a frequent cause of HO (21). Furthermore, animals that have been rendered HO show resistance to the typical effects of imipramine (22).

Subclinical Hypothyroidism

The concept of subclinical HO has been described previously, and the laboratory findings are shown in Table 4 and again in Table 5 in a broader context. The concept of subclinical HO is that it is possible to define more subtle degrees of perturbation in the direction of frank HO. Gold et al. (23) studied 250 consecutive hospitalized patients, who complained of depression or anergia, and identified two with overt HO, nine with grade 2, and ten with grade 3 HO. (The grade 4 classification was not used.) Furthermore, the prevalence of antithyroid antibodies in depressed patients has been reported by Gold et al. (24; 9%), Nemeroff et al. (25; 20%), and Haggerty et al. (26; 17%), although it is unknown whether or not the prevalence rates they reported would differ from age- and sex-matched controls (27). For some purposes, however, this question can be approached by asking another: For subclinical HO, regardless of its prevalence, does its presence make any clinically important difference?

The best-documented consequence of subclinical HO is an enhanced risk for development of overt HO (28), which has been found to pertain only to individuals with elevations in basal TSH *and* antithyroid antibodies. Another consequence may be an increased risk for coronary artery disease (29). Organic brain syndrome has also been reported in patients with subclinical

Table 5 HPT Axis Syndromes in Depression

	Standard tests (see Table 2)					Special tests (see Table 3)				
	Serum T_4	Serum T_3	T_3U	FTI	Basal TSH	Stimulated TSH	Free T_4	Free T_3	rT_3	Thyroid antibodies
Contributions to cause										
Grade 1 HO (overt)	↓	↓	↓	↓	↑	↑	↓	↓	↓	Usually +
Grade 2 HO (subclinical)	N	N	N	N	↑	↑	N	N	N	Usually +
Grade 3 HO (subclinical)	N	N	N	N	N	↑/N	N	N	N	Usually +
Grade 4 HO (subclinical)	N	N	N	N	N	N	N	N	N	±
Process of recovery										
Transient hyperthyroxinemia	↑	N	↑	↑	N or ↓	N or ↓	↑	N	N or ↑	Usually −
Adaptation to illness										
Euthyroid sick syndrome (mild)	N	↓	N	↑	N	N	↑	↓	↑	Usually −
Exhaustion of recovery process										
Blunted TSH response	N	N	N	N	N or ↓	↓	N	N	N	Usually −

N, normal.
For each syndrome the most important findings have been underscored.

HO (30). Resistance to antidepressant treatment has been associated with subclinical HO, as indicated by an increase in TSH (30,31)); the administration of a thyroid hormone has been useful in some of these patients (32). Subclinical HO has been reported in patients with rapid-cycling bipolar disorder (33); however, in a subsequent study, this syndrome appeared no more frequently than in other bipolar patients (34), and its presence could often be attributed to lithium treatment (33,34). Thyroxine has been useful in this condition (35).

Other evidence also supports the concept that slight changes in the thyroid economy, although not identified as subclinical HO, may make a substantial difference in CNS function. In an unpublished study, our group examined the relationships between initial FTI and subsequent response to tricylic antidepressant (TCA) therapy. All patients were considered EU, although the tests that might have established subclinical HO usually were not performed. About two-thirds of 80 consecutive patients had a "good" response to TCA treatment, whereas about one-third had a "poor" response. The group with a poor response had lower (but normal) FTI values than those patients with a good TCA response. In a similar study, we found that 7 of 41 hospitalized depressed patients had as their only abnormal HPT axis finding the presence of an antithyroid antibody. The patients with antibodies had worse TCA responses than those without antibodies. As a corollary, poor TCA response in an apparently EU depressed patient (a patient who does not have overt HO) may be reversed by the addition of a small dose of T_3 (36).

Transient Hyperthyroxinemia

We think that patients often reach a threshold for depression without the HPT axis having played a causal role. In such cases, the axis may be invoked in the interest of recovery. This takes the form, we think, of the syndrome of transient hyperthyroxinemia, which occurs in a variety of mental and physical illnesses (37,38) and is a common HPT axis syndrome in depressed patients (38,39). In this syndrome, T_4 is elevated, whereas T_3 is not, and TSH may be either reduced or unchanged. We believe the syndrome occurs from excessive hypothalamic drive, and that there is probably a dynamic interplay between these hormones over time. This view is supported by the findings of Baumgartner (40), who followed four patients through a psychiatric decompensation. In each patient, an *increase* in TSH was accompanied by an *increase* of T_4, or rT_3, and to a lesser extent, T_3.

If transient hyperthyroxinemia in depressed patients represents a process aimed at recovery, then patients who show this abnormality should have a better prognosis. This is supported indirectly by the work of Kirkegaard and Faber (41), who found that patients who showed relative increases in T_4, and had subsequent increases in their TSH response to TRH, had reduced relapse rates after treatment. In our studies, patients with higher (normal) FTI values had better responses to TCAs than did patients with lower (normal) values. Moreover, in earlier work, Whybrow et al. (42) found that patients with lower blood cholesterol levels or with faster ankle reflex times had a better response to TCA treatment. These measures represent, in part, tissue responses to thyroid hormones.

Euthyroid Sick Syndrome

Another response to illness is the euthyroid sick syndrome. It occurs in a variety of illnesses (43), and it has also been reported in depression (41,44,45), although depressed patients rarely exhibit the thyroid findings seen in serious medical illness. In the euthyroid sick syndrome, peripheral deiodination of T_4 to T_3 is sharply curtailed, although TSH secretion is not increased. Table 5 shows the usual findings in this syndrome when it is mild. The findings of a diminished T_3 and an elevated rT_3 indicate a pattern of thyroid hormones with diminished metabolic potency. The prognostic importance of the euthyroid sick syndrome in depressed patients is unknown. However, we would speculate that if this syndrome is an accommodation to illness, rather than a struggle against it, then its presence would augur poorly for recovery.

Blunted Thyroid-Stimulating Hormone Response

One of the most provocative HPT axis syndromes that occurs in depressed patients is the blunted TSH response to TRH injection. Definitions of blunted response vary, although most investigators have used the criterion of a < 5 μIU/mL rise in TSH to indicate a *blunted response*. The blunted TSH response in depression has been reviewed in detail (46,47), and here, only the more important findings will be highlighted, and several recent observations will be discussed.

The discovery of a reduced TSH response to TRH in some depressed patients was made in 1972 (48-50). Since then, the observation has been widely replicated (46,47), and an overall consensus exists that its prevalence is about 25%. This low sensitivity, despite a specificity of about 95% (when depressed patients are compared with normal subjects), has rendered the blunted TSH response a weak diagnostic tool. Its diagnostic value is further diminished by similar high prevalence rates in patients with alcoholism (51), borderline personality disorder (52), and panic disorder (53).

Although interest in the diagnostic usefulness of a blunted TSH response has waned, interest in its prognostic value has increased. Kirkegaard (54,55) and Langer (56) have reported a significant association between an increase in TSH response to TRH, during treatment for depression, and a reduced rate of relapse. Both groups have concluded that the TSH response to TRH is dynamically related to the neurobiological processes underlying depression, and that changes in the TSH response may indicate a normalization of underlying biological disturbances.

What causes a blunted TSH response in depressed patients? There are several possible explanations. Thyroid hormones are a powerful inhibiting influence on the TSH response, and small increases (even when within the normal range) have clear inhibitory effects (57). Early work did not adduce evidence for higher levels of T_4 or T_3 in patients with a reduced TSH response (46). However, more recent work suggests that the reduced TSH response sometimes may be related to relative increases in T_4 (38,41,58). These studies have reported reductions in T_4 levels and increases in TSH responses as depressed patients are followed through hospitalization. Clearly, this "thyroidal" explanation of the reduced TSH response requires careful testing, especially because recent reports from endocrinological studies describe patients with "preclinical hyperthyroidism," whose hormonal profiles resemble those of psychiatric patients with a blunted TSH response. However, the thyroidal explanation has not been valid in all studies. Unden et al. (59) assessed 24-hr levels of T_4 and T_3 in relation to basal TSH and the TSH response to TRH. During depression, compared with remission, the T_4 level was higher, and the levels of basal and stimulated TSH were lower. However, there was no significant relationship between the *changes* in T_4 and the *changes* in TSH. Two possible mechanisms for a blunted TSH response have been investigated and found to make no substantial contribution: excessive dopaminergic input to the pituitary (60) and hypercortisolemia (61).

A clue to the meaning of a blunted TSH response may come from a consideration of its prognostic significance. When depression abates, the blunted response can normalize, or it can persist. Thus, sometimes, it can represent an illness state-dependent marker. When it does persist and, therefore, is not an illness state marker, is it a trait marker, but if so, what does it mark? It appears to mark an increased vulnerability for relapse into depression, as noted earlier. It may be that a blunted TSH response, when it persists, is an aspect of pituitary HO. The HO is indeed mild, as is usual in pituitary HO, but it may be enough to account for the increased tendency toward depressive relapse.

Pituitary HO may be the end stage of a prolonged CNS process, of which transient hyperthyroxinemia was but the start. After transient hyperthyroxinemia subsides, the attempt at recovery nevertheless may persist. Hyperthyroxinemia probably arises from changes within the brain (i.e., from excessive TRH activity changing the set point around which thyroid hormone-TSH homeostasis is defended). In time, the excessive stimulation of pituitary thyrotrophs by TRH results in their "downregulation" and a relative refractoriness to TRH. Thus, the process of recovery that is evident in hyperthyroxinemia, and its attendant good prognosis, may fail because other contributing causes of depression are insuperable. This failure may blunt the means for fine-tuning in the HPT axis, which, in turn, contributes to a return of depression: an attempted cure, having failed, becomes a cause.

The foregoing sequence may help explain why the experience of depression makes subsequent depression more likely. This formulation also explains how it may be that both blunted TSH responses and exaggerated TSH responses to TRH are frequently encountered in depressed patients. A blunted TSH response, in the absence of other explanations, may be a sign of acquired pituitary (secondary) HO; an exaggerated TSH response is evidence of thyroidal (primary) HO, whether overt or subclinical. It is quite possible that either primary or secondary HO can contribute to the occurrence of depression, interfere with treatment response, and enhance the risk of relapse.

CONCLUSIONS

Progress in basic science as applied to thyroidology has enabled the biochemical examination of the HPT axis in fine detail. This examination, in turn, has resulted in definitions of new syndromes of HPT axis disturbance. Some of these occur frequently in depressed patients, although their relative frequencies must be established. Whatever the differential prevalence may be, the occurrence of certain of these syndromes appears to predict a difference in treatment outcome. For example, when a blunted TSH response to TRH persists after successful treatment of depression, it may predict a possible relapse. Therefore, it is useful to examine the HPT axis in depressed patients, especially in those who have had a poor response to treatment or who suffer frequent relapse. Thyroidal tests, especially the determination of basal TSH, are useful here, but they should not be relied upon exclusively. Historical and physical examinations of the patient continue to have an important role.

REFERENCES

1. DeGroot, L. J. (1979). Thyroid physiology; endocrine and neural relationships. In *Endocrinology*, Vol. 1. Edited by L. J. DeGroot, G. F. Cahill, L. Martini, D. H. Nelson, W. D. Potts, J. T. Steinberger, Jr., and A. I. Winegrad. New York, Grune & Stratton, pp. 373-386.
2. Hedge, G. A., Colby, H. D., and Goodman, R. L. (1987). *Clinical Endocrine Physiology*. Philadelphia, W. B. Saunders.
3. Martin, J. B. and Reichlin, S. (1987). *Clinical Neuroendocrinology*. Philadelphia, F. A. Davis.

4. Kannan, C. R. (1986). *Essential Endocrinology.* New York, Plenum.
5. Ingbar, S. H. (1985). The thyroid gland. In *Textbook of Endocrinology*, 7th ed. Edited by J. D. Wilson and D. W. Foster. Philadelphia, W. B. Saunders.
6. Weinberger, D., Thompson, C. C., Ong, E. S., Lebo, R., Gruol, D. J., and Evans, R. M. (1986). The c-*erb-A* gene encodes a thyroid hormone receptor. *Nature 324*:641-646.
7. Mardell, R. J. and Gamlen, T. R. (1985). *Thyroid Function Tests in Clinical Practice.* Bristol, Engl., John Wright & Son.
8. Gruhn, J. C., Barsand, C. P., and Kumar, Y. (1987). The development of test of thyroid function. *Arch. Pathol. Lab. Med. 111*:84-100.
9. Willowicz, W. Z., Chapman, R. S., Crooks, J., Day, M. E., Gossage, J., Wayne, E., and Young, J. A. (1968). Statistical methods applied to the diagnosis of hypothyroidism. *Q. J. Med. 38*:255-266.
10. Crooks, J., Murray, I. P. C., and Wayne, E. J. (1959). Statistical methods applied to the clinical diagnosis of thyrotoxicosis. *Am. J. Med. 110*:211-234.
11. Guillemin, R. (1978). Peptides in the brain: The new endocrinology of the neuron. *Science 202*:390-402.
12. Schally, A. V. (1978). Aspects of hypothalamic regulation of the pituitary gland. *Science 202*:18-28.
13. Yalow, R. S. (1978). Radioimmunoassay: A probe for the fine structure of biological systems. *Science 200*:1236-1245.
14. Evered, D. C., Ormston, B. J., Smith, P. A., Hall, R., and Bird, T. (1973). Grades of hypothyroidism. *Br. Med. J. 17*:657-662.
15. Wenzel, K. W., Meinhold, H., Raffenberg, M., Adkofer, F., and Schleusener, H. (1974). Classification of hypothyroidism in evaluating patients after radioiodine therapy by serum cholesterol, T_3 uptake, total T_4, FT_4 index, total T_3, basal TSH, and TRH test. *Eur. J. Clin. Invest. 4*:141-148.
16. Garbutt, J. C. and Haggerty, J. J., Jr. (1987). Subclinical hypothyroidism and psychiatric disorders. *Dir. Psychiatry 7*:3-7.
17. Reus, V. I., Berlant, J., Galante, M., and Becker, N. (1986). Autoimmune thyroiditis in female depressives. Abstract 39. *Soc. Biol. Psychiatry.*
18. Ham, G. C., Alexander, F. A., and Carmichael, H. T. (1951). A psychosomatic theory of thyrotoxicosis. *Psychosom. Med. 13*:18-35.
19. Ramsay, I. (1986). *A Synopsis of Endocrinology and Metabolism.* Bristol, Engl., John Wright & Son.
20. McLarty, D. G., Ratcliffe, W. A., Ratcliffe, J. G., Shaimmins, J. G., and Goldberg, A. (1978). A study of thyroid function in psychiatric inpatients. *Br. J. Psychiatry 133*:211-218.
21. Lindstedt, G., Nilsson, L.-A., Walinder, J., Scott, A., and Ohman, R. (1977). On the prevalence, diagnosis and management of lithium induced hypothyroidism. *Br. J. Psychiatry 130*:452-458.
22. Avni, J., Edelstein, E. L., Khazan, N., and Sulman, F. G. (1967). Comparative study of imipramine, amitriptyline and their desmethyl analogues in the hypothyroid rat. *Psychopharmacologia 10*:426-430.
23. Gold, M. S., Pottash, A. L. C., and Extein, I. (1981). Hypothyroidism and depression. Evidence from complete thyroid function evaluation. *JAMA 245*:1919-1922.

24. Gold, M. S., Pottash, A. L. C., and Extein, I. (1982). "Symptomless" autoimmune thyroiditis in depression. *Psychiatry Res. 6*:261-269.
25. Nemeroff, C. B., Simon, J. S., Haggerty, J. J., and Evans, D. L. (1985). Antithyroid antibodies in depressed patients. *Am. J. Psychiatry 142*:840-843.
26. Haggerty, J. J., Jr., Simon, J. J., Evans, D. L., and Nemeroff, C. B. (1987). Relationship of serum TSH concentration and antithyroid antibodies to diagnosis and DHT response in psychiatric inpatients. *Am. J. Psychiatry 144*:1491-1493.
27. Tunbridge, W. M. G., Evered, D. L., Hall, R., et al. (1977). The spectrum of thyroid disease in a community: The Whickham survey. *Clin. Endocrinol. 7*:481-493.
28. Tunbridge, W. M. G., Brewis, M., French, J. M., et al. (1981). Natural history of autoimmune thyroiditis. *Br. Med. J. 282*:258-262.
29. Fowler, P. B. S. (1977). Premyxoedema: A cause of preventable coronary heart disease. *Proc. Soc. Med. 70*:297.
30. Haggerty, J. J., Jr., Evans, D. L., and Prange, A. J., Jr. (1986). Organic brain syndrome associated with marginal hypothyroidism. *Am. J. Psychiatry 143*:785-786.
31. Baruch, P., Jousent, R., and Widlocher, D. (1985). Increased TSH response to TRH in refractory depressed women. *Am. J. Psychiatry 142*:145.
32. Targum, S. D. (1984). Thyroid hormone and the TSH stimulation test in refractory depression. *J. Clin. Psychiatry 45*:345-346.
33. Cowdry, R. W., Wehr, T. A., Zis, A. P., and Goodwin, F. K. (1983). Thyroid abnormalities associated with rapid-cycling bipolar illness. *Arch. Gen. Psychiatry 40*:414-420.
34. Wehr, T. A., Sack, D. A., Rosenthal, N. E., and Cowdry, R. W. C. (1988). Rapid cycling affective disorder: Contributing factors and treatment response in 51 patients. *Am. J. Psychiatry 145*:179-184.
35. Stancer, H. L. and Persod, E. (1982). Treatment of intractable rapid-cycling manic-depressive disorder with levothyroxine. *Arch. Gen. Psychiatry 39*:311-312.
36. Goodwin, F. K., Prange, A. J., Jr., Post, R. M., Muscellola, G., and Lipton, M. A. (1982). Potentiation of antidepressant effects by L-triiodothyronine in tricyclic nonresponders. *Am. J. Psychiatry 139*:34-38.
37. Gooch, B. R., Isley, W. C., and Utiger, R. D. (1982). Abnormalities in thyroid function tests in patients admitted to a medical service. *Arch. Intern. Med. 142*:1801-1805.
38. Spratt, D. I., Pont, A., Miller, M. B., McDonald, I. R., Bayer, M. F., and McLaughlin, W. T. (1982). Hyperthyroxinemia in patients with acute psychiatric disorders. *Am. J. Med. 73*:41-47.
39. Kirkegaard, C. and Faber, J. (1981). Altered serum levels of thyroxine, triiodothyronines and diiodothyronines in endogenous depression. *Acta Endocrinol. 96*:199-207.
40. Baumgartner, A. (1986). Central thyroid stimulation in severely ill depressed, manic and schizophrenic patients. *Biol. Psychiatry 21*:417-421.
41. Kirkegaard, C. and Faber, J. (1986). Influence of free thyroid hormone levels on the TSH response to TRH in endogenous depression. *Psychoneuroendocrinology 4*:491-497.

42. Whybrow, P. C., Coppen, A., Prange, A. J., Jr., Noguera, R., and Bailey, J. E. (1972). Thyroid function and the response to liothyronine in depression. *Arch. Gen. Psychiatry 26*:242-245.
43. Wartofsky, L. and Burman, K. D. (1982). Alterations in thyroid function in patients with systemic illness: The "euthyroid sick syndrome." *Endocr. Rev. 3*: 164-217.
44. Linnoila, M., Lamberg, B.-A., Potter, W. Z., Gold, P. W., and Goodwin, F. K. (1982). High reverse T_3 levels in manic and unipolar depressed women. *Psychiatry Res. 6*:271-276.
45. Kjellman, B. F., Ljunggren, J. G., Beck-Friis, J., and Wettenberg, L. (1983). Reverse T_3 levels in affective disorders. *Psychiatry Res. 10*:1-9.
46. Loosen, P. T. and Prange, A. J., Jr. (1982). The serum thyrotropin (TSH) response to thyrotropin releasing hormone (TRH) in depression: A review. *Am. J. Psychiatry 139*:405-406.
47. Loosen, P. T. (1985). The TRH-induced TSH response in psychiatric patients. A possible neuroendocrine marker. *Psychoneuroendocrinology 10*:237-260.
48. Prange, A. J., Jr. and Wilson, I. C. (1972). Thyrotropin releasing hormone (TRH) for the immediate relief of depression: A preliminary report. *Psychopharmacologia 26*(suppl.):82.
49. Kastin, A. J., Ehrensing, R. H., and Schalch, D. S. (1972). Improvement in mental depression with decreased thyrotropin-releasing hormone. *Lancet 2*:740-742.
50. Prange, A. J., Jr., Wilson, I. C., Lara, P. O., Alltop, L. B., and Breese, G. R. (1972). Effect of thyrotropin-releasing hormone in depression. *Lancet 2*:999-1002.
51. Loosen, P. T., Wilson, I. C., Dew, B. W., and Tipermass, A. (1983). TRH in abstinent alcoholic men. *Am. J. Psychiatry 130*:1145-1149.
52. Garbutt, J. C., Loosen, P. T., Tipermas, A., and Prange, A. J., Jr. (1983). The TRH test in borderline personality disorder. *Psychiatry Res. 9*:107-113.
53. Roy-Byrne, T. P., Uhde, T. W., Rubinow, D. R., and Post, R. M. (1986). Reduced TSH and prolactin response to TRH in patients with panic disorder. *Am. J. Psychiatry 143*:503-507.
54. Kirkegaard, C. (1981). The thyrotropin response to thyrotropin-releasing hormone in endogenous depression. *Psychoneuroendocrinology 6*:189-212.
55. Krog-Meyer, I., Kirkegaard, C., Kijne, B., Lumholtz, B., Smith, E., Lykke-Olesen, L., and Bjorum, N. (1984). Prediction of relapse with the TRH test and prophylactic amitriptyline in 39 patients with endogenous depression. *Am. J. Psychiatry 141*:945-948.
56. Langer, G., Loinig, G., Hatzinger, R., Schonbeck, G., Resch, F., Aschuer, H., Keshaven, M. S., and Sieghart, N. (1986). Response of thyrotropin to thyrotropin-releasing hormone as predictor of treatment outcome. *Arch. Gen. Psychiatry 43*:861-869.
57. Snyder, P. T. and Utiger, R. D. (1972). Inhibition of thyrotropin response to thyrotropin-releasing hormone by small quantities of thyroid hormones. *J. Clin. Invest. 51*:2077-2084.
58. Muller, B. and Boning, J. (1988). Changes in the pituitary-thyroid axis accompanying major affective disorders. *Acta Psychiatr. Scand. 77*:143-150.

59. Unden, F., Ljunggren, J.-G., Kjellman, B. F., Beck-Friis, J., and Wetterberg, L. (1986). Twenty-four hour serum levels of T_4 and T_3 in relation to decreased TSH serum levels and decreased TSH response to TRH in affective disorders. *Acta Psychiatr. Scand.* *73*:358-365.
60. Loosen, P. T., Garbutt, J. C., and Tipermas, A. (1986). The TRH test during dopamine blockade in depressed patients. *Psychoneuroendocrinology* *11*:327-336.
61. Kirkegaard, C. and Carroll, B. J. (1980). Dissociation of TSH and adrenocortical disturbances in endogenous depression. *Psychiatry Res.* *3*:253-364.

4

Use of Hypothalamic-Pituitary-Adrenal Axis Tests in Patients with Major Depression

ROGER G. KATHOL and
JERRY L. CARTER

University of Iowa Hospitals
Iowa City, Iowa

The detection of hypothalamic-pituitary-adrenal (HPA) axis abnormalities in some patients with major depression provides a physiological means of subdividing this population. It also provides a basis for telling depressed patients that they have a "chemical or hormonal imbalance" that may be related to their condition. Such an explanation often provides relief to patients who previously considered their symptoms the product of poor self-esteem or psychological weakness. In some centers, the use of HPA axis testing, has become routine for the clinical or research evaluation of patients with major depression. The clinical indications for this testing, however, are often poorly understood or vaguely stated.

This chapter will provide the clinician with information on the utilization and interpretation of HPA axis tests in patients with major depression: (1) a basic review of the HPA axis with emphasis on how it relates to findings in the depressed patient, (2) a description of how to perform endocrine tests in patients with depression, (3) data related to the clinical use of urinary free cortisol (UFC) levels and performance of the dexamethasone suppression test (DST), and (4) utilization of tests of endocrine function in differentiating major depression from Cushing's disease.

THE HYPOTHALAMIC-PITUITARY-ADRENAL AXIS

It is important to review basic information on the control of this neuroendocrine system. Since the original description of the hypophysial-portal system, several important contributions have sequentially expanded our knowledge and enhanced our appreciation of its regulation (Fig. 1). It is no longer nec-

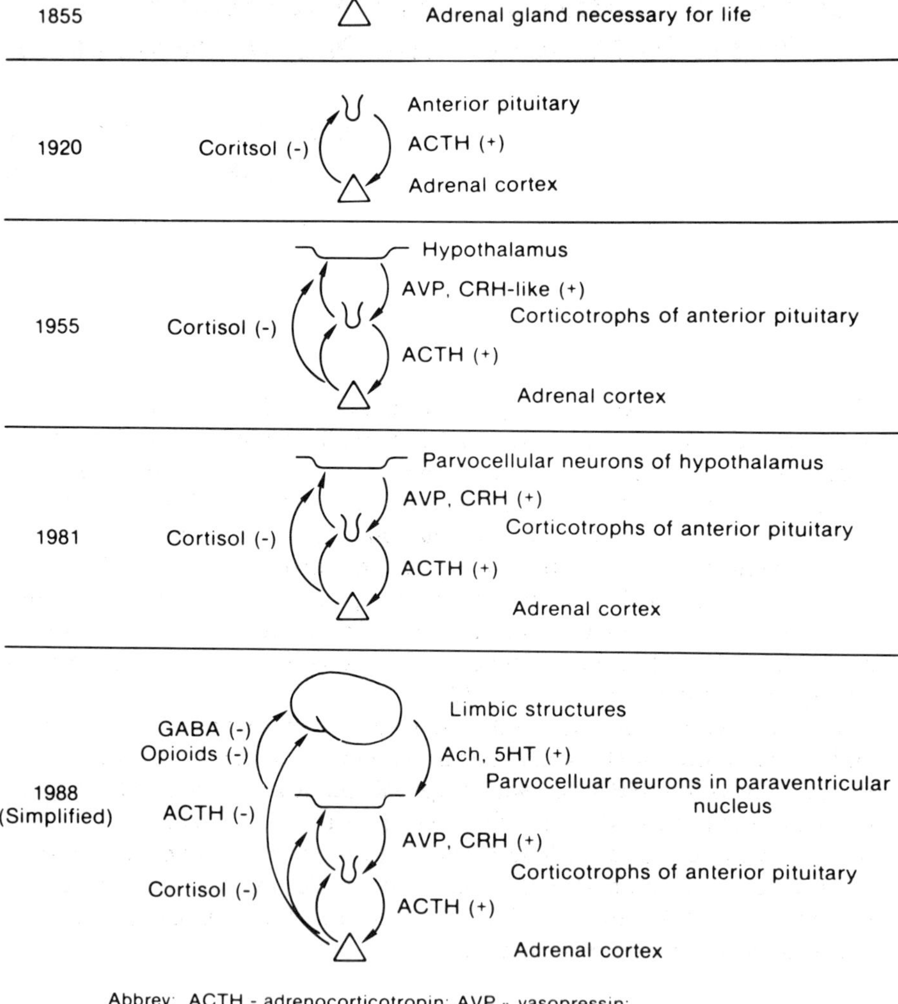

Figure 1 Historical development of our understanding of the limbic-hypothalamic-pituitary-adrenal axis.

essary, nor perhaps appropriate, to limit ourselves to discussion of the relationship of adrenocorticotropic hormone (ACTH) and cortisol in describing the pituitary-adrenal feedback loop. Although the basic tenet of the negative-feedback loop—stimulation of the adrenal cortex by ACTH and subsequent feedback by cortisol to inhibit further release of ACTH—remains true, the relationship between these two hormones may not be as closely linked as previously thought (1,2). Other factors, such as direct autonomic stimulation of the adrenal gland, variability in ACTH or glucocorticoid receptor sensitivity, metabolic changes in cortisol secretion, and alteration in the ACTH peptide configuration, may also play a substantial role in controlling cortisol levels at different times during the day or under different physiological conditions. Furthermore, central nervous system (CNS) structures, such as the parvicellular neurons in the paraventricular nucleus of the hypothalamus, are now known to play integral roles in modulating both pituitary and adrenal activity. Other limbic structures may also be involved (3,4).

Features important to our understanding of HPA axis testing include the following:

1. Cortisol levels in plasma are maintained in a fixed range with 24-hr circadian variation. The peak occurs at around 0800 hr and nadir at around midnight.
2. The limits of this range are maintained by an internal biological clock, which may be unrelated to ACTH modulation (1) and can be influenced by meals, altered sleep patterns, and stressful events.
3. Noncircadian control of cortisol production emanates from limbic structures or humoral factors not yet delineated.
4. In response to limbic or humoral stimulation, the parvicellular neurons in the paraventricular nucleus produce corticotropin-releasing hormone (CRH) and vasopressin (AVP).
5. CRH and AVP independently, or synergistically, stimulate the production of ACTH and ultimately cortisol (5).
6. CRH, AVP, and ACTH are, in turn, controlled by the negative-feedback effects of cortisol.

In addition, other factors may impinge on the interpretation of HPA axis tests in humans. For instance, some animal studies suggest that corticosterone and dexamethasone have different sites of feedback in the CNS (6). If this finding is generalizable to humans, then the finding of DST nonsuppression may not necessarily imply alteration of cortisol receptor sensitivity in depression. Nonetheless, this finding of a differential activity between dexamethasone and naturally occurring cortisol does not obviate the possibility that DST nonsuppression may represent a marker of HPA axis dysregulation in some patients with major depression.

TESTS OF HYPOTHALAMIC-PITUITARY-ADRENAL AXIS FUNCTION

General Information

Tests of HPA axis function address one of three basic questions: (1) What is the quantity of hormone being released under basal conditions? (2) Does cortisol show appropriate inhibition (negative-feedback)? and (3) Do stimulating hormones release normal amounts of pituitary or adrenal hormone under controlled conditions? The test or tests selected are based upon the aspect of HPA axis function under investigation.

Dexamethasone Suppression Test

For years the DST has been used as a standard instrument in the diagnosis of Cushing's disease (7). However, work by Carroll et al. (8) in 1968 provided a nidus for future research on HPA axis function in depression by the observation of nonsuppression of 11-hydroxycorticosteroid levels in 14 of 27 patients with major depression. Controversy still exists about the clinical usefulness of the DST in depression. Nonetheless, investigation in this area has facilitated a better understanding of the biological concomitants of major depression.

Dexamethasone is a high-potency synthetic glucocorticoid that suppresses ACTH production by binding to glucocorticoid receptors at the anterior pituitary, but also possibly at receptors in the hypothalamus and limbic structures. When Cushing's disease is suspected, the sequence of testing usually begins with a 1-mg overnight DST followed by the oral administration of 0.5 mg of dexamethasone every 6 hr for 2 days, and finally, 2 mg every 6 hr for another 2 days (the so called 2- and 8-mg DSTs). During the overnight test, 1 mg of dexamethasone is given in the late evening (about 2300 hr), and blood samples for cortisol concentration are obtained the following day at 0800 hr, 1600 hr, and 2300 hr. Individuals who do not suppress cortisol levels to below 5 μg/dL (9) are considered to have abnormal results and are called "nonsuppressors" or "early escapers." During the 2- and 8-mg tests, 24-hr urine specimens for either 17-hydroxycorticosteroids or urinary free cortisol (UFC) are collected. Few patients with major depression as the principal diagnosis will proceed to the 2- and 8-mg DST, although some continue to show cortisol nonsuppression at this stage of testing (10).

There are several mechanisms that could account for cortisol nonsuppression following DST in patients with major depression (11), which include (1) increased dexamethasone metabolism, (2) glucocorticoid receptor insensitivity, (3) adrenal hyperactivity, or (4) excessive pituitary or hypothalamic activity. The scope of this paper does not allow a complete discussion of these possibilities, although brief comments will be made about the data supporting the most likely cause of excessive cortisol secretion.

Urinary Free Cortisol

The DST does not indicate the magnitude of corticosteroid increase to which a patient is exposed. At best, the DST indirectly indicates increased levels of cortisol. Furthermore, 5-10% of the normal population shows DST non-suppression after a 1-mg DST, and this makes the assumption of hypercortisolemia in major depression less certain (12).

Furthermore, measurement of plasma cortisol levels, even at several times during the day, have not been satisfactory in differentiating patients with cortisol hypersecretion from controls. This is largely because of fluctuation in cortisol secretion from hour to hour, thereby introducing an unacceptable degree of variance. Diurnal changes in cortisol over a 24-hr period also introduce a problem in sampling because excessive cortisol secretion may occur only at specific times during the 24-hr cycle. In a comparison of depressed and control subjects, cortisol levels may differ between groups only during the night (13,14). Furthermore, it is probably the cumulative exposure of important brain receptors to cortisol that is essential in the development of HPA axis dysfunction in depression, and therefore, measurement of 24-hr urine specimens for 17-hydroxycorticosteroid (17-OHCS) or UFC levels has been used to assess daily cortisol production (15). However, measurement of UFC levels is complicated by several factors, which limit its clinical usefulness. It is cumbersome and time-consuming; the measurement relies upon the patient's self-report and the concurrent measurement of 24-hr urinary creatinine (16); and, finally, absolute UFC levels are difficult to compare between laboratories because of differences in assay procedures (17).

Despite these limitations, quantitative assessment of 24-hr cortisol secretion gives a generalized measurement of the extent of HPA axis dysfunction and may account for some of the signs and symptoms associated with cortisol excess. For instance, if circulating cortisol is elevated in patients with major depression, then one might expect to see subtle signs of insulin resistance and hypertension, both relatively early signs of corticosteroid excess. In fact, both are found with greater frequency in depressed patients with hypercortisolemia (18). Similarly, other signs of hypercortisolemia would also be expected, depending on the degree and duration of cortisol exposure.

Insulin-Induced Hypoglycemia

The insulin tolerance test (IH) has been used to further evaluate the pathological changes in HPA axis function in major depression. This test is most often used in research designs, but it has also been applied as a test to differentiate patients with Cushing's disease from those with major depression (10,19,20).

Insulin-induced hypoglycemia is a means of creating a controlled stress to which the body reacts by producing counterregulatory hormone responses. The principal hormone involved in rectifying the hypoglycemic episode is glucagon (21); however, other hormones are also secreted, including ACTH and cortisol. The HPA axis response appears to be initiated in the limbic system and other cortical structures, with neuronal messages being pass through the medial basal hypothalamus (22,23) to activate ACTH secretion through CRH (permissive) and AVP (modulatory) production (24). The importance of this test of HPA axis function is that it evaluates the entire feedback loop in response to a physiological change.

The insulin-induced hypoglycemia is accomplished by giving an intravenous bolus of 0.1-0.15 units/kg of regular insulin. Blood sugar must fall to a nadir of at least 50% of the fasting value to consistently cause a "counterregulatory" response of ACTH and cortisol (25,26). An adrenergic response (sweating, tachycardia, hunger, and weakness) usually accompanies the hypoglycemia, and this action probably stimulates an ACTH rise, which peaks at 45 min, and a cortisol rise, which peaks at 60-75 min (Fig. 2).

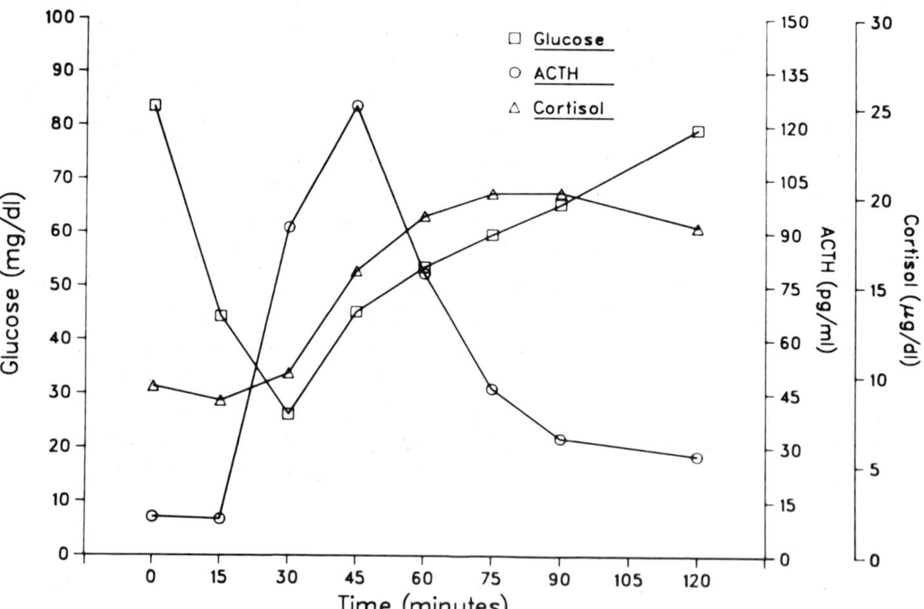

Figure 2 Glucose, ACTH, and cortisol changes after the administration of regular insulin, 0.15 units/kg, in six control subjects at 1600 hr.

The Corticotropin-Releasing Hormone Test

As suggested by its name, CRH stimulates the secretion of ACTH by acting directly on pituitary corticotroph CRH receptors (27,28). Two CRH peptides are available for human use: human (hCRH) and ovine (oCRH). The oCHR has a longer duration of action, which allows the measurement of a greater cumulative hormone response.

The CRH test has been standardized in humans by several investigators (29-34). Each CRH preparation has its own advantage, depending upon the hypotheses being tested. Both are currently being used to assess the pituitary responsiveness of ACTH and cortisol in psychiatric patients (35-38).

The CRH test also allows a systematic evaluation of both pituitary and adrenal responses to a direct CRH challenge. In contrast, the IH test presumably works through the release of endogenous CRH, the amount of which is impossible to control. Furthermore, factors such as AVP may also be involved in the ACTH response. In addition, ACTH and cortisol levels, as determined by the IH test, cannot be used to extrapolate findings from the CRH test because different pathological states produce different hormonal responses. In fact, it is just these differential responses that make these tests valuable in distinguishing Cushing's disease from major depression.

Other Tests of Hypothalamic-Pituitary-Adrenal Axis Function

A limited list of tests used to evaluate the HPA axis in normal and pathological states is presented in Table 1. The foregoing four tests were chosen

Table 1 Tests Used to Evaluate the HPA Axis

Metyrapone test
ACTH stimulation test
Circadian rhythm tests
Cortisol secretion rate
Cerebrospinal fluid CRH levels
Vasopressin stimulation test
Dexamethasone suppression tests, 2 and 8 mg
Cortisol suppression test
Clonidine stimulation test
Amphetamine stimulation test
Pyrogen stimulation test
Glucose tolerance test
Corticosteroid binding globulin levels
Glucocorticoid receptor levels
Free cortisol levels

because they are either in general clinical use or they provide the most accurate means of differentiating major depression from Cushing's disease.

URINARY FREE CORTISOL LEVELS AND DEXAMETHASONE SUPPRESSION TESTING IN PATIENTS WITH MAJOR DEPRESSION

Urinary Free Cortisol Levels

Urinary free cortisol is excreted in greater amounts in patients with major depression when compared with controls (Table 2; 39-43). Furthermore, it appears that patients who have abnormalities in HPA axis function during depression will also have elevated UFC levels after recovery, compared with age- and gender-matched controls (44). Possible correlations between UFC excretion and clinical variables have not been investigated. In fact, few studies have examined the UFC elevation in other psychiatric conditions (45-47).

Two studies have investigated the relationship between UFC levels and DST nonsuppression (41,43). Both have reported that many patients with DST nonsuppression do not demonstrate UFC elevation, although there is an overall association between the two. Additionally, patients who are DST suppressors show consistently lower UFC levels than do patients who are DST nonsuppressors. These data suggest that UFC levels are less sensitive than DST results in identifying patients with HPA axis abnormalities; hence, there currently is no clinical reason to order this test in patients with major depression unless the differential diagnosis includes Cushing's syndrome.

The Dexamethasone Suppression Test

Carroll (48) and Arana et al. (49) have extensively reviewed DST nonsuppression in psychiatric disorders other than depression. These reviews and

Table 2 Mean Urinary Free Cortisol Levels in Patients with Major Depression

	Major depression	Control	
Study (Ref.)	UFC level (N)	UFC level (N)	P
Carroll et al. (39)	90 (60)	49 (35)	0.0001
Milln et al. (40)	110 (24)	69 (30)	0.02
Vandewalle et al. (41)	87 (14)	75 (11)	NS
Rosenbaum et al. (63)	195 (24)	66 (22)	0.001
Rubinow et al. (42)	75 (28)	57 (31)	
Stokes et al. (43)	130 (98)	70 (70)	0.001

Table 3 Specificity of the DST in Major Depression vs Other Diagnoses

Comparison diagnosis	No. of subjects	Specificity (%)
Normal controls	687 (8 AM)	96
	1144 (4 PM)	93
	434 (11 PM)	94
Chronic pain	33	100
Acute grief	21	91
Obsessive compulsive	27	93
Anxiety/panic/phobia	76	88
Schizophrenia[a]	275	87
Alcoholism[a]	355	80
Dysthymic disorder	240	77
Acute/atypical psychosis	98	65
Dementia	180	57
Mania	163	52
Bulemia[a]	179	44
Anorexia	38	5
Alcohol withdrawal	133	95
Opiate withdrawal	23	96
Mental retardation	68	81
Stroke	33	70

[a]Secondary depression not necessarily deleted.

others (12,50-53) illustrate the variable specificity of the DST in several psychiatric disorders when compared with depression (Table 3). This factor seriously limits the clinical usefulness of the DST as a diagnostic or prognostic test in patients with major depression; therefore, the DST is usually

Table 4 Treatment Response as It Relates to DST Status

	Rate of successful treatment	
Study	DST (+)	DST (−)
Brown and Shuey (64)	4/8	14/38
Coryell (65)	21/21	18/21
Schlesser and Rush (66)	36/43	9/18
Amsterdam et al. (67)	4/12	20/28
Ettigi et al. (68)	10/11	3/7
Fraser (69)	10/22	8/11
Green and Kane (70)	13/18	21/27
Greden et al. (71)	17/21	10/10
Lipman et al. (72)	20/26	9/12
Total (%)	140/185 (76)	112/162 (69)

Table 5 Relapse after Clinical Recovery in DST Nonsuppressors

Study	Number relapsed	
	DST normal	DST abnormal
	(At recovery)	
Goldberg (73)	0/5	3/3
Greden et al. (74)	1/10	4/4
Yerevanian et al. (75)	1/4	10/10
Holsboer et al. (76)	0/16	4/4
Coryell and Zimmerman (77)	8/9	1/7
Peselow et al. (78)	6/20	4/9
Total (%)	16/20 (25)	26/37 (70)

neither necessary nor indicated for most of these patients. Carroll (50), however, suggests that the DST is still useful for clinical discrimination when diagnostic uncertainty exists. This approach is justified when one is trying to distinguish depression from conditions with few false-positive DST results, such as the anxiety disorders or schizophrenia (see Table 3). Needless to say, these differential diagnoses rarely present difficulties and, thus, limit the role of the DST in most patients with major depression.

Many studies have investigated the role of the DST in predicting response to treatment. A review of those studies that were well controlled suggests that there is a marginal difference in response rate between suppressors and nonsuppressors (Table 4).

One clinical indication for the DST is its possible prognostic value for predicting early relapse after successful treatment with an antidepressant. Several studies suggest that those patients with DST nonsuppression after clinical recovery are at higher risk for relapse than those who revert to suppressor status (Table 5). If further studies confirm this relationship, the DST could be of use when discontinuation or alteration of treatment is being contemplated.

ASSESSMENT FOR CUSHING'S DISEASE IN PATIENTS WITH MAJOR DEPRESSION

Cushing's syndrome is characterized by signs and symptoms of hypercortisolemia, including truncal obesity, moon facies, hypertension, hirsutism, acne, pink stria, proximal muscle weakness, thin skin, and glucose intolerance, among others. The syndrome can arise from a variety of causes (Fig. 3); however, Cushing's disease (pituitary adenoma) accounts for as many as 80% of the cases (10).

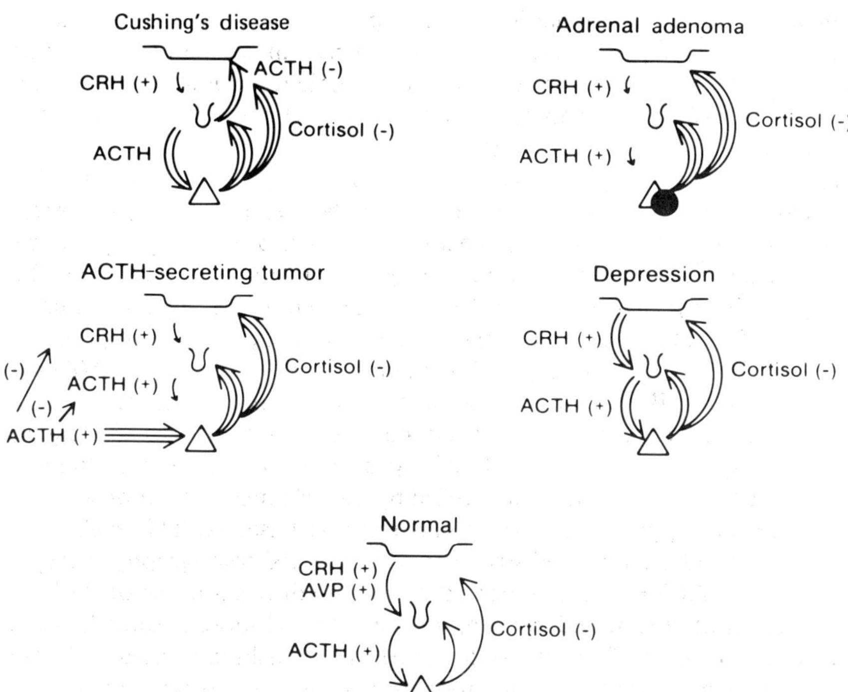

Figure 3 Hypothalamic, pituitary, and adrenal secretory relationships in normal persons and in those with various causes of hypercortisolemia.

For a number of years it was uncertain whether these pituitary adenomas occurred spontaneously or were the result of suprehypophysial stimulation by CRH, AVP, or both. With the advent of CRH stimulation testing and measurement of CRH in the cerebrospinal fluid, it now appears that Cushing's disease is most likely due to an autonomous pituitary adenoma (20, 54).

Approximately 60% of patients with Cushing's syndrome demonstrate affective symptoms (55), of which, 20% require psychiatric attention because of severity of symptoms.

Occasionally, the question arises of whether a patient has primary major depression or the psychiatric symptoms of Cushing's syndrome. This occurs when patients present with major depression accompanied by obesity, stria, hypertension, or other early signs of cortisol excess. The DST is helpful in distinguishing between these syndromes only if it results in cortisol suppression, because this effectively rules out Cushing's syndrome. On the other hand, DST nonsuppression further confuses the clinical picture.

The approach to the evaluation of these patients should be conservative, but systematic. The obvious initial step is to perform a thorough endocrine examination for Cushing's syndrome. These patients should have a 2- and 8-mg DST, followed by computed tomography of the sella tursica if the dexamethasone tests are abnormal.

When there is a moderate index of suspicion for Cushing's syndrome after the endocrine examination, the patient should be treated for major depression. If psychiatric symptoms resolve and other signs of Cushing's syndrome persist, endocrine evaluation should be pursued. Factors supporting the validity of this approach include the fact that major depression is usually episodic and of relatively short duration and has a high rate of response to treatment (70-80%). If the depression resolves and the abnormal DST normalizes, then the likelihood of Cushing's syndrome is diminished.

Even with this conservative approach, occasional patients will still require further testing to differentiate Cushing's syndrome from depression. In most cases, adrenal adenoma can be identified by the presence of high-dose dexamethasone nonsuppression, low or undetectable basal ACTH levels, and changes in the adrenal glands' structure on computed tomography. Ectopic production of ACTH is characterized by very high basal levels of ACTH, electrolyte disturbances, and nonsuppression with high-dose dexamethasone.

More problematic discrimination occurs with Cushing's disease. These patients can present with mild symptoms; show cortisol nonsuppression after a 2-mg DST, but not after an 8-mg DST; have normal to slightly elevated UFC and basal ACTH; and have an undetectable pituitary microadenoma on magnetic resonance or computed tomographic scans. Similarly, these findings can also be compatible with major depression.

The IH test has been suggested as a means of distinguishing Cushing's disease from nonendocrine causes of hypercortisolemia (10,56). After IH, patients with Cushing's disease demonstrate a blunted cortisol and absent ACTH response, whereas patients with depression have a blunted (not absent) ACTH response and a normal cortisol response (57). However, there remains the exceptional depressed or Cushing's patient who makes this test imperfect (58-60). Despite these limitations, cortisol response to IH remains a useful clinical test to improve diagnostic certainty in differentiating borderline cases of Cushing's disease and major depression.

Two newer tests that may prove useful are the CRH stimulation test and cerebrospinal fluid (CSF) CRH levels. Both are presently used in research settings; however, they offer promise for the future (20,51,54,61,62).

SUMMARY

The development and application of laboratory techniques are enhancing our ability to localize and define abnormalities of neuroendocrine function in major depression and Cushing's disease. For example, application of these techniques suggests that the heightened cortisol secretion found in many patients with depression is the result of hypersecretion of CRH, AVP, or both, either autonomously or in response to signals from the limbic system or higher cortical structures.

In contrast, in patients with Cushing's disease, the stimulus for cortisol production is probably the result of autonomous secretion of ACTH from a pituitary adenoma. This view is supported by studies demonstrating that there is an augmented ACTH response to CRH and vasopressin.

Although tests of HPA axis function have established a clearly defined role in the investigation of the pathophysiology of major depression, there are few situations in which their performance is clinically useful for everyday practice. Nevertheless, there may be indications when these tests are useful in the differentiation of major depression from Cushing's syndrome and the prediction of early relapse after successful antidepressant treatment. With these exceptions, neither the DST nor other tests of neuroendocrine function appear to improve diagnostic accuracy or predict response to treatment in patients with major depression.

Neuroendocrine tests have not yet found wide applicability in psychiatric clinical practice. However, their theoretical implications are substantial. Many of these findings suggest that CNS dysfunction results in chronic intermittent hypersecretion of cortisol which, in turn, influences the affective state (the HPA axis is not merely affected by, but integrally involved in the manifestation of the syndrome of major depression). Substantiation of this possibility could be far-reaching for prophylaxis, monitoring, and treatment. Medications that alter ACTH and cortisol secretion could effectively treat acute depression and act prophylactically in patients with abnormal HPA axis function. Furthermore, such techniques as monitoring absolute UFC or salivary cortisol levels may more effective predict relapse potential, thereby allowing early intervention and possibly avoid the clinical syndrome.

ACKNOWLEDGMENTS

This chapter received partial support from CRC Grant RR59 and NIMH Grant No. MH40174.

The authors gratefully acknowledge the assistance of Betty Stevens in the preparation this manuscript.

REFERENCES

1. Fehm, H. L., Klein, E., Holl, R., and Voigt, K. H. (1984). Evidence for extrapituitary mechanisms mediating the morning peak of plasma cortisol in man. *J. Clin. Endocrinol. Metab.* *58*:410-414.

2. Sherman, B. M., Schlechte, J. A., and Pfohl, B. M. (1984). Dissociation of plasma cortisol and ACTH responses to dexamethasone in healthy subjects. *Horm. Res. 20*:157-165.
3. Antoni, F. A. (1986). Hypothalamic control of adrenocorticotropin secretion: Advances since the discovery of 41-residue corticotropin-releasing factor. *Endocr. Rev. 7*:351-378.
4. Holsboer, F. (1987). Psychoneuroendocrine strategies. *Adv. Psychosom. Med. 17*:185-233.
5. DeBold, C. R., Sheldon, W. R., DeCherney, G. S., Jackson, R. V., Alexander, A. N., Vale, W., Rivier, J., and Orth, D. N. (1984). Arginine vasopressin potentiates adrenocorticotropin release induced by ovine corticotropin-releasing factor. *J. Clin. Invest. 73*:533-538.
6. McEwen, B. S., DeKloet, E. R., and Rostene, W. (1986). Adrenal steroid receptors and actions in the nervous system. *Physiol. Rev. 66*:1121-1187.
7. Liddle, G. W. (1960). Tests of pituitary-adrenal suppressibility in the diagnosis of Cushing's syndrome. *J. Clin. Endocrinol. Metab. 20*:1539-1560.
8. Carroll, B. J., Martin, F. I. R., and Davies, B. (1968). Resistance to suppression by dexamethasone of plasma 11-O.H.C.S. levels in severe depressive illness. *Br. Med. J. 3*:285-287.
9. Meltzer, H. Y. and Fang, V. S. (1983). Cortisol determination and the dexamethasone suppression test: A review. *Arch. Gen. Psychiatry 40*:501-505.
10. Besser, G. M. and Edwards, C. R. W. (1972). Cushing's syndrome. *Clin. Endocrinol. Metab. 1*:451-490.
11. Kathol, R. G., Jaeckle, R. S., Lopez, J. F., Meller, W. H. (1989). Pathophysiology of hypothalamic-pituitary-adrenal axis abnormalities in patients with major depression: An update. *Am. J. Psychiatry 146*:311-317.
12. Zimmerman, M. and Coryell, W. (1987). The dexamethasone suppression test in healthy controls. *Psychoneuroendocrinology 12*:245-251.
13. Pfohl, B., Sherman, B., Schlechte, J., and Winokur, G. (1985). Differences in plasma ACTH and cortisol between depressed patients and normal controls. *Biol. Psychiatry 20*:1055-1072.
14. Linkowski, P., Mendlewicz, J., Leclercq, R., Brasseur, M., Hubain, P., Golstein, J., Copinschi, G., and Van Cauter, E. (1985). The 24-hour profile of adrenocorticotropin and cortisol in major depressive illness. *J. Clin. Endocrinol. Metab. 61*:429-438.
15. Hsu, T. H. and Bledsoe, T. (1970). Measurement of urinary free corticoids by competitive protein-binding radioassay in hypoadrenal states. *J. Clin. Endocrinol. 30*:433-448.
16. Cryer, P. E. and Sode, J. (1970). Variation in urinary creatinine excretion and its relationship to measurement of urinary 17-hydroxycorticosteroids. *Clin. Chem. 16*:1012-1015.
17. Murphy, B. E. P., Okouneff, L. M., Klein, G. P., and Ngo, S. C. (1986). Lack of specificity of cortisol determination in human urine. *J. Clin. Endocrinol. Metab. 53*:91-99.
18. Lewis, D. A., Kathol, R. G., Sherman, B. M., Winokur, G., and Schlesser, M. A. (1983). Differentiation of depressive subtypes by insulin insensitivity in the recovered phase. *Arch. Gen. Psychiatry 40*:167-170.

19. James, V. H. T., Landon, J., Wynn, V., and Greenwood, F. C. (1968). A fundamental defect of adrenocortical control in Cushing's disease. *J. Endocrinol.* *40*:15-28.
20. Gold, P. W., Kling, M. A., Khan, I., Calabrese, J. R., Kalogeras, K., Post, R. M., Avgerinos, P. C., Loriaux, D. L., and Chrousos, G. P. (1987). Corticotropin releasing hormone: Relevance to normal physiology and to the pathophysiology and differential diagnosis of hypercortisolism and adrenal insufficiency. In *Hypothalamic Dysfunction in Neuropsychiatric Disorders.* Edited by D. Nerozzi, F. K. Goodwin, and E. Costa. New York, Raven Press, 1987.
21. Gerich, J., Davis, J., Lorenzi, M., Rizza, R., Bohannon, N., Karam, J., Lewis, S., Kaplan, R., Schultz, T., and Cryer, P. (1979). Hormonal mechanisms of recovery from insulin-induced hypoglycemia in man. *Am. J. Physiol.* *236*:E380-E385.
22. Aizawa, T., Yasuda, N., and Greer, M. A. (1981). Hypoglycemia stimulates ACTH secretion through a direct effect on the basal hypothalamus. *Metabolism* *30*:996-1000.
23. Jozova, D., Kvetnansky, R., Kovacs, K., Oprsalova, Z., Vigas, M., and Makara, G. B. (1987). Insulin-induced hypoglycemia activates the release of adrenocorticotropin predominantly via central and propranolol insensitive mechanisms. *Endocrinology 120*:409-415.
24. Plotsky, P. M., Bruhn, T. O., and Vale, W. (1985). Hypophysiotropic regulation of adrenocorticotropin secretion in response to insulin-induced hypoglycemia. *Endocrinology 117*:323-329.
25. Keller-Wood, M. E., Shinsako, J., Keil, L. C., and Dallman, M. F. (1981). Insulin-induced hypoglycemia in conscious dogs: I. Dose-related pituitary and adrenal responses. *Endocrinology 109*:818-824.
26. Lewis, D. A. and Sherman, B. M. (1985). Stimulus-response relationship of hypoglycemia and anterior pituitary hormone secretion. *Clin. Res. 33*:28A.
27. Reisine, T. and Hoffman, A. (1983). Desensitization of corticotropin-releasing factor receptors. *Biochem. Biophys. Res. Commun. 1*:919-925.
28. Hauger, R. L., Millan, M. A., Catt, K. J., and Aguilera, G. (1987). Differential regulation of brain and pituitary corticotropin-releasing factor receptors by corticosterone. *Endocrinology 120*:1527-1533.
29. Orth, D., Jackson, R., De Cherney, G., De Bold, C., Alexander, A., Island, D., Rivier, J., Spiess, J., and Vale, W. (1983). Effect of synthetic ovine corticotropin-releasing factor: Dose response of plasma adrenocorticotropin and cortisol. *J. Clin. Invest. 71*:587.
30. Hermus, A. R. M. M., Pieters, G. F. F. M., Smals, A. G. H., Benraad, T. J., and Kloppenborg, P. W. C. (1984). Plasma adrenocorticotropin, cortisol, and aldosterone responses to corticotropin-releasing factor: Modulatory effect of basal cortisol levels. *J. Clin. Endocrinol. Metab. 58*:187-191.
31. De Cherney, G. S., De Bold, C. R., Jackson, R. V., Sheldon, W. R., Jr., Island, D. P., and Orth, D. N. (1985). Diurnal variation in the response of plasma adrenocorticotropin and cortisol to intravenous ovine corticotropin-releasing hormone. *J. Clin. Endocrinol. Metab. 61*:273-279.
32. Muller, O. A., Stalla, G. K., and von Werder, K. (1987). Corticotropin-releasing factor in humans: II. CRF stimulation in patients with diseases of the hypothalamo-pituitary-adrenal axis. *Horm. Res. 25*:185-198.

33. Oelkers, W., Boelke, T., and Bahr, V. (1988). Dose-response relationships between plasma adrenocorticotropin (ACTH), cortisol, aldosterone, and 18-hydroxycorticosterone after injection of ACTH-(1-39) or human corticotropin-releasing hormone in man. *J. Clin. Endocrinol. Metab. 66*:181-186.
34. Vale, W., Spiess, J., Rivier, C., and Rivier, J. (1981). Characterization of a 41-residue ovine hypothalamic peptide that stimulates secretion of corticotropin and beta-endorphin. *Science 213*:1394-1397.
35. Holsboer, F., von Bardeleben, U., Gerken, A., Stalla, G. K., and Muller, O. A. (1984). Blunted corticotropin and normal cortisol response to human corticotropin-releasing factor in depression. *N. Engl. J. Med. 311*:1127.
36. Gold, P. W., Loriaux, D. L., Roy, A., Kling, M. A., Calabrese, J. R., Kellner, C. H., Nieman, L. K., Post, R. M., Pickar, D., Gallucci, W., Avgerinos, P., Paul, S., Oldfield, E. H., Cutler, G. B., Jr., and Chrousos, G. P. (1986). Responses to corticotropin-releasing hormone in the hypercortisolism of depression and Cushing's disease: Pathophysiologic and diagnostic implications. *N. Engl. J. Med. 314*:1329-1336.
37. Holsboer, F., von Bardeleben, U., Wiedemann, K., Muller, O. A., and Stalla, G. K. (1987). Serial assessment of corticotropin-releasing hormone response after dexamethasone in depression: Implications for pathophysiology of DST nonsuppression. *Biol. Psychiatry 22*:228-234.
38. Amsterdam, J. D., Maislin, G., Winokur, A., Kling, M., and Gold, P. (1987). Pituitary and adrenocortical responses to the ovine corticotropin releasing hormone in depressed patients and healthy volunteers. *Arch. Gen. Psychiatry 44*: 775-781.
39. Carroll, B. J., Curtis, G. C., Davies, B. M., Mendels, J., and Sugerman, A. A. (1976). Urinary free cortisol excretion in depression. *Psychol. Med. 6*:43-50.
40. Milln, P., Bishop, M., and Coppen, A. (1981). Urinary free cortisol and clinical classification of depressive illness. *Psychol. Med. 11*:643-645.
41. Vandewalle, J., Charles, G., Mardens, Y., and Mendlewicz, J. (1983). Dexamethasone resistance and cortisol secretion in depressive illness. *Biol. Psychiatry 18*:385-389.
42. Rubinow, D. R., Post, R. M., Savard, R., and Gold, P. W. (1984). Cortisol hypersecretion and cognitive impairment in depression. *Arch. Gen. Psychiatry 41*:279-283.
43. Stokes, P. E., Stoll, P. M., Koslow, S. H., Maas, J. W., Davis, J. M., Swann, A. C., and Robins, E. (1984). Pretreatment DST and hypothalamic-pituitary-adrenocortical function in depressed patients and comparison groups: A multicenter study. *Arch. Gen. Psychiatry 41*:257-267.
44. Kathol, R. G. and Gehris, T. (1986). Peak amplitude and frequency of urinary free cortisol excretion in patients with a history of major depressive disorder. *Chronobiol. Int. 3*:281-287.
45. Persky, H. (1962). Adrenocortical function during anxiety. In *Physiological Correlates of Psychological Disorders*. Edited by R. Roessler and N. S. Greenfield. Madison, University of Wisconsin Press.
46. Kathol, R. G., Noyes, R., Jr., Lopez, A. L., and Reich, J. H. (1988). Relationship of urinary free cortisol levels in patients with panic disorder to symptoms of depression and agoraphobia. *Psychiat. Res. 24*:211-221.

47. Mason, J. W., Giller, E. L., Kosten, T. R., Ostroff, R. B., and Podd, L. (1986). Urinary free-cortisol levels in posttraumatic stress disorder patients. *J. Nerv. Ment. Dis. 174*:145-149.
48. Carroll, B. J. (1985). Dexamethasone suppression test: A review of contemporary confusion. *Clin. Psychiatry 46*:13-24.
49. Arana, G. W., Baldessarini, R. J., and Ornsteen, M. (1985). The dexamethasone suppression test for diagnosis and prognosis in psychiatry: Commentary and review. *Arch. Gen. Psychiatry 42*:1193-1204.
50. Walsh, B. T., Lo, E. S., Cooper, T., Lindy, D. C., Roose, S. P., Gladis, M., and Glassman, A. H. (1987). Dexamethasone suppression test and plasma dexamethasone levels in bulimia. *Arch. Gen. Psychiatry 44*:797-800.
51. Kennedy, S. H. and Garfunkle, P. E. (1987). In *Handbook of Clinical Psychoneuroendocrinology.* Edited by C. B. Nemeroff and P. T. Loosen. New York, Guilford Press, pp. 143-159.
52. Ruedrich, S. L., Wadle, C. V., Sallach, H. S., Hahn, R. K., and Menolascino, F. J. (1987). Adrenocortical function and depressive illness in mentally retarded patients. *Am. J. Psychiatry 144*:597-602.
53. Lipsey, J. R., Robinson, R. G., Pearlson, G. D., Rao, K., and Price, T. R. (1985). The dexamethasone suppression test and mood following stroke. *Am. J. Psychiatry 142*:318-323.
54. Tomori, N., Suda, T., Tozawa, F., Demura, N., Shizume, K., and Mouri, T. (1983). Immunoreactive corticotropin-releasing factor concentrations in cerebrospinal fluid from patients with hypothalamic-pituitary-adrenal disorders. *J. Clin. Endocrinol. Metab. 57*:1305-1307.
55. Kathol, R. G. (1985). Etiologic implications of corticosteroid changes in affective disorder. In *Psychiatric Medicine*, Vol. 3, no. 2. Edited by R. C. W. Hall. New York, SP Medical & Scientific Books, pp. 135-162.
56. Scott, R. S., Espiner, E. A., and Donald, R. A. (1979). Intermittent Cushing's disease with spontaneous remission. *Clin. Endocrinol. 11*:561-566.
57. Lopez, J., Kathol, R. G., Jaeckle, R. S., and Meller, W. (1987). The HPA axis response to insulin hypoglycemia in depression. *Biol. Psychiatry 22*:153-166.
58. Demura, R., Demura, H., Nunokawa, T., Hideyuki, B., and Miura, K. (1972). Responses of plasma ACTH, GH, LH and 11-hydroxycorticosteroids to various stimuli in patients with Cushing's syndrome. *J. Clin. Endocrinol. 34*:852-859.
59. Carroll, B. J. (1969). Hypothalamic-pituitary function in depressive illness: Insensitivity to hypoglycaemia. *Br. Med. J. 3*:27-28.
60. Winokur, A., Amsterdam, J., Caroff, S., Snyder, P. J., and Brunswick, D. (1982). *Am. J. Psychiatry 139*:39-44.
61. Banki, C. M., Bissette, G., Arato, M., O'Connor, L., and Nemeroff, C. B. (1987). CSF corticotropin-releasing factor-like immunoreactivity in depression and schizophrenia. *Am. J. Psychiatry 144*:873-877.
62. Roy, A., Pickar, D., Paul, S., Doran, A., Chrousos, G. P., and Gold, P. W. (1987). CSF corticotropin-releasing hormone in depressed patients and normal control subjects. *Am. J. Psychiatry 144*:641-645.
63. Rosenbaum, A. H., Maruta, T., Schatzberg, A. F., Orsulak, P. J., Jiang, N., Cole, J. O., Schildkrant, J. J. (1983). Toward a biochemical classification of

depressive disorders. VII. Urinary free cortisol and urinary MHP in depression. *Am. J. Psychiatr. 140*:314-318.
64. Brown, W. A., and Shuey, I. (1980). Response to dexamethasone and subtype of depression. *Arch. Gen. Psychiatry 37*:747-751.
65. Coryell, W. (1982). Hypothalamic-pituitary-adrenal axis abnormality and ECT response. *Psychiatry Res. 6*:283-291.
66. Schlesser, M. and Rush, J. (1982). DST Status in relation to desipramine response. 37th Annual Meeting, Bio Psych at Toronto. p. 79 (Abstr. 48).
67. Amsterdam, J. D., Winokur, A., Bryant, S., Larkin, J., and Rickels, K. (1983). The dexamethasone suppression test as a predictor of antidepressant response. *Psychopharmacology 80*:43-45.
68. Ettigi, P. G., Hayes, P. E., Narasimhachari, N., Hamer, R. M., Goldberg, S., and Secord, G. J. (1983). d-Amphetamine response and dexamethasone suppression test as predictors of treatment outcome in unipolar depression. *Biol. Psychiatry 18*:499-504.
69. Frazer, A. R. (1983). Choice of antidepressant based on the dexamethasone suppression test. *Am. J. Psychiatry 140*:786-787.
70. Green, H. S., and Kane, J. M. (1983). The dexamethasone suppression test in depression. *Clin. Neuropharmacol. 6*:7-24.
71. Greden, J. F., Gardner, R., King, D., Grunhaus, L., Carroll, B. J., and Kronfol, Z. (1983). Dexamethasone suppression test in antidepressant treatment of melancholia. The process of normalization and test-retest reproducability. *Arch. Gen. Psychiatry 40*:493-500.
72. Lipman, R. S., Backup, C., Bobrin, Y., Delaplane, J. M., Doeff, J., Gittleman, S., Joseph, R., and Kanefield, M. (1986). Dexamethasone suppression test as a predictor of response to electroconvulsive therapy. I. Inpatient treatment. *Conv. Ther. 2*:151-160.
73. Goldberg, I. K. (1980). Dexamethasone suppression test as an indicator of safe withdrawal of antidepressant therapy (letter). *Lancet 1*:376.
74. Greden, J. F., Albala, A. A., Haskett, R. F., James, N. McI., Goodman, L., Steiner, M., and Carroll, B. J. (1980). Normalization of the dexamethasone suppression test: a laboratory index of recovery form endogenous depression. *Biol. Psychiatry 15*:449-458.
75. Yerevanian, B. I., Olafsdotter, H., Milanese, E., Russotto, J., Mullon, P., Baciewicz, G., and Sagi, E. (1983). Normalization of dexamethasone tests at discharge from hospital: its prognostic value. *J. Aff. Disord. 5*:191-197.
76. Holsboer, F., Liebl, R., and Hofschuster, E. (1982). Repeated dexamethasone suppression test during depressive illness: normalization of test results compared with clinical improvement. *J. Aff. Disord. 4*:93-101.
77. Coryell, W., and Zimmerman, M. (1983). The dexamethasone suppression test and ECT outcome: a six month follow-up. *Biol. Psychiatry 18*:21-27.
78. Peselow, E. D., Baxter, N., Fieve, R. R., Barouche, F. (1987). The dexamethasone suppression test as a monitor of clinical recovery. *Am. J. Psychiatry 144*:30-35.

5

Tricyclic Antidepressants

GEORGE M. SIMPSON and HARDEEP SINGH

Medical College of Pennsylvania/Eastern Pennsylvania Psychiatric Institute
Philadelphia, Pennsylvania

INTRODUCTION

Since imipramine hydrochloride was introduced in the 1950s, many attempts have been made to determine which patients should be treated with tricyclic antidepressants (TCAs). The earliest reports (1,2) suggested that imipramine was most effective in the treatment of "endogenous depressions" and less effective for the "reactive depressions." More recently, several variables have been shown to be predictive of response or nonresponse to imipramine and amitriptyline. For example, the predictive value of age is unclear from the available evidence (3), and several groups have shown that patients with neurotic, hypochondriacal, or hysterical personality traits respond no better to TCAs than to placebo. One study (4) demonstrated that responders to amitriptyline seldom had a history of neurotic symptoms when compared with nonresponders. In addition, several studies (3) have demonstrated that past history variables are predictive of TCA response, in that the number of prior episodes is inversely related to a positive treatment outcome with TCAs. Two studies (5,6) have shown that insidious onset appears to predict a favorable response to TCAs, whereas a sudden onset is associated with a poor response. However, the relationship between duration of illness and TCA response remains unclear (3). It appears that endogenomorphic symptoms of the DSM-III-R subtype of melancholic depression are one of the best clinical predictors of a positive response to TCAs. These include pervasive loss of interest and pleasure in all, or almost all, activities, lack of reactivity to normally pleasurable stimuli, depression regularly worse in the morning, early-morning awakening (at least 2 hr before usual time of awakening), psychomotor retardation or agitation, significant anorexia or weight loss (e.g., more than 5% of body weight in 1 month), and a diurnal mood swing that is worse in the morning. In addition, there is usually no significant personality disturbance before the depressive episode, one or more previous episodes were followed by complete or nearly complete recovery, and patient previously had a good response to antidepressant therapy. Finally, a family history of depression, as well as a prior history of multiple depressive episodes with normal interepisode functioning predict a good response to TCAs (7).

Three studies (8-10) have reported that delusional depressed patients do not respond well to TCAs alone, and this observation has been recently confirmed by several other authors (11-13). In these studies, only 34% of the delusionally depressed patients responded to treatment with a TCA alone. However, several studies have suggested that a combination of a TCA and an antipsychotic drug is superior to treatment with either drug alone (11, 12,14-16), and these results were recently confirmed in a double-blind study (17). The reason for the synergistic effect of the TCA plus antipsychotic drug is not clear, and there is controversy over whether the presence of delusions represents a distinct depressive illness or greater illness severity. Symptomatically, delusional depressive patients appear to have significantly more psychomotor retardation or agitation, guilt feelings, ruminating self-referential thinking, and affect-congruent delusions and hallucinations. They respond poorly to antidepressants alone and should be treated by combining a TCA and neuroleptic agent.

The choice of TCA treatment for depression is based not only upon a detailed diagnostic evaluation, but also on the severity of illness (7). Mildly depressed patients often do not require medication and do well with supportive psychotherapy. Moderately depressed patients often do best with a combination of psychotherapy and a TCA. For severely depressed patients, antidepressants along with supportive psychotherapy is the treatment of choice. Electroconvulsive therapy (ECT) is usually the treatment of choice when there is a high risk of suicidal behavior, or in medically ill patients who could not tolerate TCA treatment. Recovery from ECT may be followed by treatment with TCAs to prevent a depressive relapse.

In addition to patients with major depression, favorable outcome to TCA therapy has also been suggested for a subgroup of patients with DSM-III-R (18) dysthymic disorder (7). These chronic depressive patients seem to manifest a subclinical form of major depression and phenomenologically exhibit some endogenomorphic features such as anhedonia, guilt, and hypersomnia. The practicing clinician should be aware that dysthymic disorder can precede a major depressive episode, or can coexist with a major depressive episode (double depression) (19). Additionally, patients whose major depressive disorder is accompanied by a preexisting chronic dysthymic disorder are at a higher risk for repeated episodes of major depression. Recent findings also indicate that patients with double depression should receive preventive TCA treatment after recovery from the episode of major depressive disorder because it appears that they are predisposed to rapid relapse by the continued existence of the chronic preexisting depression (19).

Among the biological predictors of treatment outcome, cortisol response after dexamethasone suppression (DST), and some of the sleep electroencephalographic (EEG) parameters appear to be promising. Thus, it was recently reported that depressed patients with less than 80% sleep efficiency respond favorably to TCAs, whereas rapid eye movement (REM) latency of less than 20 min is associated with poor TCA response (7).

Abnormal DST results (i.e., cortisol levels above 5 μg/dL) have been associated with a positive response to TCAs. Studies by some authors have indicated that more than 90% of cortisol nonsuppressors after DST have a complete recovery following treatment with TCAs (7).

Evidence from an increasing number of double-blind placebo-controlled studies support the earlier reports that monoamine oxidase inhibitor (MAOI) drugs are effective antidepressants for the subsets of patients who are described as nonendogenous, atypical, or neurotic depressives (20,21). Conversely, the conventional idea that TCAs are not useful for nonendogenous or atypical depression is also being questioned (20). For example, Sovner (22) reported treatment success with TCAs in an open study of 15 patients with atypical depressive symptoms including hyperphagia, hypersomnia, and excessive anxiety. Two large-scale double-blind studies comparing tricyclic with MAOI drugs for patients with nonendogenous depression found both classes of antidepressants to be equally effective, although in both studies patients with prominent anxiety symptoms tended to respond better to the MAOI (23,24). Thus, the clinical impression that MAOI drugs have a special efficacy for atypical depression appears to hold in controlled studies, but perhaps only for those patients with prominent anxiety or panic attacks.

PHARMACOKINETICS

At least 70% of depressed patients are helped by antidepressants. Despite 30 years of basic and clinical research on antidepressants, about 30-40% of depressed patients fail to improve on single trials. Undoubtedly, some of the patients who are not helped are suffering from a form of depression unresponsive to that class of drugs. However, other patients do not respond for clinical or pharmacologic reasons (7).

Only four drugs marketed in this country have been subjected to a significant number of clinical trials in which blood level measurements of the drug were compared with the clinical outcome. These include imipramine, desmethylimipramine, nortriptyline, and amitriptyline.

There are many factors relating to absorption, distribution, metabolism, and elimination of TCAs that can influence their average plasma level. In general, TCAs have complicated kinetic (metabolic) properties. A single plasma level measurement is difficult to interpret in relationship to clinical effects without specifying specific values for the drug that is being used and measured (25).

Routes of Administration

The bioavailability of TCAs depends on the routes of administration. In general, TCAs have a low and variable availability when given orally. This relates to what is called the first-pass effect (i.e., the time needed to reach the general circulation) with concurrent metabolism in the liver (26). When amitriptyline is administered intramuscularly (IM), it is presumed that the antidepressant effects may appear more rapidly than with oral administration because the first-pass metabolic effect is eliminated. On the other hand, plasma levels of nortriptyline were similar with IM and oral administration of the drug, and the major metabolite (10-hydroxynortriptyline) was also found in similar concentrations after both routes of administration (27). In one study, lower levels of desipramine were found after parenteral, compared with oral, administration of imipramine (28).

There is considerable intersubject and interdrug variability in the first-pass metabolic effect and, therefore, in the amount of available drug in the plasma. For the tertiary amine TCAs, like imipramine and amitriptyline, the "excess" *N*-demethylation observed between oral and parenteral pharmacokinetic parameters accounts for most of the "first-pass" effect. Furthermore, the amount of TCA actually available has varied between 13 and 90% among subjects. Thus, the first-pass effect may be of major importance for determining the magnitude of the steady-state drug concentration, as well as the dosage necessary for optimal clinical response.

METABOLISM AND ACTIVE METABOLITES

The TCAs are divided into two broad groups according to their chemical structure. The tertiary amine group includes imipramine, amitriptyline, trimipramine, and doxepin, whereas the secondary amine group includes desmethylimipramine, nortriptyline, and protriptyline. The tertiary amine TCAs are demethylated in the liver into secondary methylamine derivatives, and these compounds are subsequently eliminated through hydroxylation and glucuronidation. Consequently, patients treated with tertiary amine tricyclics will also be exposed to their corresponding secondary amine metabolites. In some subjects, the extent of this conversion is so great that the predominant pharmacologically active compound in the plasma will be the secondary amine metabolite. For example, the ratio of amitriptyline to its demethylated metabolite, nortriptyline, varies from less than 0.25 to more than 3.0, whereas for imipramine, the ratio with its metabolite desipramine ranges from 0.1 to 3.0 (29,30). Because the demethylation reaction is almost certainly not reversible, patients treated with a secondary amine TCA are exposed to only this compound and not to any corresponding tertiary metabolite.

The hydroxy metabolites of TCAs (e.g., 2-OH-imipramine, 2-OH-desmethylimipramine, 10-OH-amitriptyline, 10-OH-nortriptyline) cross the blood-brain barrier and are effective in neuronal reuptake blockade of 5-hydroxytryptamine and norepinephrine; they also may be therapeutically active. They are present in significant concentrations in plasma, urine, and cerebrospinal fluid and are freely bound to glucuronic acid, the conjugate being present in two- to fourfold excess (31-33). They are not routinely measured, and their contribution to the therapeutic effect of the TCA is subject to debate. Some of the hydroxy metabolites are highly cardiotoxic, which, in part, may explain the presence of cardiac side effects at relatively low serum levels of the parent compound.

PROTEIN BINDING

The TCAs are lipid-soluble, and this property facilitates the intestinal absorption, circulatory dispersion, and eventual accumulation in tissues such as the brain. The free, unbound (to protein) concentration in plasma is assumed to reflect the concentration available for binding to receptors at the cell membrane. The routine practice of measuring the sum of the protein-bound and free TCA concentration, and not specifically measuring the free concentration, in part, may explain some of the conflicting observations between plasma drug levels and clinical response (34-36). Under conditions of rigorous pH control, unbound fractions of TCAs equaled 7.8 ± 1% for amitriptyline, 11.0 ± 1.2% for nortriptyline, 11.5 ± 1.4% for imipramine, and 15.3 ± 1.5% for desipramine (37,38). These binding values were unaffected by gender or by the use of estrogen hormones in women. Interindividual variations in protein-binding values may also be partially explained by fluctuations of plasma lipoprotein levels.

CEREBROSPINAL FLUID LEVELS

Antidepressant concentration in the cerebrospinal fluid (CSF) may more closely approximate the TCA level at neuronal receptor sites in the brain, and, thus, may correlate better with therapeutic outcome. However, some studies have suggested that CSF concentrations of imipramine may not be readily correlated with drug concentrations in the plasma (39,40). This may have implications for studies attempting to correlate blood TCA levels with clinical outcome, and more research will be needed before definitive statements can be made concerning the relationship between TCA blood levels and drug efficacy.

INTERINDIVIDUAL VARIATIONS OF STEADY-STATE LEVELS

The TCA plasma concentrations reach *steady-state* when the amount of drug eliminated daily equals the dose consumed. Thus, the steady-state concentration is an index of the total amount of drug in the body and, for a given individual, is directly dependent upon the daily dosage. In general, steady-state TCA levels are reached within 5 to 7 days after a consistent daily dosage regimen.

Numerous researchers have demonstrated marked interindividual differences in steady-state TCA levels, ranging from 5- to 36-fold, and occasionally, higher for nortriptyline and desipramine, after a fixed daily dosage (41,42). The most important factor that contributes to differences in steady-state TCA levels appears to be genetic. Individuals differ widely in their ability to metabolize certain drugs. In addition, there are also environmental factors such as diet, smoking, and the use of other medications (30,43).

These variations in steady-state TCA plasma levels indicate that the dose must be individualized to achieve an optimum TCA blood level.

DRUG INTERACTIONS

Chronic use of alcohol, barbiturates, and other sedative-hypnotics induce hepatic microsomal enzymes that increase the metabolic breakdown of TCAs, thereby reducing the plasma concentrations (44,45). Methylphenidate increases TCA levels (46) and, therefore, may enhance the antidepressant effect. Neuroleptic drugs can increase plasma TCA levels (47-50), possibly contributing to their efficacy in psychotic depression. In contrast, thyroid hormones appear to potentiate TCAs by altering the ratio of protein binding of the TCA (51), rather than by increasing plasma TCA levels (52).

No pharmacokinetic interactions have been seen between modest doses of benzodiazepines and TCAs (53) or between MAOIs and TCAs (54).

Cigarette smoking is thought to induce hepatic enzymes and, consequently, to increase the rate of drug metabolism. One study (42) found a significant difference in the steady-state levels of imipramine and desipramine in smokers compared with nonsmokers treated with equal doses of medication. However, other studies have found no correlations between cigarette smoking and plasma nortriptyline levels (55,56).

RENAL DISEASE

Dawling et al. (57) studied the pharmacokinetics of a single dose of nortriptyline in 20 patients with chronic renal failure, eight of whom were receiving hemodialysis. They reported a tenfold interindividual variability in nortriptyline half-life and a 15-fold variability in clearance. These variations closely resemble observations in physically healthy subjects. No differences were observed between the dialyzed and the nondialyzed groups. The authors concluded that chronic renal failure was not associated with a significant change in nortriptyline metabolism as measured by its half-life or clearance rate. However, TCAs should be used with caution in these patients and monitored closely.

PHARMACODYNAMICS

A relationship between plasma levels of TCAs and clinical efficacy or side effects have been extensively studied since 1962. Most studies have suggested a lower limit for a favorable clinical response, but higher plasma levels may not necessarily lead to a better clinical response. The debate over whether or not there is a threshold or "therapeutic window" for the plasma concentration of the various TCAs is far from resolved (58).

Imipramine

The relationship between plasma levels and clinical outcome is clearest with impramine. As early as 1971, Walter (59) reported that all patients responding favorably to imipramine had plasma levels above 20 ng/mL. Gram and Christiansen (60) reported that 11 of 12 patients who responded to imipramine had plasma levels greater than 45 ng/mL of imipramine and 75 ng/mL of desipramine. Olivier-Martin et al. (61) reported a significant correlation between the degree of clinical improvement and total imipramine plus desipramine levels or desipramine levels alone, but not to levels of imipramine alone. Perel et al. (42) reported that imipramine responders had levels exceeding 180 ng/mL, in contrast with nonresponders, who had levels less than 180 ng/mL. Glassman et al. (9) found a linear relationship between imipramine plus desipramine plasma levels and therapeutic effects in a study in which 21 of 29 nonresponders had levels less than 180 ng/mL; whereas, 22 of 31 responders had total plasma levels of more than 180 ng/mL. Response rate was 93% for patients with plasma levels greater than 225 ng/mL; 64% for patients with levels of 150-225 ng/mL; and 20% for patients with levels less than 150 ng/mL. An earlier report by these authors (62) claimed that therapeutic levels for imipramine ranged between 200 and 250 ng/mL, which was about double the concentration Asberg et al. (63) reported for nortriptyline (i.e., 50-150 ng/mL). Reisby et al. (64) found that a threshold imipramine plus desmethylimipramine level of 240 ng/mL was needed for good response to imipramine, whereas Perel et al. (30) suggested a therapeutic response range for imipramine of 150-240 ng/mL, although there was no indication for the presence of a therapeutic window.

Simpson et al. (10) conducted a trial using two doses of imipramine in severely depressed inpatients and consistently found that the 300-mg regimen produced more improvement than the 150-mg regimen. This observation has important clinical implications for treating patients who appear refractory to conventional doses of a TCA, and it seems justifiable to increase the dose in patients who do not respond to modest doses of imipramine (and probably other TCAs as well). Treatment should not be regarded as having failed unless there is no improvement with the maximum recommended daily dosage of 300 mg of imipramine for several weeks.

In conclusion, studies of imipramine agree that (1) interindividual metabolic differences do influence therapeutic outcome; (2) the percentage of patients responding favorably increases as imipramine blood levels increase to 200-250 ng/mL (although some patients may show favorable response at lower levels); (3) plasma levels in excess of 250 ng/mL can produce more side effects, but in five of the six studies, no change in clinical response was seen—the effect of blood levels in excess of 750 ng/mL on clinical outcome has not been systematically examined; and (4) the maximum recommended daily dosage of imipramine is 300 mg, given for at least several weeks.

Nortriptyline

Nortriptyline has received extensive pharmacokinetic investigation. Asberg and co-workers (63) initially reported a curvilinear plasma level-response relationship (50-150 ng/mL) in 29 patients with endogenous depression. Subsequently, she showed that in patients randomly assigned to nortriptyline, 25 mg t.i.d. or 50 mg t.i.d. regimen, most subjects had steady-state plasma levels within the therapeutic range when taking 50 mg t.i.d. (65), and many of the patients receiving 25 mg t.i.d. were below the threshold of 50 ng/mL. Asberg recommended that patients for whom blood determinations were not readily available should be given 50 mg t.i.d., and those not responding should have their dosage decreased, rather than increased. Other studies have confirmed the presence of a therapeutic window of 50-140 ng/mL for nortriptyline (66), whereas several have failed to confirm this relationship.

Table 1 Suggested Dosage Regimen Based on 24-hr Blood Levels After Ingestion of 50 mg Nortriptyline

Blood level (ng/mL)	Suggested dosage regimen
< 12	50 mg t.i.d.
13-19	50 mg b.i.d.
20-24	25 mg t.i.d.
25-34	25 mg b.i.d.
35-40[a]	10 mg t.i.d.
> 41[a]	10 mg b.i.d.

[a]These ranges are calculated by extrapolation of the regression line ($y = a + bx$) calculated for these experimental data.

These negative findings have been attributed to heterogeneous groups of depressed patients and large interindividual variations in steady-state plasma levels, perhaps related to problems with the assay. Why this window effect exists for nortriptyline is still unclear, but it is not related to drug toxicity at plasma levels in excess of 150 ng/mL.

Alexanderson (27) demonstrated the ability to predict steady-state plasma levels of nortriptyline by determining the plasma clearance rate from a single oral dose of nortriptyline. The correlation between this rate and the steady-state plasma level was 0.93. Cooper and Simpson (46) subsequently described a technique enabling physicians to determine a patient's dosage requirements for nortriptyline from a single 24-hr blood sample after a 50-mg dose of nortriptyline. By using this technique, one can potentially predict the precise dosage requirements for each patient (Table 1). Thus, with a 24-hr predictive plasma level of nortriptyline, a patient can be started on medication immediately (e.g., the dose rapidly increase to 150 mg/day) and the dosage adjusted when laboratory data become available. The patient can be kept on this adjusted regimen for 4 weeks, and if therapeutic response is not achieved then there seems little point in changing from the optimum dosage. Cooper and Simpson (46) emphasized that this observation applies only to patients with endogenous depression, and a relationship between drug plasma level and clinical efficacy in nonendogenous depression has not been established.

Desmethylimipramine

Early studies measured desmethylimipramine as the primary metabolite in imipramine-treated patients (9,67). There are fewer data available specifically examining the relationship between plasma levels of desmethylimipramine and clinical outcome when desmethylimipramine itself is used as the TCA.

Only four studies have been published, and one of these examined only five patients (68). Khalid et al. (69) and Nelson et al. (70) described a linear relationship between drug concentration and outcome. In the Nelson et al. study, 32 unipolar, melancholic, nondelusional patients were examined, and they found that plasma concentrations above 125 ng/mL were significantly more effective than lower blood levels. The absence of a curvilinear response was also supported by two other studies (71,72). In contrast, Simpson et al. (25) found no obvious relationship between plasma desmethylimipramine levels and clinical outcome in 31 depressed inpatients suffering from major affective disorder, and this is in agreement with the study by Stewart et al. (72) who found that responders had blood levels that ranged from 160 to 877 ng/mL.

Amitriptyline

In 1972, Braithwaite et al. (73) reported a positive correlation between plasma levels of amitriptyline and its metabolite, nortriptyline and clinical response in 15 depressed patients. Patients who had plasma concentrations of amitriptyline plus nortriptyline less than 120 ng/mL showed a poor clinical response. A subsequent reanalysis of the data showed that the best therapeutic effect occurred at intermediate plasma levels, between 70 and 180 ng/mL (74,75), whereas Montgomery et al. (41) also reported the best outcome in those patients with intermediate plasma levels (ie., a mean ± SD amitriptyline and nortriptyline of 137 ± 60.2 ng/mL). Zeigler (76) found that patients with amitriptyline plus nortriptyline levels above 95 ng/mL fared better than those with lower levels. Improvements increased continuously as the plasma levels reached 240 ng/mL, indicating a linear relationship. Kupfer et al. (77) also reported a linear relationship between total levels of amitriptyline plus nortriptyline and the clinical response. In contrast, Volmat et al. (78) reported a curvilinear relationship for plasma levels and therapeutic response, with the best results occurring between 60 and 220 ng/mL of amitriptyline plus nortriptyline. Furlong et al. (79) also reported the possibility of a therapeutic window for amitriptyline, with most responders having mean blood levels of 63 ng/mL at a maintenance dose of 150 mg/day.

Coppen et al. (80) conducted a multicenter study that failed to demonstrate any relationship between steady-state amitriptyline plus nortriptyline plasma levels and therapeutic efficacy. Approximately one-third of their patients recovered completely, one-third improved somewhat, and one-third remained the same, regardless of blood levels. However, these negative findings have been attributed to the overall poor efficacy of the antidepressant in the group of patients studied (81). Thus, three studies have now shown a linear relationship, three have demonstrated a curvilinear relationship similar to that seen with nortriptyline, and four studies have found no relationship at all between blood levels and outcome (66).

Protriptyline

In 1973, Moody et al. (82) administered 25-105 mg/kg of protriptyline to nine depressed patients and found plasma levels ranging between 89 and 292 ng/mL. Later studies showed that patients taking 10-70 mg/day of protriptyline had plasma levels ranging from 24-434 ng/mL (83), and two different therapeutic blood level ranges for protriptyline were suggested: 189-270 ng/mL (84) and 70-170 ng/mL (85), respectively.

Other Tricyclic Antidepressants

Very limited information is available concerning maprotiline and doxepin, and even less is known about the other antidepressants marketed in the United States. There is tentative suggestion that 75 mg of trimipramine may be equal to or better in efficacy than 150 mg daily in outpatients with major depression (86).

BLOOD LEVELS AND SIDE EFFECTS

Studies of the relationship between plasma TCA levels and side effects have not generally found consistent results; however, plasma levels will change with dosage reduction within patients, and side effects often improve, implying an indirect association between side effects and plasma drug levels. There is an important element of individual susceptibility, which appears to be independent of blood levels. However, Asberg et al. (64) and Simpson et al. (25) have observed a significant positive correlation between plasma levels of nortriptyline and subjective side effects in depressed patients and healthy volunteers given nortriptyline.

BLOOD LEVELS AND OVERDOSE

Because TCAs have relatively long half-lives, serious medical complications may be prolonged for many patients who overdose with large quantities of a TCA. Reduction of cardiac contractility has been demonstrated with TCA blood levels as low as 50-100 ng/mL, and at levels over 500 ng/mL the incidence of serious cardiac toxicity is increased significantly. Above 1000 ng/mL, there is often severe and sometimes fatal cardiac and central nervous system side effects (17,87). In this regard, Bailey and Shaw (88) measured TCA levels in the blood, liver, and epicardium of 29 decedents with a fatal TCA overdose and reported that the drug was more highly concentrated in liver than in myocardium, but more concentrated in myocardium than in blood. As the concentration of TCA in myocardium may account for cardiotoxicity, which is closely associated with risk of fatality in a TCA overdose, great caution must be exercised in interpreting plasma level results in such cases. Patients should have continuous cardiac monitoring for several days if any serious TCA overdose is suspected, regardless of blood levels.

TREATMENT OF DEPRESSION WITH TRICYCLIC ANTIDEPRESSANTS

Major depression without melancholic features can be treated by both drugs and brief psychotherapy, and one study found the combined treatment to be superior (89). In the choice of a TCA, the family or past history of response to a specific TCA can provide a useful guide. Otherwise one generally begins a TCA treatment with a modest nighttime dose of imipramine or amitriptyline (50 mg) and, if well tolerated, increases to 100 mg hs on the third day and 150 mg on the fifth day. After 1 week, the dose is adjusted to 200 mg/day or, in some patients, up to 250 mg/day as a single or b.i.d. dosage. A slower rate of increase may be used (e.g., weekly increments) which may reduce side effects, but this will also reduce the speed of response. On the other hand, it may help define subjects who respond at low dosages of TCAs. The systematic recording of the baseline pulse and the postural blood pressure (taken both lying and 30 sec after standing) can be helpful in determining dosage adjustments. A bedtime (hs) dosing regimen is often easier for the patient to remember and, thus, improves compliance. A b.i.d. dosage can be used if toxicity at peak plasma levels after once-daily dosing is of particular concern. Steady-state plasma levels are reached within 1-2 weeks and are usually not helpful before this time. Most commonly, plasma drug levels at steady-state are measured after the patient has been receiving a fixed dose of the drug for at least 7 days.

CONCLUSION

Pharmacokinetic properties of TCAs provide information that may be related to pharmacodynamic effects. Measurements of TCA blood levels are not only useful for research purposes, but also for a variety of clinical situations. For example, plasma level measurements are useful in patients who do not respond to the usual oral doses of medication, or are at high risk of toxic effects because of age (elderly and children) or concurrent medical illness, who are suspected of poor compliance, and finally, in case of unwanted side effects. The rational use of plasma level monitoring in patients taking TCAs can often improve therapeutic efficacy with reduced risk of unwanted adverse effects.

REFERENCES

1. Kuhn, R. (1958). The treatment of depressive states with G22355 (imipramine hydrochloride). *Am. J. Psychiatry 115*:459-464.
2. Lehmann, H. E., Cahn, M. D., and DeVertevil, R. L. (1958). The treatment of depressive conditions with imipramine. *Can. Psychiatr. Assoc. J. 3*:115-164.
3. Bielski, R. J. and Friedel, R. O. (1976). Prediction of tricyclic antidepressant response. A critical review. *Arch. Gen. Psychiatry 33*:1479-1489.
4. Deykin, E. Y. and DiMascio, A. (1972). Relationship of patient background characteristics to efficacy of pharmacotherapy in depression. *J. Nerv. Ment. Dis. 155*:209-215.
5. Kiloh, L. G., Ball, J. R. B., and Garside, R. F. (1962). Prognostic factors in treatment of depressive states with imipramine. *Br. Med. J. 1*:1225-1227.
6. Raskin, A., Schulterbrandt, J. G., Reatig, N., et al. (1970). Differential response to chlorpromazine, imipramine and placebo. *Arch. Gen. Psychiatry 23*:164-173.
7. Georgotas, A. (1985). Affective disorders: Pharmacotherapy. In *Comprehensive Textbook of Psychiatry/IV*. Edited by H. I. Kaplan and B. J. Sadock. Baltimore, Williams & Wilkins, pp. 821-833.
8. Glassman, A. H., Kantor, S. J., and Shostak, M. (1975). Depression, delusions, and drug response. *Am. J. Psychiatry 132*:716-719.
9. Glassman, A. H., Perel, J. M., Shostak, M., et al. (1977). Clinical implications of imipramine plasma levels for depressive illness. *Arch. Gen. Psychiatry 34*: 197-204.
10. Simpson, G. M., Lee, J. H., Cucilic, Z., and Kellner, R. (1976). Two dosages of imipramine in hospitalized endogenous and neurotic depressives. *Arch. Gen. Psychiatry 33*:1093-1102.
11. Minter, R. E. and Mandel, M. R. (1979). The treatment of psychotic major depressive disorder with drugs and ECT. *J. Nerv. Ment. Dis. 167*:726-733.
12. Kaskey, G. B., Nasr, S., and Meltzer, H. Y. (1980). Drug treatment in delusional depression. *Psychiatry Res. 1*:267-277.
13. Frances, A., Brown, R. P., Kocsis, J. H., et al. (1981). Psychotic depression: A separate entity? *Am. J. Psychiatry 138*:831-833.
14. Nelson, J. C. and Bowers, M. B. (1978). Delusional unipolar depression: Description and drug response. *Arch. Gen. Psychiatry 35*:1321-1328.
15. Minter, R. E. and Mandel, M. R. (1979). A prospective study of the treatment of psychotic depression. *Am. J. Psychiatry 136*:1470-1472.
16. Charney, D. S. and Nelson, J. C. (1981). Delusional and nondelusional unipolar depression: Further evidence for distinct subtypes. *Am. J. Psychiatry 138*:328-333.
17. Spiker, D. J., Weiss, J. C. et al. (1985). The pharmacological treatment of delusion and depression. *Am. J. Psychiatry 142*:430-436.

18. American Psychiatric Association (1987). *Diagnostic and Statistical Manual of Mental Disorders*, 3rd ed, revised. Washington, D. C., American Psychiatric Association.
19. Keller, M. B., Labori, B. W., et al. (1983). Double depression: Two-year follow up. *Am. J. Psychiatry 140*:689-694.
20. Aarons, S. F., Frances, A. J., and Mann, J. J. (1983). Atypical depression: A review of diagnosis and treatment. *Hosp. Commun. Psychiatry 35*:275-282.
21. Liebowitz, M. R., Quitkin, F. M., Stewart, J. W., McGrath, P. J., Harrison, W. M., Markowitz, J. S., Rabkin, J. G., Tricamo, E., Goetz, D. M., and Klein, D. F. (1988). Antidepressant specificity in atypical depression. *Arch. Gen. Psychiatry 45*:129-137.
22. Sovner, R. D. (1981). The clinical characteristics and treatment of atypical depression. *J. Clin. Psychiatry 42*:285-289.
23. Ravaris, C. L., Robinson, D. S., Ives, J. O., et al. (1980). Phenelzine and amitriptyline in the treatment of depression. *Arch. Gen. Psychiatry 37*:1075-1080.
24. Rowen, P. R., Paykel, E. S., Parker, R. R., et al. (1981). Tricyclic antidepressants and MAOIs: Are there differential effects? In *Monoamine Oxidase Inhibitors: The State of the Art*. Edited by M. B. H. Youdin and E. S. Paykel. New York: John Wiley & Sons.
25. Simpson, G. M., Pi, E. H., and White, K. (1983). Plasma drug levels and clinical response to antidepressants. *J. Clin. Psychiatry 44*:27-34.
26. Alexanderson, B. (1972). Pharmacokinetics of desmethylimipramine and nortriptyline in man after single and multiple oral doses—a cross-over study. *Eur. J. Clin. Pharmacol. 5*:7-10.
27. Alexanderson, B. (1972). Pharmacokinetics of nortriptyline in man after single and multiple oral doses: The predictability of steady-state plasma concentrations from single-dose plasma-level data. *Eur. J. Clin. Pharmacol. 4*:82-91.
28. Nagy, A. and Johansson, R. (1975). Plasma levels of imipramine and desipramine in man after different routes of administration. *Naunyn Schmiedebergs Arch. Pharmacol. 290*:145-160.
29. Perel, J. M., Shostak, M., Gann, E., et al. (1976). Pharmacodynamics of imipramine and clinical outcome in depressed patients. In *Pharmacokinetics of Psychoactive Drugs*. Edited by L. A. Gottschalk and S. Merlis. New York: Spectrum Publ.
30. Perel, J. M., Stiller, R. L., and Glassman, A. H. (1978). Studies on plasma level/ effect-relationships in imipramine therapy. *Commun. Psychopharmacol. 2*:429-439.
31. Javaid, J. L., Perel, J. M., and Davis, J. M. (1979). Inhibition of biogenic-amine uptake by imipramine, desipramine, 2-hydroxy-imipramine and 2-hyroxy-desipramine in rat brain. *Life Sci. 24*:21-28.
32. Potter, W. Z., Calil, H. M., and Manian, A. A. (1979). Hydroxylated metabolites of TCA: Preclinical assessment of activity. *Biol. Psychiatry 14*:601-613.
33. DeVane, C. L. and Wolin, R. E. (1981). Excessive plasma concentrations of TCAs resulting from usual doses: A report of 6 cases. *J. Clin. Psychiatry 42*:143-147.
34. Borga, O., Azarnoff, D. L., Forshell, G. P., et al. (1969). Plasma protein binding of tricyclic antidepressants in man. *Biochem. Pharmacol. 18*:2135-2143.

35. Borga, O. (1973). Studies on the protein binding and pharmacokinetics of nortriptyline in man [Dissertation]. Karolinska Institute, Stockholm.
36. Gram, L. F. (1977). Plasma level monitoring of tricyclic antidepressant therapy. *Clin. Pharmacokinet. 2*:237-251.
37. Brinkschulte, M. and Breyer-Pfaff, U. (1979). Binding of tricyclic antidepressants and perazine to human plasma: Methodology and findings in normals. *Naunyn Schmiedebergs Arch. Pharmacol. 308*:1-7.
38. Brinkschulte, M. and Breyer-Pfaff, U. (1980). The role of lipoproteins in the binding of tricyclic antidepressants and perazine to human plasma. In *Proceedings 4th International Symposium on Phenothiazines and Related Drugs.* Amsterdam: Elsevier/North-Holland.
39. Sathananthan, G. L., Gershon, S., Almeida, M., et al. (1976). Correlation between plasma and cerebrospinal levels of imipramine. *Arch. Gen. Psychiatry 33*:1109-1110.
40. Elwan, O. and Adam, H. K. (1980). Relationship between blood and cerebrospinal levels of the antidepressant agent viloxazine. *Eur. J. Pharmacol. 17*:179-182.
41. Montgomery, S., Braithwaite, R., and Coppen, A. (1975). The relationship between plasma concentrations of amitriptyline and therapeutic response. Presented at *Br. Acad. Psychopharmacol.* London, July 1, 1975.
42 Perel, J. M., Shostak, M., Gann, E., et al. (1976). Pharmacodynamics of imipramine and clinical outcome in depressed patients. In *Pharmacokinetics of Psychoactive Drugs.* Edited by L. A. Gottschalk and S. Merlis. New York, Spectrum Publishers.
43. Burrows, G. D., Turecek, L. R., Davies, B., et al. (1977). Plasma nortriptyline and clinical response—a study using changing plasma levels. *Psychol. Med. 7*: 87-91.
44. Burrows, G. D. and Davies, B. (1971). Antidepressants and barbiturates. *Br. Med. J. 4*:113.
45. Moody, J. P., Whyte, S. F., MacDonald, A. J., et al. (1977). Pharmacokinetic aspects of protriptyline plasma levels. *Eur. J. Clin. Pharmacol. 11*:41-46.
46. Cooper, T. B. and Simpson, G. M. (1978). Prediction of individual dosage of nortriptyline. *Am. J. Psychiatry 135*:333-335.
47. Moody, J. P., Tait, A. C., and Todrick, A. (1967). Plasma levels of imipramine and desmethylimipramine during therapy. *Br. J. Psychiatry 113*:183-193.
48. Gram, L. F. and Over, K. F. (1972). Drug interaction: Inhibitory effect of neuroleptics on metabolism of tricyclic antidepressants in man. *Br. Med. J. 1*:463-465.
49. Vandel, B., Vandel, S., Allers, G., et al. (1979). Interaction between amitriptyline and phenothiazine in man: Effects on plasma concentration of amitriptyline and its metabolite nortriptyline and correlation with clinical response. *Psychopharmacology 65*:187-190.
50. Nelson, J. C. and Jatlow, P. I. (1980). Neuroleptic effect on desipramine steady-state plasma concentration. *Am. J. Psychiatry 137*:1232-1234.
51. Wilson, I. C., Prange, A. J., Jr., and McClure, T. K. (1970). Thyroid hormone enhancement of imipramine in non-retarded depressions. *N. Engl. J. Med. 282*: 1063-1067.

52. Feighner, J. P., King, L. J., Schuckit, M. A., et al. (1972). Hormonal potentiation of imipramine and ECT in primary depression. *Am. J. Psychiatry 128*:1230-1238.
53. Gram, L. F., Over, K. F., and Kirk, L. (1974). Influence of neuroleptics and benzodiazepines on metabolism of tricyclic antidepressants in man. *Am. J. Psychiatry 131*:863-866.
54. Snowdon, J. and Braithwaite, R. (1974). Combined antidepressant medication. *Br. J. Psychiatry 125*:610-611.
55. Alexanderson, B., Price Evans, D. A., and Sjoqvist, F. (1969). Steady-state plasma levels of nortriptyline in twins: Influence of genetic factors and drug therapy. *Br. Med. J. 4*:764-768.
56. Norman, T. R., Burrows, G. D., Maguire, K. P., et al. (1977). Cigarette smoking and plasma nortriptyline levels. *Clin. Pharmacol. Ther. 21*:453-456.
57. Dawling, S., Lynn, K., Rosser, R., et al. (1981). The pharmacokinetics of nortriptyline in patients with chronic renal failure. *Br. J. Clin. Pharmacol. 12*:39-45.
58. Cooper, T. B., Simpson, G. M., and Lee, J. H. (1976). Thymoleptic and neuroleptic drug plasma levels in psychiatry: Current status. *Int. Rev. Neurobiol. 19*: 269-309.
59. Walter, C. J. S. (1971). Clinical significance of plasma imipramine levels. *Proc. R. Soc. Med. 64*:282.
60. Gram, L. F. and Christiansen, J. (1975). First-pass metabolism of imipramine in man. *Clin. Pharmacol. Ther. 17*:555-563.
61. Oliver-Martin, R., Marzin, D., Buschenschutz, E., et al. (1975). Concentrations plasma tiques de l'imipramine et de la desmethylimipramine et effet antidepresseur au coms d'un traitement controle. *Psychopharmacologia 41*:187-195.
62. Glassman, A. H. (1981). Blood level measurements of tricyclic drugs as a diagnostic tool. *Psychiatr. Ann. 11*:14-26.
63. Asberg, M., Cronholm, B., Sjoqvist, F., et al. (1971). Relationship between plasma level and therapeutic effect of nortriptyline. *Br. Med. J. 3*:331-334.
64. Reisby, N., Gram, L. F., Bech, B., et al. (1977). Imipramine: Clinical effects and pharmacokinetic variability. *Psychopharmacology 54*:263-272.
65. Asberg, M. (1976). Treatment of depression with tricyclic drugs pharmacokinetic and pharmacodynamic aspects. *Pharmacopsychiatria 9*:18-26.
66. APA Task Force Report (1985). Tricyclic antidepressants, blood level measurement and clinical outcome. *Am. J. Psychiatry 142*:155-162.
67. Gram, L. F., Reisby, N., Ibsen, I., et al. (1976). Plasma levels and antidepressant effect of imipramine. *Clin. Pharmacol. Ther. 19*:318-324.
68. Amin, M. M., Cooper, R., Khalid, R., et al. (1978). A comparison of desipramine and amitriptyline plasma levels and therapeutic response. *Psychopharmacol. Bull. 14*:45-46.
69. Khalid, R., Amin, M. M., and Ban, T. A. (1978). Desipramine plasma levels and therapeutic response. *Psychopharmacol. Bull. 14*:43-44.
70. Nelson, J. C., Jatlow, P., Quinlan, D. M., et al. (1982). Desipramine plasma concentration and antidepressant response. *Arch. Gen. Psychiatry 39*:1419-1422.
71. Watt, D. C., Crammer, J. L., and Elkes, A. (1972). Metabolism, anticholinergic effects, and therapeutic outcome of desmethylimipramine in depressive illness. *Psychol. Med. 2*:397-405.
72. Stewart, J. W., Quitkin, F., Fyer, A., et al. (1980). Efficacy of desipramine in endogenomorphically depressed patients. *J. Affect. Disord. 2*:165-176.

73. Braithwaite, R. A., Goulding, R., Theano, G., et al. (1972). Plasma concentration of amitriptyline and clinical response. *Lancet 1*:1297-1300.
74. Gravstad, M. (1973). Plasma levels of antidepressants and clinical response. *Lancet 1*:95-96.
75. Kane, J., Rifkin, A., Quitkin, F., et al. (1976). Antidepressants in drug blood levels: Pharmacokinetics and clinical outcome. In *Progress in Psychiatric Drug Treatment,* Vol. 2. Edited by D. F. Klein and R. Gittleman-Klein. New York, Brunner Mazel.
76. Ziegler, V. E., Clayton, P. J., Taylor, J. R., et al. (1976). Nortriptyline plasma levels and therapeutic response. *Clin. Pharmacol. Ther. 20*:458-463.
77. Kupfer, F. J., Hanin, I., Spiker, D. G., et al. (1977). Amitriptyline plasma levels and clinical response in primary depression. *Clin. Pharmacol. Ther. 22*:904-911.
78. Volmat, R., Bechtel, P., Allers, G., et al. (1977). Determination of the plasma concentration and antidepressive effects of amitriptyline. *Therapie 32*:309-319.
79. Furlong, F. W., Sellers, E. M., and Kapur, B. M. (1977). Amitriptyline blood levels and relapse. *Can. Psychiatr. Assoc. J. 22*:275-284.
80. Coppen, A., Montgomery, S., Ghose, K., et al. (1978). Amitriptyline plasma concentration and clinical effect—World Health Organization Collaborative Study. *Lancet 1*:63-66.
81. Potter, W. Z. and Goodwin, F. K. (1978). Antidepressant drug levels and clinical response. *Lancet 1*:1049-1059.
82. Moody, J. P., Whyte, S. F., and Naylor, G. J. (1973). A simple method for the determination of protriptyline in plasma *Clin. Chim. Acta 43*:355-359.
83. Biggs, J. T., Holland, H. W., and Sherman, W. R. (1975). Steady-state protriptyline levels in an outpatient population. *Am. J. Psychiatry 132*:960-962.
84. Whyte, S. F., MacDonald, A. J., Naylor, G. J., et al. (1976). Plasma concentrations of protriptyline and clinical effects in depressed women. *Br. J. Psychiatry 128*:384-390.
85. Biggs, J. T. and Ziegler, V. E. (1977). Protriptyline plasma levels and antidepressant response. *Am. J. Psychiatry 22*:269-273.
86. Simpson, G. M., Pi, E. H., Gross, L., Baron, D., and November, M. (1988). Plasma levels and therapeutic response with trimipramine treatment of endogenous depression. *J. Clin. Psychiatry 49*:113-116.
87. Petit, J. M. (1977). Tricyclic antidepressant plasma levels and adverse effects after overdose. *Clin. Pharmacol. Ther. 21*:47.
88. Bailey, D. N. and Shaw, F. F. (1979). Tricyclic antidepressants: Interpretation of blood and tissue levels in fatal overdose. *J. Anal. Toxicol. 3*:43.
89. Klerman, G. L. (1983). Psychotherapies and somatic therapies in affective disorders. *Psychiatr. Clin. North Am. 6*:85-103.

6

Monoamine Oxidase Inhibiting Drugs

NEIL M. KURTZ

CNS Clinical Research, Miles Inc.
West Haven, Connecticut

HISTORICAL OVERVIEW OF MONOAMINE OXIDASE INHIBITOR DEVELOPMENT

Monoamine oxidase inhibitors (MAOIs) were introduced early in the modern era of psychopharmacology and have an important place in its history. As is true of many scientific breakthroughs, astute clinical observation and serendipity played a significant role in their discovery. Nonpsychiatric physicians observed that patients treated with iproniazid for tuberculosis experienced a sense of well-being, even when there was no bacteriologic improvement. The subsequent discovery of iproniazid's enzyme inhibition properties contributed to an already emerging hypothesis that monoamines play a role in regulating mood (1). In 1958 Kline and co-workers (2) conducted the first clinical trials with an MAOI in a psychiatric patient population. Their results suggested that iproniazid had "activating" properties in depressed patients, and they inferred from this that MAOIs would be effective treatment for affective disorders. This prompted pharmaceutical companies to synthesize a number of MAOIs, of which currently available agents in the United States are listed in Table 1.

After the initial enthusiasm, MAOIs fell rapidly into relative disuse in the United States. Iproniazid was withdrawn from United States markets because of reports of hepatotoxicity. In hindsight, this may have been an unfortunate

Table 1 Classification of MAOI Drugs Approved for Use in the United States

MAOI	Recommended therapeutic dose in depression (mg/day)
Hydrazine	
Phenelzine (Nardil)	60-90 mg (1 mg/kg)
Isocarboxazid (Marplan)	30 mg
Procarbazine (Matulane)[a]	
Nonhydrazine	
Tranylcypromine (Parnate)	20-30 mg
Pargyline (Eutonyl)[a]	
Molindone (Moban)[a]	

[a]Not marketed for antidepressant indication: procarbazine is a cancer chemotherapeutic agent; pargyline, a relatively selective MAO_B inhibitor marketed for hypertension; and molindone is an antipsychotic, which at higher doses may selectively inhibit MAO_A.

and hasty decision because iproniazid-induced hepatotoxicity was dose-related, with the most cases occurring at daily dosages over 150 mg (considerably above the recommended dose). In addition, the rash of reports of liver toxicity emanated from large mental institutions in which viral and amebic hepatitis were also endemic. Concerns about hepatotoxicity have lingered for all MAOIs; however, a recent literature search indicated little if any risk for phenelzine (Nardil) and tranylcypromine (Parnate) (3).

The side effect that caused the most controversy for the MAOIs was the "cheese reaction," or severe hypertension after ingestion of food high in tyramine content or after consuming certain vasoactive drugs. Although relatively rare, this side effect represents a medical emergency. Before the cause was recognized, numerous hypertensive reactions were reported. However, it is now evident that a reliable patient, observing modest dietary restrictions, has only a slight risk of this untoward event. Understandably, fear of these reactions, coupled with the overly restrictive diet, led to an abrupt decline in the popularity of MAOIs. Finally, a 1965 British study indicated that phenelzine was no more effective than placebo for treating severely depressed patients (4), thereby suggesting a relatively high risk for marginal benefit compared with the newly marketed, and clearly efficacious, tricyclic antidepressants (TCAs). Subsequently, MAOIs remained interesting scientific tools for use in psychopharmacologic research, but were thought to be of relatively little practical value, except in a few countries. Ironically, the United Kingdom was one such.

The precise clinical usefulness of the MAOIs has only recently been suggested. They have now gained widespread acceptance as effective alternatives to TCAs, and their therapeutic efficacy is documented in several psychiatric disorders (5,6). In retrospect, it is now clear that experimental design deficiencies contributed, in large part, to the premature conclusion that MAOIs were ineffective (8,9). Many of the early efficacy studies of MAOIs lacked adequate statistical power or knowledge of the therapeutic dose range. Instead of advancing their clinical utility, these studies contributed to a delay in the understanding of the unique therapeutic properties of these agents. Recent studies have now demonstrated that, when used in proper dosage, MAOIs are among the most efficacious treatments for both endogenous and nonendogenous depression, as well as other disorders.

MONOAMINE OXIDASE ENZYME SUBTYPES

In 1968, Johnstone described two forms of MAO enzyme on the basis of a bimodal pattern of tyramine deamination inhibition with the MAOI, clorgyline (9). He proposed the existence of two distinct enzyme subtypes: MAO_A and MAO_B. Varying ratios of MAO_A and MAO_B activities have been described in brain, kidney, liver, intestine, and platelets, and both forms have been extensively characterized for electrophoretic mobility of radiolabeled subunits, immunological and chromatographic characteristics, and monoamine substrate specificities (10-12). However, attempts to purify, sequence, and delineate the primary structure of these enzymes have proved unsuccessful. Therefore, it is premature to state definitively that MAO_A and MAO_B are distinct isoenzymes.

There are apparently large species differences in the ratio of MAO A and B isoenzymes (13,14). Human brain is believed to be predominantly MAO_B (70-75%), whereas nonhuman primates may have even higher levels. Only limited data concerning regional brain levels of enzyme activity are available.

The enzyme subtypes exhibit substrate specificity. Therefore, it is possible to synthesize MAOIs with high selectivity toward one form or the other. Table 2 summarizes the current understanding of substrate and inhibitor specificities for each subtype.

Consistent with the catecholamine hypothesis of depression, the MAO_A-specific inhibitors appear to have utility in the treatment of affective disorders. Pharmaceutical companies are currently developing specific inhibitors of the MAO_A enzyme, with several compounds in early clinical trials. Clorgyline, a specific MAO_A inhibitor, has been efficacious in treating depression (5). However, evidence for efficacy in depression of the specific MAO_B inhibitor L-deprenyl is less convincing. Although L-deprenyl has been reported to be effective in treating endogenous depression (15,16), a review of the doses used reveals that most patients exceeded 15 mg/day. Preclinical data suggest that at high doses, specificity for MAO_B may be lost and MAO_A also inhibited.

Table 2 Substrates and Inhibitors for MAO Subtypes

Enzyme subtype	Substrate	Inhibitors
MAO_A	Serotonin	Clorgyline[c]
	Norepinephrine	Amiflamine[d]
		Moclobenide[c]
		CGP-11305A[c]
		Harmaline[c]
		Lilly 51641[c]
MAO_B	Phenylethyamine	Pargyline
	Phenylethanolamine	L-Deprenyl[c]
	tele-Methylhistamine	Lilly 54781[c]
	Benzylamine	MD 72145[c]
	o-Tyramine	
MAO_A and MAO_B	Dopamine[a]	Phenelzine
	Tyramine	Tranylcypromine
	Typramine	Procarbazine
		Isocarboxazid
		Sercloremine[b,c]
		Iproniazid[d]
		Nialamid[d]

[a]Human brain dopamine may be preferentially deaminated by MAO_B.
[b]Sercloremine is an investigational, nonspecific reversible inhibitor of MAO.
[c]These investigational agents are not approved for use in the United States.
[d]Drug withdrawn from United States market.

The degree of scientific interest in selective MAOIs reflects their value as tools for elucidating the neurochemical basis of various psychological disturbances and in enhancing our understanding of the pathophysiology of MAOI-responsive disorders.

METABOLISM OF MONOAMINE OXIDASE INHIBITORS

Acetylation was originally thought to be a major metabolic pathway for the degradation of hydrazine MAOIs, such as phenelzine and isocarboxazid (see Table 1). Slow acetylator patients were initially thought to show greater improvement and more side effects. However, subsequent studies failed to confirm this association (17,18), and acetylation was ultimately found to play a minor role in the metabolism of hydrazine MAOIs. In humans, phenelzine is rapidly converted to phenylacetic acid with ring hydroxylation, and acetylated metabolites are undetectable in plasma or urine (19).

Phenelzine, an irreversible inhibitor of MAO, exhibits nonlinear pharmacokinetics. This property explains, in part, the brief metabolic half-life of the drug and the longer pharmacodynamic half-life that has been reported after single doses of phenelzine. Although a detailed discussion of the implications of nonlinear pharmacokinetics is beyond the scope of this chapter, one should appreciate that this property makes the choice of dosage critical. Many patients will have an all or none response to MAOIs.

Measurement of platelet MAO inhibition is a useful pharmacologic marker in establishing the therapeutic dose. A relatively simple and convenient assay, based on a high or low percentage of platelet MAO inhibition (20), can show a differential clinical response to phenelzine. The optimal daily dosage of phenelzine approximates 1 mg/kg of body weight, which translates to 60-90 mg/day for most adults. By 2 weeks at this dosage, platelet MAO inhibition generally attains 80%. Patients with lower inhibition percentages respond less well to phenelzine.

In summary, pharmacokinetic studies indicate that MAOIs are cleared rapidly from the systemic circulation, whereas their biological effects persist much longer. The unique pharmacokinetic and pharmacodynamic actions of MAOIs derive from irreversible binding of the drug to the enzyme, with resultant nonlinear pharmacokinetics. This must be considered when evaluating therapeutic response. In addition, irreversible inhibition means that the pharmacodynamic effects of MAOIs will persist for as long as 2 weeks after the drug is discontinued.

SAFETY PROFILE OF MONOAMINE OXIDASE INHIBITORS

As indicated in the foregoing, uncertainty exists about the precise nature and prevalence of the side effects and toxicities of MAOIs. Issues surrounding possible hepatotoxicity, dietary constraints, and hypertensive crises, as well as information about side effects with long-term therapy have plagued the clinical acceptance of these agents. The reemergence of the drugs over the past decade has prompted an impetus for a definitive assessment of their safety profile.

Hypertensive Crisis

Dietary indiscretions can result in a hypertensive reaction that is considered a medical emergency. Recent experience now suggests that modest dietary restrictions by reliable patients should almost entirely avoid this risk. In studies involving several hundred phenelzine-treated patients, the incidence of hypertensive reactions was less than 1% (Robinson, D. S. and Kayser, A., unpublished data).

The hypertensive reaction is a result of too much dietary tyramine or dopamine. The mechanisms by which an MAOI may affect the cardiovascular response to the pressor agents are varied and complex. (Reviewed in Ref. 21). Table 3 lists foods, beverages, and medications that should be avoided by patients receiving irreversible MAOIs. The clinician should learn to recognize the characteristic signs and symptoms of hypertensive reactions, which generally develop within 2 hr after ingestion of foods with high tyramine or dopamine content. Patients may complain of severe occipital or temporal headaches, with occasional photophobia. Sensations of palpitations, choking, and a feeling of "dread" are common. Marked systolic and diastolic increases in blood pressure occur, sometimes with marked neck stiffness. The degree of the hypertension appears to be directly related to the amount of systemically available tyramine. Dose-response studies have suggested that

Table 3 Instructions for MAOI Therapy

Foods with high tyramine content: must be avoided	
	Unpasteurized, strong, or aromatic cheese (cheddar, Camembert, blue cheese)
	Yeast extract (some packet soups)
	Smoked herring
	Fermented meats (salami, pepperoni, summer sausage)
	Fava beans
	Red wines (chianti, burgundy, cabernet sauvignon)
Foods with moderate tyramine content: limited amounts allowed	
	Avocado, banana
	Ales and beers
	Most white wines, champagne
	Caffeinated coffee, chocolate, cola
Foods with low tyramine content: permissable	
	Pasteurized cheeses (cream, cottage, ricotta)
	Distilled spirits (in moderation)
Drugs absolutely contraindicated	
	Stimulants: amphetamine, cocaine, anorectic drugs
	Decongestants: sinus, hay fever, and cold tablets
	Antihypertensives: methyldopa, guanethidine, reserpine
	Antiparkinson: L-dopa
Drugs markedly potentiated	
	Narcotics: meperidine (pethidine)
	Sympathomimetics: epinephrine, norepinephrine, dopamine
	General anesthetics
Drugs potentiated	
	Narcotics: morphine, codeine, etc.
	Sedatives: barbiturates, alcohol
	Local anesthetics with vasoconstrictors

at least 6 mg of tyramine (given intravenously) are required to produce a moderate rise in blood pressure (22), and progressive blood pressure increases are seen with up to 10 mg of tyramine. Ingestion of more than 20 mg invariably produces a severe hypertensive reaction in patients taking MAOIs. Although some MAOIs, particularly tranylcypromine, are thought to carry greater risk, it should be assumed that all currently marketed MAOIs may produce this reaction. Food and beverages with high tyramine or dopamine content are risky and should be avoided. Medications containing both direct- and indirect-acting sympathomimetic amines should also be avoided. Furthermore, these restrictions should be maintained for at least 14 days after stopping the MAOI.

Hypertensive crises can be treated with an α_1-adrenergic blocking drug, such as phentolamine 5 mg intravenously, although parenteral chlorpromazine is also effective. Because of phentolamine's short elimination half-life, the response may be short-lived, and repeated doses may be necessary. Pharmaceutical firms are currently trying to develop MAOIs that are free of this liability, and some evidence suggests that reversible inhibitors of MAO may offer promise.

Hepatotoxicity

The early association of MAOIs with hepatotoxicity derived from the iproniazid experience; however, current evidence does not substantiate a propensity for hepatotoxicity (3). Therefore, the clinician need not routinely monitor hepatic function, except in patients at increased risk for hepatotoxicity (e.g., elderly patients). Psychopharmacologic drugs, including the MAOIs, that undergo a high percentage of first-pass metabolism through the liver are known to transiently elevate hepatic enzymes, as high as two to three times normal. Such borderline elevations are not, of themselves, sufficient justification for discontinuing MAOI treatment, because they are generally transient and not clinically significant.

Other Side Effect Profiles of Monoamine Oxidase Inhibitors

Recent studies have provided a more accurate assessment of the true prevalence of MAOI side effects (23,24). Table 4 lists the more frequent side effects of phenelzine, with an estimate of their frequency. Most patients experience some sleep abnormalities, usually difficulty falling asleep, with increased awakenings and reduced sleep time. For some, daytime drowsiness becomes a problem. Paradoxically, some patients report improvement in sleep when the dose of MAOI is concentrated in the later part of the day; however, most experience less insomnia and daytime drowsiness when the daily dosage is concentrated in the morning.

Table 4 Drug Side Effects Associated with Phenelzine Therapy

Side effects	Estimated frequency (%)	Impaired liability
Sleep disturbances	50	Usually tolerated, frequently involves sleep initiation; most common reason for discontinuation
Symptomatic orthostatic hypotension	10	Sometimes disabling; may respond to dose reduction
Dry mouth	20-30	Mild
Daytime sedation	20	Rarely impairing
Impaired sexual response	20 (men) 5 (women)	May respond to dose reduction; generally presents in women as anorgasmia
Hyperphagia with weight gain	20-30	Often marked carbohydrate craving; may respond to dose reduction
Myoclonic jerking	10	Mild; most common at sleep onset; can be exacerbated by abrupt drug withdrawal
Bipedal edema	<5	Infrequent; refractory to diuretics

Other side effects include orthostatic hypotension, excessive weight gain and hyperphagia, impotence, anorgasmia, hypomania, and bipedal edema. Less common side effects include myoclonic twitching during sleep onset, joint pains and, rarely, pyridoxine deficiency with neuropathy. Abrupt discontinuation of MAOI treatment can result in an excerbation of sleep-onset myoclonic movements, which appear to be associated with REM rebound. Therefore, it is best to taper the MAOI when discontinuing treatment.

The lack of significant anticholinergic side effects make MAOIs attractive for use in the elderly (25). Unlike TCAs and related drugs, MAOIs lack direct cardiac effects, and in geriatric patients with cardiovascular disease, MAOIs may represent a safe alternative treatment (26).

Although both the MAOIs and TCAs cause postural hypotension, MAOIs are more likely to lower supine blood pressure, and this may imply a potential advantage in the treatment of the depressed hypertensive patient. Furthermore, MAOIs do not increase the resting heart rate, which is important for patients with angina; nor do they slow cardiac conduction, which is an advantage in patients with conduction delays. In contrast, the quinidinelike effect of TCAs suppress ventricular ectopic beats and may make them a better choice for patients with ventricular dysrhythmias. Neither the TCAs nor the MAOIs significantly depress myocardial contractility.

Recently, long-term studies have assessed the value of maintenance antidepressant treatment, including adverse experiences during long-term MAOI use. These data are of obvious importance because of a growing trend to routinely treat depressive episodes for periods up to a year or longer. A recent 2-year maintenance treatment study with phenelzine indicated that of 79 patients treated for an episode of major depression, 25% ultimately discontinued treatment for side effects, despite an initial favorable response (27). A smaller study involving 14 patients receiving long-term phenelzine treatment reported similar results.

Monoamine Oxidase Inhibitor Overdose

An MAOI overdose produces a characteristic toxic syndrome characterized by altered mental status, hyperpyrexia, and hyperreflexia, which progresses to metabolic acidosis, seizures, and cardiovascular collapse. Treatment is primarily nonspecific and supportive and includes measures to reduce or retard further drug absorption.

An interesting case report described a patient who ingested at least 1000 mg of phenelzine, resulting in coma, metabolic acidosis, and fever up to 41 °C (29). The patient responded rapidly to intravenous dantrolene administration, a treatment successfully used for malignant hyperthermia and the neuroleptic malignant syndrome. Although the mechanism of action of dantrolene is unclear, its ability to reverse the hyperthermia may be associated with an inhibitory action on release of cytoplasmic calcium ions.

DRUG-MONOAMINE OXIDASE INHIBITOR INTERACTIONS

Narcotics

Care must be exercised when using any narcotic with an MAOI. The opiate agonists—meperidine and morphine—and the agonist/antagonists—pentazocine, butorphanol, or buprenophine—should be avoided. The meperidine-MAOI interaction is particularly serious and fatalities have been reported. The clinical picture is characterized by shivering, agitation, hyperthermia, circulatory collapse, and death. The etiology may be interference with the hepatic metabolism by meperidine, and treatment involves acidification of the urine, α_1-adrenergic drugs, and supportive measures. Codeine in reduced doses, although not entirely without risks, is the narcotic of choice for patients receiving MAOI therapy.

Antihypertensives

Many antihypertensive drugs produce serious reactions in combination with MAOIs. Agents such as methyldopa, clonidine, reserpine, guanethidine, and high-dose β-blockers should be avoided. To date, there is no consensus on whether or not angiotensin-converting enzyme inhibitors (enalapril, lisonopril, and captopril) pose less risk in combination with MAOIs.

Insulin

Symptomatic hypoglycemia has occurred in patients receiving insulin and MAOI treatment, although the precise mechanism for this is not well understood. It has been suggested that MAOIs interfere with the adrenergically mediated compensatory reaction to hypoglycemia. The use of oral hypoglycemic agents appears to be safer in MAOI-treated diabetic patients.

Anesthesia

It is advisable to discontinue MAOIs for at least 2 weeks before elective surgery. If emergency surgery is required, it is essential that the anesthesiologist and surgeon be aware of the MAOI therapy. A principal concern is the development of hypotension. If hypotension develops, pressor agents should be avoided, and fluid expansion should be relied upon. There are reports of prolonged apnea in patients exposed to succinylcholine who are also receiving concomitant phenelzine therapy. However, a report of a series of patients receiving MAOIs before undergoing general anesthesia indicates that, with proper management, MAOIs can be safe even in the emergent situation (30).

Sympathomimetic Agents

Over-the-counter products for asthma, cough, colds, and appetite suppression that contain sympathomimetic amines should be avoided. Because of their pressor effects, medication containing isoproterenol, phenylephrine, ephedrine, amphetamine, methamphetamine, methylphenidate, or dopa may produce severe hypertension. In this context, local anesthetics are safe when they do not contain vasoconstrictors such as epinephrine. Antihistamines appear to be safe in combination with MAOIs and, when used without decongestants, pose little risk of drug interaction.

THE ROLE OF MONOAMINE OXIDASE INHIBITORS IN DEPRESSIVE DISORDERS

The precise role that MAOIs should play in the treatment of depressive illness is still being defined. West and Dally (31) described a profile of symptoms they termed "atypical depression" that appeared to predict a favorable response to MAOIs. It was not until the 1970s that well-controlled trials further clarified their efficacy in patients with atypical depression (8,32). In spite of these data, there is still controversy over whether or not MAOIs are effective in the treatment of classic endogenous depressions (33). In an open-label study (34), phenelzine was particularly effective in major depressive disorder with melancholia (35) and MAOIs used in adequate doses were as efficacious as the TCAs in a variety of severe depressive disorders. However, more work in this area is still needed.

Atypical Depression

Much of the recent research in the patient category of atypical depression has been done by the Columbia University group in New York, who categorize these patients by the presence of reactive mood, rejection sensitivity, and vegetative atypical features such as overeating, oversleeping, lethargy, or "leaden paralysis" (36). Other clinical features include multiple psychophysiological complaints including reverse diurnal variation in mood, agoraphobia, chronic anxiety, and dysphoria. These patients differ from those with melancholic depression in that there is an absence of intense guilt. In a recent trial comparing phenelzine (60-90 mg/day), imipramine (200-300 mg/day), and placebo in atypical depression, the MAOI was superior to both placebo and imipramine (37). However, in a study employing a similar design, Davidson (38) was unable to show superiority for MAOIs, with both active treatments being superior to placebo.

Depressed patients with panic attacks (with or without agoraphobia) respond particularly well to phenelzine (6). Although the overall efficacy of MAOIs and TCAs may be equivalent, patients with major depression and panic symptoms, phobic avoidance, or prominent somatic anxiety symptoms may respond better to phenelzine.

Phenelzine appears to be the most popular MAOI for treatment of depression. A potentially important finding is that patients can be started at full therapeutic doses without untoward effects (34). Such a "loading-dose" technique might accelerate therapeutic response and, once improvement has been achieved, an individualized maintenance dose can be utilized. However, lowering the dose of the MAOI to a "maintenance" level in a fashion similar to TCAs is not recommended with MAOIs.

In summary, evidence suggests that the MAOIs and TCAs have similar efficacy in treating endogenous depressions, whereas MAOIs may be superior for subgroups of depressive illness with atypical features, panic symptoms, or excessive anxiety symptoms. The MAOIs are not recommended as the primary treatment, but should be held in reserve to treat those patients who are refractory to prior TCA treatments.

CONCOMITANT THERAPY WITH OTHER ANTIDEPRESSANT DRUGS

It has been a widely held belief that MAOIs and TCAs should not be given concomitantly because of alterations in biogenic amine metabolism that might result in adverse effects, such as hypertensive crises. It is now generally felt that combined TCAs and MAOIs can be used for resistant depression, provided certain precautions are observed (40). The TCA and MAOI may be started simultaneously, or the MAOI added to TCA therapy with safety, although adding a TCA to ongoing MAOI therapy is not recommended. A drug-free interval of 2-3 weeks after MAOI use is prudent before starting TCA therapy. Anecdotal evidence suggests that tranylcypromine may possess greater risks when used in combination with TCAs when compared with other MAOIs. Antidepressants that are selective serotonin-uptake inhibitors, such as fluvoxamine, fluoxetine, citalopram, and sertraline, should be avoided; noradrenergic-uptake inhibitors are preferred.

The toxic syndrome that occasionally can result with MAOI-TCA combination includes hyperthermia, agitation, delirium, convulsions, and coma. The clinical picture suggests a serotonergic mechanism and resembles antidepressant overdose. Interestingly, the clinical picture does not resemble the hypertensive crisis seen with tyramine ingestion (see section on hypertensive crisis).

Clinical guidelines for the combined use of MAOIs and TCAs have been reviewed (41,42). The most common reason for initiating combination MAOI and TCA therapy is for the treatment of resistant depression, although controlled studies that demonstrate an advantage for the combination are lacking. However, it has been argued (43) that ". . . patients with treatment resistant depression, who do not respond to standard methods [of treatment] have a moral and legitimate right to innovative therapy" and that combined treatment may be justified in such cases. These authors report successful treatment of resistant depression with the combination of MAOI and TCA.

OTHER CLINICAL INDICATIONS FOR MONOAMINE OXIDASE INHIBITORS

There is growing evidence that MAOIs may be efficacious for the treatment of panic disorder. In a large sample of patients meeting DSM-III (35) criteria for panic disorder, Sheehan et al. (44) found both phenelzine (45 mg/day) and imipramine (150 mg/day) superior to placebo, with a trend for phenelzine to be superior to imipramine. In a subsequent study, Sheehan and associates (45) compared higher doses of phenelzine to imipramine and alprazolam, a triazolobenzodiazepine with antipanic properties, and found that phenelzine was superior in measures of disability from avoidance behavior.

Phenelzine's advantage may lie not only in its ability to block the panic attacks, but also in its ability to reduce the accompanying anticipatory anxiety and phobic avoidance behavior.

The MAOIs have also been effective in treating phobic avoidance behavior associated with both mood and anxiety disorders. Tyrer et al. (46) showed that phenelzine (60 mg/day) was effective in treating patients with agoraphobia, and Johnstone and Marsh (32) reported that patients with neurotic depression and phobic avoidance behavior improved more than did patients treated with placebo. Solyom et al. (47) compared three types of behavioral treatment in combination with phenelzine or placebo in phobic patients and concluded that phenelzine was equivalent to the most effective behavioral treatment and more economical. Liebowitz et al. (48) reported that phenelzine, independent of any antidepressant properties, may also be effective in the treatment of social phobias.

Evidence suggests that there may be an association between bulimia and affective disorder. Pheneline and isocarboxazid have been reported to be effective in the treatment of bulimia (49), and Walsh et al. (50) found that five of nine bulimic patients treated with phenelzine stopped binging, and the remainder experienced at least a 50% reduction in binging. This contrasted sharply with placebo therapy, which failed to show any significant antibinging activity.

Davidson and Raft (51) found phenelzine superior to both placebo and imipramine in the treatment of patients with chronic pain syndrome and depression. The presence of atypical vegetative symptoms, including changes in appetite, weight, and libido, seemed to correlate with the analgesic response to phenelzine. This suggested that some of these patients might be suffering from atypical depression as part of the pain syndrome and that it is important to elicit atypical depressive features that may predict a response to MAOIs.

In a small open trial of eight patients with obsessive-compulsive disorder, Jenike et al. (52) reported a rapid and sustained response in four with either phenelzine or tranylcypromine. This finding needs replication in controlled studies to assess the possible role for MAOIs in obsessive-compulsive illness.

Finally, in recent years, there has been extensive interest in the morbidity that can result from unusual or overwhelming stress. In a small open-pilot study, Davidson (53) reports that phenelzine appeared promising for the treatment of posttraumatic stress disorders. These findings are still speculative and require confirmation, but they do suggest another potential application of MAOIs in psychiatry.

NEW MONOAMINE OXIDASE INHIBITORS

The discovery of selective MAO isoenzyme inhibitors offers exciting possibilities for safer and more effective drugs, as well as for new research tools for studying the pathophysiology of affective disorders. For example, MAO_A preferentially deaminates norepinephrine and serotonin, whereas MAO_B preferentially acts on dopamine and phenylethylamine. It is believed that the norepinephrine effects mediate the increased sensitivity to tyramine and are prerequisite to hypertensive crisis. A selective MAO_B inhibitor, therefore, would not be expected to carry this liability.

It seems probable that MAO_A inhibition is a necessary component for antidepressant activity. Unfortunately, selective irreversible MAO_A inhibitors do not offer added safety benefits, and research has been directed toward developing reversible MAO inhibitors. All currently available compounds are irreversible enzyme inhibitors. Theoretically, reversible inhibitors might avoid the undesirable cheese reaction, and drugs such as RO-11-1163 or moclobemide, MD780515, and fla336(+), are currently under investigation as rapidly reversible, selective MAO_A inhibitors (54). In open studies involving 300 patients, RO-11-1163 showed preliminary evidence of antidepressant activity in nonpsychotic unipolar endogenous depression, with few side effects. Over 500 patients have now been treated, with no reports of hypertensive crisis, and there have now been nine controlled trials comparing RO-11-1163 with placebo or a TCA, with results that support its efficacy in severe depression.

A particularly innovative approach is the new MAOI, MDL72145, which acts as a prodrug (54), crossing the blood-brain barrier, where it is selectively taken up by aminergic neurons and decarboxylated into a specific irreversible MAO_B inhibitor. Because tyramine is primarily deaminated in the periphery, the prodrug approach could obviate troublesome side effects that result from inhibition of MAO in intestine and liver, thereby reducing the risk of hypertensive crisis and easing the need for dietary restrictions.

REFERENCES

1. Schildkraut, J. J. (1965). The catecholamine hypothesis of affective disorder: A review of supporting evidence. *Am. J. Psychiatry 122*:505-518.
2. Loomer, H. P., Saunders, J. C., and Kline, N. D. (1958). A clinical and pharmacodynamic evaluation of iproniazid as a psychic energizer. *Am. Psychiatr. Assoc. Res. Rep. 8*:129.
3. Robinson, D. S. and Kurtz, N. M. (1986). Is phenelzine hepatotoxic? *J. Clin. Psychopharmacol.* (in press).
4. British Medical Research Council (1965). Clinical trial of the treatment of depressive illness. *Br. Med. J. 1*:881-886.
5. Quitkin, F., Rifkin, A., and Klein, D. F. (1979). Monoamine oxidase inhibitors: A review of antidepressant effectiveness. *Arch. Gen. Psychiatry 36*:749-760.
6. Robinson, D. S., Kayser, A., Corcella, J., Laux, D., Yingling, K., and Howard, D. (1985). Panic attacks in outpatients with depression: Response to antidepressant treatment. *Psychopharmacol. Bull. 21*:562-567.

7. Greenblatt, M., Grossner, G. H., and Wechsler, H. (1964). Differential response of hospitalized depressed patients to somatic therapy. *Am. J. Psychiatry 120*:935-943.
8. Robinson, D. S., Nies, A., Ravaris, C. L., and Lamborn, K. R. (1973). The monoamine oxidase inhibitor phenelzine in the treatment of depressive-anxiety states. *Arch. Gen. Psychiatry 29*:407-413.
9. Johnstone, J. P. (1968). Some observations upon a new inhibitor of monoamine oxidase in brain tissue. *Biochem. Pharmacol. 17*:1285-1297.
10. Archee, F. M., Gabay, S., and Tipton, K. F. (1977). Some aspects of monoamine oxidase activity in brain. *Prog. Neurobiol. 8*:325-348.
11. Denny, R. M., Fritz, R. R., Patel, N. T., and Abel, S. W. (1982). Human liver MAO-A and MAO-B separated by immunoaffinity chromatography with MAO-B specific monoclonal antibody. *Science 215*:1400-1403.
12. Denny, R. M., Fritz, R. R., Patel, N. T., Widen, S. G., and Abell, S. W. (1983). Use of a monoclonal antibody for comparative studies of monoamine oxidase B in mitochondrial extracts of human brain and peripheral tissues. *Mol. Pharmacol. 24*:60-68.
13. Murphy, D. L., Garrick, N. A., Aulakh, C. S., and Cohen, R. M. (1984). New contributions from basic science to understanding the effects of monoamine oxidase inhibiting antidepressants. *J. Clin. Psychiatry 45*:37-43.
14. Garrick, N. A. and Murphy, D. L. (1980). Species differences in the deamination of dopamine and other substrates for monoamine oxidase in brain. *Psychopharmacology 72*:27-33.
15. Mann, J. J., Frances, A., Kaplan, R. D., Kocsis, J., Peselow, E. D., and Gershon, S. (1982). The relative efficacy of L-deprenyl, a selective monoamine oxidase type B inhibitor, in endogenous and nonendogenous depression. *J. Clin. Psychopharmacol. 2*:54-57.
16. Mendlewicz, J. and Youdim, M. B. H. (1983). L-Deprenyl, a selective monoamine oxidase type B inhibitor in the treatment of depression. *Br. J. Psychiatry 142*:508-511.
17. Davidson, J., McLeod, M. N., and Blum, M. R. (1978). Acetylation phenotype, platelet monoamine oxidase inhibition and the effectiveness of phenelzine in depression. *Am. J. Psychiatry 135*:467-469.
18. Robinson, D. S., Nies, A., Ravaris, C. L., Ives, J. O., and Bartlett, D. (1978). Clinical pharmacology of phenelzine. *Arch. Gen. Psychiatry 35*:629-635.
19. Robinson, D. S., Cooper, T. B., Jindal, S. R., Corcella, J., and Lutz, T. (1985). Pharmacokinetics and metabolism of phenelzine. *J. Clin. Psychopharmacol. 5*: 333-337.
20. Robinson, D. S., Lovenberg, W., Keiser, H., and Sjoerdsma, A. (1968). Effects of drugs on human blood platelet and plasma amine oxidase activity in vitro and in vivo. *Biochem. Pharmacol. 17*:109-119.
21. Simpson, G. M. and White, K. (1984). Tyramine studies and the safety of MAOI drugs. *J. Clin. Psychiatry 45*:59-61.
22. Blackwell, B., Marley, E., and Price, J. (1967). Hypertensive interactions beween monoamine oxidase inhibitors and foodstuff. *Br. J. Psychiatry 113*:349.
23. Rabkin, J., Quitkin, F., Harrison, W., Tricano, E., and McGrath, P. (1984). Adverse reactions to monoamine oxidase inhibitors Part I. A comparative study. *J. Clin. Psychopharmacol. 4*:270-278.

24. Ravaris, C. L., Robinson, D. S., Ives, J. O., Nies, A., and Barlett, D. (1980). A comparison of phenelzine and amitriptyline in the treatment of depression. *Arch. Gen. Psychiatry 37*:1075-1080.
25. Georgotas, A., McCue, R. E., Friedman, E., Hapworth, W. E., Kim, O. M., Welkowitz, J., and Cooper, T. B. (1986). Comparative efficacy and safety of MAOIs versus TCAs in treating depressed elderly (in press).
26. Goldman, L. S., Alexander, R. C., and Luchins, D. J. (1986). Monoamine oxidase inhibitors and tricyclic antidepressants: Comparison of their cardiovascular effects. *J. Clin. Psychiatry 47*:225-29.
27. Robinson, D. S., Kayser, A., Bennett, B., Devereaux, E., Lerfald, S., Albright, D., Laux, D., and Corcella, J. (1986). Maintenance phenelzine treatment of depression: An interim report. *Psychopharmacol. Bull.* (in press).
28. Source unknown.
29. Kaplan, R. F., Feinglass, N. G., Webster, W., and Mudra, S. (1986). Phenelzine overdose treated with dantroline sodium. *JAMA 225*:642-644.
30. El-Ganzouri, A. R., Ivankovich, A. D., Braverman, B., and McCarthy, R. (1985). Monoamine oxidase inhibitors: Should they be discontinued preoperatively? *Anesth. Analg. 64*:592-596.
31. West, E. D. and Dally, P. J. (1959). Effects of iproniazid in depressive syndromes. *Br. Med. J. 1*:1491-1494.
32. Johnstone, E. C. and Marsh, W. (1973). Acetylator status and response to phenelzine in depressed patients. *Lancet 1*:567-570.
33. Pare, C. M. B. (1985). The present status of monoamine oxidase inhibitors. *Br. J. Psychiatry 146*:576-584.
34. McGrath, P. J., Quitkin, F. M., Harrison, W., and Stewart, J. W. (1984). Treatment of melancholia with tranylcypromine. *Am. J. Psychiatry 14*:288-289.
35. American Psychiatric Association (1980). *Diagnostic and Statistical Manual of Mental Disorders*, 3rd ed. Washington, D.C., American Psychiatric Association.
36. Quitkin, F. M., Harrison, W., Liebowitz, M., McGrath, P., Rabkin, J. G., Stewart, J., and Markowitz, J. (1984). Defining the boundaries of atypical depression. *J. Clin. Psychiatry 45*:19-21.
37. Liebowitz, M. R., Quitkin, F. M., Stewart, J. W., McGrath, P. J., Harrison, W., Rabkin, J., Tricamo, E., Markowitz, J. G., and Klein, D. F. (1985). Effect of panic attacks on the treatment of atypical depressives. *Psychopharmacol. Bull. 21*:558-561.
38. Davidson, J. and Pelton, S. (1986). Forms of atypical depression and their response to antidepressant drugs. *Psychiatry Res. 17*:87-95.
39. Robinson, D. S. (1986). New perspectives on long-standing issues: The monamine oxidase inhibitors. *Psychopharmacol. Bull. 1*:12-16.
40. Anath, J. and Luchins, D. (1977). A review of combined tricyclic and MAOI therapy. *Compr. Psychiatry 18*:221-230.
41. Lader, M. (1983). Combined use of tricyclic antidepressant and monoamine oxidase inhibitors. *J. Clin. Psychiatry 44*:20-24.
42. White, K. and Simpson, G. (1984). The combined use of MAOIs and tricyclics. *J. Clin. Psychiatry 45*:67-69.

43. Feighner, J. P., Herbstein, J., and Damloiji, N. (1985). Combined MAOI-TCA and direct stimulant therapy of treatment resistant depression. *J. Clin. Psychiatry 46*:206-209.
44. Sheehan, D. V., Ballenger, J., and Jacoban, G. (1980). Treatment of endogenous depression anxiety with phobic hysterial and hypochondriacal symptoms. *Arch. Gen. Psychiatry 37*:51-59.
45. Sheehan, D. V., Barry, J., Claycomb, M. D., Surman, O. S., Gelles, L., Gallo, J., and LeGros, B. S. (1984). The relative efficacy of alprazolam, phenelzine and imipramine in treating panic attacks and phobia. *Syllabus and Proceedings from the 137th Annual Meeting of the American Psychiatric Association*, p. 32.
46. Tyrer, P., Candy, J., and Kelly, D. (1973). Phenelzine in phobic anxiety: A control trial. *Psychopharmacologia 32*:237-254.
47. Solyom, C., Solyom, L., LaPierre, Y., Pecknold, J., and Morton, L. (1981). Phenelzine and exposure in the treatment of phobias. *Biol. Psychiatry 16*:239-247.
48. Liebowitz, M. R., Fyer, A. J., Gorman, J. M., Compeas, R., and Levin, A. (1986). Phenelzine in social phobia. *J. Clin. Psychopharmacol. 6*:93-97.
49. Kennedy, S. H., Piran, N., and Garfinkel, P. E. (1985). Monoamine oxidase inhibitor therapy for anorexia nervosa and bulimina: A preliminary trial of isocarboxazid. *J. Clin. Psychopharmacol. 5*:279-285.
50. Walsh, B. T., Steward, J. W., Roose, S. P., Glades, M., and Glassman, A. H. (1984). Treatment of bulimia with phenelzine. A double-blind, placebo-controlled trial. *Arch. Gen. Psychiatry 41*:1105-1109.
51. Davidson, J. and Raft, D. (1985). Monoamine oxidase inhibitors in inpatients with chronic pain. *Arch. Gen. Psychiatry 42*:635-636.
52. Jenike, M. A., Surman, O. S., Cassem, N. H., Zusky, P., and Anderson, W. H. (1983). Monoamine oxidase inhibitors in obsessive-compulsive disorder. *J. Clin. Psychiatry 44*:131-132.
53. Davidson, J. (1987). A pilot study of phenelzine in the treatment of post-traumatic stress disorder. *Br. J. Psychiatry 150*:252-255.
54. Zreika, M., McDonald, I. A., Bay, P., and Palfreyman, M. G. (1984). MDL 72163, an enzyme-activated irreversible inhibitor with selectivity for monoamine oxidase type B. *J. Neurochem. 43*:448-454.
55. Zreika, M., McDonald, I. A., Bay, P., and Palfreyman, M. G. (1984). MDL 72163, an enzyme-activated irreversible inhibitor with selectivity for monoamine oxidase type B. *J. Neurochem. 43*:448-454.

7

The Clinical Application of Lithium

JAMES W. JEFFERSON and JOHN H. GREIST

University of Wisconsin Center for Health Sciences, Madison, Wisconsin

Lithium does not readily come to mind when the term "antidepressant" is used; indeed, it does not have Food and Drug Administration (FDA)-labeling approval for use as an antidepressant. The American Psychiatric Association Task Force on Lithium recently concluded, "Experimental results are not sufficiently conclusive to permit a clear definition of the value of lithium in acute depression. It should not be considered standard treatment but in selected cases may be considered if the usual methods fail" (1). However, other research evidence is considerably less pessimistic (2). Seven of nine studies have found lithium to be a more effective antidepressant than placebo, and three of four studies have showed it to be equivalent to a tricyclic antidepressant. When categorized by diagnosis, a favorable response to lithium was observed in 42% of unipolar patients, 65% of bipolar II depressives, and 65% of depressed patients with unspecified bipolar disorders. Because the sample size in each group was fewer than 100, broad generalizations concerning the antidepressant effect of lithium should be made with some caution.

LITHIUM, DEPRESSION, AND ANTIDEPRESSANT DRUGS

Lithium and Antidepressant Drug-Induced Mania

In some bipolar patients, lithium may be used to prevent tricyclic-induced mania. Wehr and Goodwin have suggested the possibility that "antidepressants cause mania and worsen the course of affective illness'' (3). Although the experimental data are less substantial than clinical case observations would suggest, these authors conclude: ''On balance, the available evidence suggests that some bipolar patients become manic, and a few experience rapid cycling, when they are treated with antidepressants. The prevention of these responses will require further research on risk factors and on the antimanic efficacy of coadministered lithium or other mood stabilizers.''

Lithium and Bipolar Depression

The issue of combining lithium with other antidepressants was reviewed in terms of its potential merits and drawbacks (4). In drug-free depressed bipolar patients, clinical circumstances will often determine which of two approaches should be taken. For example, lithium can be administered alone for several weeks to allow the subgroup of lithium-responsive depressives to be identified and to avoid potential side effects from using a conventional antidepressant. Alternatively, therapy with lithium and an antidepressant can be started simultaneously, with the goal of preventing antidepressant-induced mania and, perhaps, potentiating the antidepressant action of each compound in a synergistic fashion.

LITHIUM AUGMENTATION

In unipolar depressed patients, drugs other than lithium are usually the treatment of choice. However, lithium may act as an ''augmenter'' when a patient fails to respond to an adequate trial of treatment with an antidepressant. As early as 1976, synergistic effects were reported when lithium was added to the treatment regimen of a tricyclic antidepressant in treatment-resistant psychotic depression (5). It was not until 1981, however, that lithium augmentation became more universally accepted, when DeMontigny et al. reported that eight unipolar depressed patients responded rapidly (within 48 hr) to the addition of lithium (6). Since then, this observation has been supported by many case reports in patients with unipolar, bipolar, psychotic, and nonpsychotic depression. Furthermore, response does not appear limited to the addition of lithium to tricyclic antidepressants, but synergism has also been reported with other heterocyclic and MAO inhibitor antidepressants, as well as alprazolam (7). Nor does age does not appear to be a limiting factor, because safe and effective lithium augmentation has also been shown in elderly patients (8).

Lithium augmentation is usually initiated at a dosage of 300 mg t.i.d. Although age and other factors may necessitate a lower dose. If a robust response does not occur in the first few days, then dosage adjustment should be made based on the serum lithium level (range 0.6-1.0 mEq/L). If no response has occurred in 2-3 weeks, more lengthy lithium treatment is unlikely to be effective. Response to augmentation may be complete or partial, and a worsening of depression has also been described (9). Paradoxically, the appearance of manic symptoms has rarely been observed following the addition of lithium to an antidepressant regimen (10,11). Overall, lithium augmentation has become an accepted therapeutic intervention for many clinicians who utilize it as the next step in the treatment of resistant depression. This approach represents an effective and safe treatment that is far less time-consuming than switching from one to another antidepressant.

Lithium Maintenance

In contrast with its relatively limited role as an antidepressant, lithium has become more widely accepted for its prophylactic effect in preventing mood swings in individuals with bipolar and unipolar affective disorder. Interestingly, the FDA has not given formal approval for the prophylactic use of lithium in preventing recurrent depressive episodes: "Lithium is also indicated as a maintenance treatment for individuals with a diagnosis of Bipolar Disorder. Maintenance therapy reduces the frequency of manic episodes and diminishes the intensity of those episodes which may occur" (12). On the other hand, many clinicians and investigators have found that lithium is of value in reducing the severity and frequency of depressive episodes in patients with bipolar and unipolar disorder. Because of its effectiveness in mania, lithium is the preferred long-term treatment for bipolar patients. Although its effect on the depressive component may be less well studied, it is often of substantial benefit in preventing depressive episodes. Maintenance therapy with antipressants alone in bipolar patients is not wise, because these compounds do not prevent (and may even increase) manic episodes and may precipitate rapid cycling (3). Although the combination of lithium and an antidepressant may have theoretical appeal in maintenance for bipolar illness, controlled studies have failed to substantiate any advantages over lithium alone. Nonetheless, many patients are maintained on the combination of lithium and an antidepressant, and some patients do benefit to a greater extent than they have from either drug alone.

Most studies of maintenance therapy for unipolar affective disorder have found lithium to be at least as effective as conventional antidepressants (13), although a multicenter study showed lithium to be less effective than imipramine, especially following episodes of severe depression (14). For maintenance treatment of major unipolar depression, the combination of lithium with an antidepressant has not been shown to be of greater benefit than either drug alone. Again, there may be exceptions that are recognized in clinical practice but get lost in the statistical convolutions of research studies. The issue of whether to use lithium or a conventional antidepressant for maintenance treatment in unipolar depression is usually resolved by continuing the drug that effectively treated the initial depressive episode. Lithium, therefore, can be considered a "backup" for use when conventional antidepressants are ineffective or not well tolerated.

Breakthrough Depression

Maintenance therapy with lithium is often less than perfect for affective recurrences (15). For example, Schou estimates that perhaps 40-50% of bipolar patients will require additional treatment and that only 20% will have a "strikingly good treatment effect . . ." (16). Although there may be exceptions, several studies (14,17,18) have not found additional protection from maintenance therapy with lithium and imipramine combined, when compared with lithium alone.

There is some evidence that affective morbidity may be reduced in patients maintained as a lower serum lithium level. Coppen et al. (19), in a 1 year prospective, double-blind study compared patients maintained at serum lithium levels between 0.45 and 0.79 mEq/L(mean 0.63) with another group maintained between 0.8 and 1.2 mEq/L (mean 0.92). In addition to a reduction in side effects, the lower dosage group demonstrated no increase in affective morbidity, and the unipolar patients had a statistically significant reduction in affective morbidity.

On the basis of clinical observation, Kukopulos and Reginaldi (20) described three distinct courses that unipolar depression may take during maintenance lithium therapy. First, although "real depressive episodes" may not recur, persistent depressive symptoms (fatigue, sleep disturbance, reduced concentration, aches and pains) can be present. These investigators suggest that the ". . . use of antidepressant drugs in moderate doses and a lower serum lithium level help the patient improve quickly. When he is well again, lithium must be increased to prophylactic levels and antidepressants gradually suspended." Second, clear-cut depressive episodes may occur, which are usually less severe, of shorter duration, and more responsive to antidepressants than the depressive episodes were before lithium. In such situations, they have suggested avoiding supplementary antidepressants ". . . because these short depressive episodes disappear in a few months under continuous lithium treatment." Finally, Kukopulos and Reginaldi note that if ". . . lithium is started during a depression and serum lithium levels are kept above 0.60 mmol/1 the depression may last a long time, though gradually becoming less severe" (20). They suggest that reducing or temporarily stopping the lithium might terminate the prolonged depressive episodes (20).

These suggestions are in keeping with the observations of Himmelhoch and Neil (21) who stated "... our experience suggests that lithium levels effective in the management of mania may be too high for either the acute or maintenance treatment of lithium sensitive depression."

If "breakthrough" depression occurs, thyroid function should also be evaluated by measuring serum TSH, because lithium-induced hypothyroidism can cause symptoms similar to major depression. If thyroid function is normal and the depression is not severe, continued treatment with lithium alone may be adequate. There is some evidence that the risk of a depressive relapse decreases with increasing time on lithium. For example, in bipolar II patients Dunner et al. found lithium to be equal to placebo at 15 months, but more effective at 33 months, in preventing depressive recurrence (22). Adjusting the lithium dose may also be helpful in dealing with breakthrough depression with more support for the potential benefit of dosage reduction than dosage increase. Obviously, clinical judgment must be exercised here.

If these approaches are ineffective, or if the depressive episode is severe, then the addition of an antidepressant drug is appropriate. The tricyclics remain the most commonly used agents for treating breakthrough bipolar or unipolar depression, although some clinicians feel that MAO inhibitors, especially tranylcypromine, are more effective for a bipolar depression (23). If supplemental antidepressants are used, there is the possibility of inducing rapid-cycling, lithium-resistant postdepression mania, or an increased susceptibility to side effects.

Response Prediction

Efforts to predict which patients will respond favorably to lithium's antidepressant effect have been unsuccessful. Investigators have examined the serum calcium/magnesium ratio, visual-evoked response, catecholamine and indolamine metabolite levels, red blood cell/plasma lithium ratio, and psychological tests without finding any to be predictively useful. Similar efforts to predict responsiveness to lithium maintenance therapy in bipolar and unipolar patients have met with limited success. At present, "... clinicians must still rely on empirical trials to determine which patients will respond to lithium therapy" (13).

LITHIUM THERAPY

Pharmacology

Unlike other psychiatric medications, lithium is an element, with an atomic number of 3 and an atomic weight of 6.94. It enters and leaves the body intact, and excretion is almost entirely by the kidneys. It has no metabolites, is essentially not protein-bound, and is easily measured in the serum by a variety of laboratory techniques.

In the United States, lithium is most readily available as tablets and capsules in the form of lithium carbonate. There is, however, a liquid preparation of lithium citrate also available. Dosage formulations include 150-, 300-, and 600-mg capsules and 300-mg tablets of standard-release lithium carbonate. These preparations are rapidly absorbed from the gastrointestinal tract and reach peak serum levels within 1/2 to 3 hr. In addition, there are 300 mg and 450 mg slow or controlled release tablets which are just as completely absorbed but take longer to reach peak serum levels. The liquid formulation contains 8.0 mEq of lithium per 5 mL of solution, so that the amount of lithium present is similar to that in a 300-mg tablet or capsule. Most patients can be effectively managed by standard preparations and by adjusting dosage in 300-mg increments. The 150-mg capsules should be useful in elderly patients who require lower doses and for whom breaking scored 300-mg tablets may be difficult. The slow-release preparations are better tolerated by some patients and may produce less initial stomach upset.

Lithium has traditionally been given in divided doses, and the package insert still suggests this approach. Doses of controlled-release lithium are usually given b.i.d. at approximately 12-hr intervals (12). Despite these recommendations, more recent research has shown that single daily dosing may be as effective as divided dosing and be associated with fewer renal and urinary tract side effects, such as polyuria. Unless the total daily dosage is very large, most people tolerate the immediate-release preparations on a twice or once daily basis. Three, four, or more daily doses can often create compliance problems in many patients. The main disadvantage of once-daily dosing is that the standardized 12-hr serum lithium level may be substantially higher than that seen with similar doses given on a divided basis. One reasonable compromise would be to utilize a twice-daily dosage schedule of conventional or slow-release lithium and alter this regimen only if the patient is unable to tolerate the prescribed dose, in which case, a thrice daily dosage regimen might be more appropriate. The pharmacokinetics of all permutations of dosage schedule and form have not been studied, and this, coupled with interindividual variability, precludes accurate mathematical adjustment of 12-h serum lithium levels to compensate for changes in dosage schedule and form (13).

Serum Lithium Levels

Serum lithium levels should serve as treatment guidelines. In recent years, the trend has been toward lower levels (0.8-1.2 mEq/L for acute mania and 0.6-0.8 mEq/L for maintenance therapy without any apparent decrease in overall efficacy (13). In treating depression, improvement usually occurs at lithium levels between 0.6 and 1.0 mEq/L, although higher levels may be necessary in some individuals. Unlike the rapid response that sometimes occurs when lithium is used to augment another antidepressant, the onset of therapeutic action when lithium is used alone is often delayed at least 2-3 weeks. Unfortunately, no tests are yet available that can predict an effective serum lithium level for a given individual. Consequently, the practitioner must proceed based upon careful clinical observation and repeated lithium level monitoring. A recent prospective study found a relapse rate 2.6 times higher in patients maintained between 0.4-0.6 mEq/L compared to those maintained at 0.8-1.0 mEq/L (Gelenberg AJ, Kane JM, Keller MB, et al: N Engl J Med 1989; 321:1489-93). In some individuals, the serum lithium level may be influenced by mood state, with higher levels during depression and lower levels during mania (24). Consequently, measuring the serum lithium level at the onset and termination of an affective episode can be extremely important.

The usual starting dosage of lithium carbonate is 300 mg three times daily or 600 mg twice daily. Although there are a number of dose prediction methods that promise to shorten the time required to reach a desirable serum level, none of these have gained widespread acceptance, and most practitioners adjust dosage based on clinical observation and sequential serum lithium determinations (13).

Dosage adjustments can most effectively be made if they are based on *steady-state lithium levels* obtained on morning blood samples drawn at approximately 12 hr after the last dose. Because at least 4 days at a specific dose is necessary to achieve steady-state levels, a dosage increase before this time is likely to result in an excessive lithium level. Furthermore, if sampling intervals are not *standardized*, serum lithium levels can "appear" quite inconsistent, being too high shortly after a dose and too low long after a dose. Therefore, the sampling interval of 12 hr is the standard against which therapeutic lithium ranges have been established.

Baseline Testing

Before starting lithium therapy, a thorough medical history is necessary. This, in turn, will determine the extent of additional evaluation and testing. Factors such as advanced age, associated major illnesses, special diets, and other medications, are cause for added concern. All patients should have thyroid and renal function tests performed. Thyroid disorders, such as hypothyroidism and apathetic thyrotoxicosis, may be mistaken for major depression. Furthermore, lithium treatment may adversely affect thyroid function, and pretreatment testing of thyroxine (T_4), triiodothyronine (T_3) uptake, and thyrotropin (thyroid-stimulating hormone; TSH) should suffice for most patients. A thyrotropin-releasing hormone (TRH) stimulation test is seldom, if ever, necessary before initiating lithium therapy.

Because lithium is almost entirely excreted by the kidneys and because lithium can adversely affect renal function, baseline testing is essential. For most patients, measurement of serum creatinine and perhaps, a urinalysis is usually adequate. Even in the elderly in whom serum creatinine is a less sensitive reflection of glomerular filtration rate, a 24-hour creatinine clearance is usually not necessary. Additional laboratory tests, such as blood chemistries, hematology profile, electrocardiogram, and electroencephalogram, can be obtained if clinically indicated.

Ongoing Treatment

During the course of lithium therapy, periodic clinical evaluation and laboratory testing are necessary. The frequency of these evaluations should be individualized. In selected patients, after a period of clinical stability, good compliance, stable lithium levels, and an absence of troublesome side effects and extenuating circumstances, visits every 3, 4 or even 6 months may suffice at which time serum lithium level, serum creatinine and other indicated testing can be done. In less stable patients, more frequent testing should be obtained. Patients should be encouraged to contact their physician between appointments to discuss changes in affective state, intercurrent medical illness, the use of other medicines, side effects, and special diets. Written educational materials can be helpful in addressing many of these questions (25, 26).

Stopping Lithium Therapy

The length of time one remains on a lithium therapeutic regimen depends on a number of factors, including efficacy, type of affective illness, severity of illness, and whether lithium is to be used as an adjunctive medication or for long-term maintenance therapy.

Nonresponders

If the depressive illness has not responded to an adequate trial of lithium therapy for 4 weeks, further treatment with lithium alone is unlikely to be effective. In patients already receiving another antidepressant, a 2-week trial of lithium augmentation should be administered, although Price et al. advocate a 3-week trial (9). Evaluating responsiveness to maintenance lithium therapy is often more difficult because the duration of an adequate trial also depends on the frequency and type of pretreatment episodes. For example, a disorder characterized by fewer affective episodes may require a longer period of evaluation to determine overall efficacy. In addition, that treatment efficacy may improve over time with continued lithium therapy suggests the need for perseverance.

Responders

If long-term lithium therapy is not considered, then the guidelines for stopping lithium therapy are similar to those for conventional antidepressants. Some data have indicated that the risk of relapse can be minimized by maintaining treatment for at least 4-5 months after resolution of depressive symptoms (27).

In the case of successful lithium augmentation, there is some controversy over which drug to discontinue first. DeMontigny et al. described some patients who remained well on a tricyclic alone after only 48 hr of lithium augmentation (28). Most clinicians, however, would be more likely to continue both drugs for several months, unless side effects were intolerable. In bipolar patients, the antidepressant should be stopped first, although in unipolar patients the decision is less clearly defined.

When, or even if, to discontinue maintenance therapy is a difficult decision. Some evidence suggests that, after discontinuation of successful lithium maintenance, the risk of affective recurrence is similar to that of the pretreatment period. However, this observation has been difficult to establish with certainty, given the marked variation in the course of affective illness during an individual's lifetime. It is clear that lithium does not cure these conditions. Other factors to be considered include the pattern of onset (gradual or abrupt) and severity of previous episodes, how well the drug is tolerated and the availability of more affective and safer treatment alternatives. Furthermore, there are as yet no tests that can reliably predict which patient will have a substantial risk of relapse.

The issue of whether abrupt discontinuation of lithium is associated with an increased risk of early relapse also is not resolved. The conclusion of our review was "The majority of patients do not experience withdrawal symptoms or rebound phenomenon [sic] upon cessation of long-term lithium therapy. In view of the occasional reports of sudden relapse occurring with abrupt discontinuation, gradual withdrawal under close supervision may be wise, especially for patients who continue to show mood lability during maintenance lithium therapy" (13).

SPECIAL SITUATIONS

Children and Adolescents

Lithium has also been useful in the treatment of bipolar disorder in children and adolescents. Delong and Aldershof recently reported a 66% success rate in the long-term lithium treatment of childhood manic-depression (29). Their results with unipolar depression were far less promising with only a 17% overall success rate. Although lithium is not a well-established treatment in this age group, especially in preadolescents, it does appear to be quite effective in carefully selected individuals (13).

Geriatric Patients

Advanced age does not appear to diminish to efficacy of lithium in preventing affective episodes. Although it has been far less extensively studied in geriatric patients, the indications for lithium are similar to those for younger individuals (13,30). Whether the elderly actually respond to lower serum lithium levels or whether similar levels would be as effective in younger patients is not clear. However, susceptibility to side effects and toxicity from lithium does seem to increase in older persons. In addition, reduced renal clearance does result in both higher serum levels and a longer time to reach steady-state serum lithium concentrations for a given dose. The safe and effective use of lithium in geriatric patients requires closer monitoring. Schulman et al. reported that a once-daily dosage regimen of lithium carbonate (average 408 mg/day) in 93% of 43 patients, with a mean age of 74 years, produced a mean 12-hr lithium level of 0.5 mmol/L (30). With an average follow-up duration of 23 months (range 3-44), these investigators observed a substantially higher relapse rate in patients with bipolar (67%) compared with those with unipolar (13%) depression. As a result, they suggested that a serum lithium level of 0.5 mmol/L (mEqL) might seem most reasonable. If the drug is given in divided dose, the amount to reach this level will be somewhat larger. Although higher blood levels may ultimately be necessary in some patients, the lithium dose should be increased only if lower serum levels were ineffective.

Pregnancy

The risk of fetal malformation, especially cardiovascular abnormalities, is increased by use of lithium during the first trimester. Consequently, its use should be avoided during this period if at all possible. As pregnancy progresses, physiological changes in the mother make treatment with lithium more complicated (although not impossible). While frequent small doses have been advocated, no research has been done to verify the merit of this approach. If lithium therapy is unavoidable during pregnancy, then the drug should be stopped shortly before delivery to reduce the risk of toxicity in the newborn.

Because women with affective disorders are at higher risk for developing a postpartum affective disturbance, consideration should be given to restarting lithium shortly after delivery. Breast-feeding is usually discouraged if the mother is taking lithium. Both patient and physician guidelines regarding lithium and pregnancy are available from the Lithium Information Center (13).

ADVERSE INTERACTIONS

Concomitant Medications

The combined use of lithium and antidepressants is generally well tolerated, with a slight increase in some side effects from both drugs. Case reports of idiosyncratic reactions have been published, but should not discourage the use of lithium in combination with other antidepressants (13). Neurotoxicity has been reported with the combination of lithium and neuroleptics. Whether this is merely an additive effect of two central nervous system active drugs or a synergism (as has been suggested with haloperidol) has not been established. As a consequence, we suggest avoiding the simultaneous use of large doses of both drugs when treating mania and keeping close observation of these patients for neurotoxic symptoms (13).

Other drugs that can interact with lithium are thiazide (and possibly potassium-sparing) diuretics and most nonsteroidal anti-inflammatory drugs. These compounds can produce a reduced renal clearance of lithium, with increased serum lithium levels and possible lithium toxicity. Nevertheless, lithium can be safely used with these drugs, but a dosage reduction in lithium may be necessary when they are added, and a subsequent dosage increase given when they are discontinued. Lithium interactions have been described with many other medications, although these reports tend to be anecdotal and their clinical significance unclear (13,31).

Diet

Restricting dietary sodium intake results in increased renal retention of sodium *and* lithium and, consequently, serum lithium levels rise and the risk of lithium intoxication increases. A low-sodium diet, however, is not contraindicated with lithium therapy, but a lower lithium dose may be required. Dietary extremes should be avoided during lithium therapy because marked alterations in hydration can destabilize serum lithium levels.

Electroconvulsive Therapy

Electroconvulsive therapy (ECT) has a well-established role in the treatment of depression. There have been several reports of neurotoxicity occurring when ECT was given to patients receiving lithium and, therefore, the following suggestions have been made: ". . . discontinuation of lithium at least 48 hr before ECT; serum levels below 0.5 mEq/L at the time of ECT; and resumption of lithium 48 hr after ECT" (13). The cause of the interaction between lithium and ECT is not clear, because ECT does not alter renal lithium clearance, serum lithium level, or brain lithium concentration (in animals). Furthermore, lithium does not appear to alter the seizure thresholds for ECT. Although there are no data supporting an enhanced clinical benefit from the combination of lithium and ECT, there may be some circumstances when continuation of lithium is necessary to prevent ECT-induced mania. In a review, Rudorfer and Linnoila concluded that there is no substantial advantage to combining lithium with ECT (32). However, following ECT, lithium maintenance has been shown to successfully reduce the risk of relapse and would be indicated in the continued treatment of bipolar patients and some unipolar depressed patients.

SIDE EFFECTS AND TOXICITY

Most persons taking lithium experience some transient or lasting side effects. However, most patients consider these to be mild and tolerable. An extensive review of the subject is beyond the scope of this chapter, but more comprehensive information can be obtained from several resources (13,33, and the Lithium Information Center). The remainder of this section will focus on some of the more prominent adverse reactions to lithium treatment.

Neurological

Complaints such as a lack of spontaneity, dysphoria, intellectual dullness, reduced creativity, impaired concentration and memory may be encountered in patients taking lithium. Because these symptoms are also associated with depression, it is important to know if they predate lithium therapy or if they appear during the course of treatment whether they represent symptoms of "breakthrough" depression or lithium-induced hypothyroidism. If these symptoms are caused by lithium, a reduction in dosage often provides symptomatic relief.

Tremor

Tremor is a common side effect and is seldom incapacitating. It resembles essential tremor and may be aggravated by the associated use of tricyclic antidepressant drugs. Although improvement often occurs spontaneously, tremors can often be treated by dosage reduction, switching to a slow-released preparation, discontinuation of additional antidepressants, or intermittent treatment with a β-blocker such as propranolol. A tremor that increases in severity or generalizes beyond the upper extremities suggests impending lithium intoxication, and a serum lithium level measurement and dosage reduction should be initiated.

Intoxication

Lithium intoxication is primarily characterized by symptoms of neurotoxicity, although other organ systems (gastrointestinal, renal, cardiac, and respiratory) may also be involved. The severity of symptoms is related to the duration and amount of lithium exposure, as well as to individual sensitivity. Early manifestation, such as dysarthria and ataxia, can progress to neuromuscular irritability, seizures, coma. and eventually irreversible neurological damage (especially cerebellar) and death. More milder cases of lithium intoxication can be treated by discontinuing the drug and applying gastric lavage (for acute overdose), hydration, and forced diuresis with osmotic diuretics and/or furosemide. Severe intoxication should be aggressively treated with hemodialysis. When to dialyze is a matter of medical judgment based on the patient's clinical condition and the serum lithium level (13). Cases with poor outcomes are commonly faulted for (1) failure to dialyze, (2) delay in dialysis, and (3) inadequate dialysis in terms of frequency or duration.

Thyroid

"Abnormal thyroid function tests may occur in 5-15% of patients receiving long-term lithium therapy. However, clinical manifestations are rare. Regular monitoring of TSH levels every 6-12 months and awareness of the clinical signs of hypothyroidism (lethargy, fatigue, voice and skin changes, weight gain, cold intolerance, constipation, mental sluggishness) are recommended. Supplemental thyroid medication should not be started on the basis of a single deviant thyroid value unless these clinical signs are present" (34,35). Asymptomatic, milder abnormalities of thyroid function usually normalize over time with continued lithium therapy, and as a consequence only the more severe alterations should be treated with supplemental thyroid hormone. Because symptoms of hypothyroidism and depression may mimic one another, testing of thyroid function (serum TSH is the most sensitive readily available test) is encouraged at the slightest clinical provocation. Restricting testing to an arbitrary interval of every 6 or 12 months may delay diagnosis and appropriate treatment. Although the aggressive treatment of subclinical thyroid abnormalities is not encouraged, a trial of supplemental thyroid hormone should be considered in suggestive clinical situations. Exogenous thyroid hormone has been useful in some cases of otherwise treatment resistant depression and rapid-cycling bipolar disorder (see Chaps. *20* and *21*).

Weight

Weight gain is not uncommon during the course of lithium therapy. Contributing factors include a genetic predisposition, mood stabilization, a high caloric fluid intake, hypothyroidism, and the direct metabolic effects of lithium. Because depressive illness per se, as well as the use of tricyclic antidepressants can cause weight gain, it is often difficult to determine the real factor in lithium-induced weight gain. "Treatment of this side effect should begin with preventive education, good dietary habits, regular exercise, and routine monitoring of weight" (33).

Kidney Function

Lithium therapy may cause an impaired renal concentrating ability, a modest reduction in glomerular filtration rate (GFR), increase urine volume (sometimes to the point of nephrogenic diabetes insipidus), and morphological abnormalities, including focal interstitial fibrosis, tubular atrophy and glomerular sclerosis (36). Hence, periodic monitoring of renal function is imperative and, for most patients, this includes measuring serum creatinine along with the serum lithium level and total urine volume if polyuria seems excessive. When there is concern of possible lithium-induced nephrotoxicity, 24-hr creatinine clearance is a more accurate measure of GFR. If altered kidney function is suspected, more sophisticated renal tests and a nephrology consult should be obtained.

Renal lithium clearance does not appear to be substantially altered by antidepressant drugs (37). Whether the combined use of lithium and antidepressants increases the risk of lithium-induced renal complications, compared with the use of lithium alone, is not known, although there is currently little support for such an interaction.

Reducing the likelihood of kidney complications is essential to the successful long-term use of lithium. Maintaining the lowest effective serum lithium level will do much to attain this goal. Animal and human evidence continues to accumulate that single daily dose may be associated with fewer renal abnormalities than divided dose (36). Finally, if polyuria cannot be effectively reduced by a lower daily lithium dosage or single daily dose, the careful administration of a thiazide and/or potassium-sparing diuretic should be considered (33).

RESOURCES

Well over 19,000 medical articles have been published about lithium in medicine. Staying abreast of this literature is a time-consuming task. Books (13, 25) and journal articles do much to meet those informational needs but cannot always keep abreast of the explosion of information.

The Lithium Information Center (Department of Psychiatry, University of Wisconsin Center for Health Sciences, 600 Highland Avenue, Madison,

Wisconsin 53792, 608/263-6171) maintains a computerized data base of lithium articles and is able to meet the informational needs of professionals and lay persons throughout the world (38). The Center, which is accessible by telephone, mail, or direct computer link, can provide timely and comprehensive information about all aspects of lithium and medicine.

The recent development of self-help groups promises much in the way of support and education for individuals with affective disorders. The National Depressive and Manic-Depressive Association (NDMDA), an organization of over 61 groups throughout the United States and Canada, provides personal support and direct service to persons with clinical depression or manic-depression and their families, and public education concerning the nature and management of affective disorders. The NDMDA mailing address is NDMDA, Merchandise Mart, Box 3395, Chicago, Illinois 60654; (312) 446-9009.

REFERENCES

1. Cohen, I. M., Bunney, W. E., Cole, J. O., Fieve, R. R., Gershon, S., and Prien, R. F. (1975). The current status of lithium therapy: Report of the APA Task Force. *Am. J. Psychiatry 132*:997-1001.
2. Fieve, R. R. and Peselow, E. D. (1983). Clinical applications. In *Drugs in Psychiatry*, Vol. 1, *Antidepressants*. Edited by G. D. Burrows, T. R. Norman, and B. Davies, Amsterdam, New York, Elsevier, pp. 277-321.
3. Wehr, T. A. and Goodwin, F. K. (1987). Can antidepressants cause mania and worsen the course of affective illness? *Am. J. Psychiatry 144*:1403-141.
4. Jefferson, J. W. and Ayd, F. J. (1983). Changing lithium and antidepressants. *J. Clin. Psychopharmacol. 3*:303-307.
5. Neubauer, H. and Bermingham, P. (1976). A depressive syndrome responsive to lithium: An analysis of 20 cases. *J. Nerv. Ment. Dis. 163*:276-281.
6. DeMontigny, C., Grunberg, F., Mayer, A., and Deschenes, J.-P. (1981). Lithium induces rapid relief of depression in tricyclic antidepressant drug nonresponders. *Br. J. Psychiatry 138*:252-256.
7. Cerra, D., Meacham, T., and Coleman, J. (1986). A possible synergistic effect of alprazolam and lithium carbonate. *Am. J. Psychiatry 143*:552.
8. Kushnir, S. L. (1986). Lithium-antidepressant combinations in the treatment of depressed, physically ill geriatric patients. *Am. J. Psychiatry 143*:378-379.
9. Price, L. H., Charney, D. S., and Heninger, G. R. (1986). Variability of response to lithium augmentation in refractory depression. *Am. J. Psychiatry 143*:1387-1392.
10. Price, L. H., Charney, D. S., and Heninger, G. R. (1984). Manic symptoms following addition of lithium treatment to antidepressant treatment. *J. Clin. Psychopharmacol. 4*:361-362.
11. Louie, A. K. and Meltzer, H. Y. (1984). Lithium potentiation of antidepressant treatment. *J. Clin. Psychopharmacol. 4*:316-321.
12. *Physicians' Desk Reference.* Oradell, N. J., Medical Economics, 1988.

13. Jefferson, J. W., Greist, J. H., Ackerman, D. L., and Carroll, J. A. (1987). *Lithium Encyclopedia for Clinical Practice*, 2nd ed. Washington, D. C., American Psychiatric Press, pp. 1-744.
14. Prien, R. F., Kupfer, D. J., Mansky, P. A., Small, J. G., Tuason, V. B., Voss, C. B., and Johnson, W. E. (1984). Drug therapy in the prevention of recurrences in unipolar and bipolar affective disorders. *Arch. Gen. Psychiatry 41*:1096-1104.
15. Prien, R. F. (1983). Long-term prophylactic pharmacologic treatment of bipolar illness. In *Psychiatry Update*, Vol. 2. Edited by L. Grinspoon. Washington, D. C., American Psychiatric Press, pp. 303-318.
16. Schou, M. (1980). *Lithium Treatment of Manic-Depressive Illness: A Practical Guide*. Basel, New York, Karger, pp. 213-215.
17. Quitkin, F. M., Kane, J., Rifkin, A., Ramos-Lorenzi, J. R., and Nayak, D. V. (1981). Prophylactic lithium carbonate with and without imipramine for bipolar I patients. *Arch. Gen. Psychiatry 38*:902-907.
18. Quitkin, F., Rifkin, A., Kane, J., Ramos-Lorenzi, J. R., and Klein, D. F. (1978). Prophylactic effect of lithium and imipramine in unipolar and bipolar II patients: A preliminary report. *Am. J. Psychiatry 135*:570-572.
19. Coppen, A., Abou-Saleh, M., Milln, P., Bailey, J., and Wood, K. (1983). Decreasing lithium dosage reduces morbidity and side effects during prophylaxis. *J. Affect. Disord. 5*:353-362.
20. Kukopulos, A. and Reginaldi, D. (1980). Recurrences of manic-depressive episodes during lithium treatment. In *Handbook of Lithium Therapy*. Edited by F. N. Johnson. Lancaster, Engl., MTP Press, p. 109-117.
21. Himmelhoch, J. M., and Neil, J. F. (1980). Lithium therapy in combination with other forms of treatment. In *Handbook of Lithium Therapy*. Edited by F. N. Johnson. Lancaster, Engl., MTP Press, pp. 51-67.
22. Dunner, D. L., Stallone, F., and Fieve, R. R. (1982). Prophylaxis with lithium carbonate: An update. *Arch. Gen. Psychiatry 39*:1344-1345.
23. Himmelhoch, J. M., Mallinger, A. G., and Fuchs, C. Z. (1987). Tranylcypromine versus imipramine in manic depression. *New Res. Abstr.* American Psychiatric Association 139th Annual Meeting, Washington, D. C., p. 78.
24. Kukopulos, A., Minnai, G., and Muller-Oerlinghausen, B. (1985). The influence of mania and depression on the pharmacokinetics of lithium. *J. Affect. Disord. 8*:159-166.
25. Bohn, J. and Jefferson, J. W. (1982). *Lithium and Manic Depression: A Guide*, 1st ed. Madison, Wis., Lithium Information Center, pp.1-35. (revised 1990)
26. Schou, M. (1983). *Lithium Treatment of Manic-Depressive Illness: A Practical Guide*, 2nd ed. Basel, New York, Karger, pp. 1-49.
27. Prien, R. F. and Kupfer, D. J. (1986). Continuation drug therapy for major depressive episodes: How long should it be maintained? *Am. J. Psychiatry 143*: 18-23.
28. DeMontigny, C., Cournoyer, G., Morissette, R., Langlois, R., and Caille, G. (1983). Lithium carbonate addition in tricyclic antidepressant resistant unipolar depression. *Arch. Gen. Psychiatry 40*:1327-1334.

29. Delong, G. R. and Aldershof, A. L. (1987). Long-term experience with lithium treatment in childhood: Correlation with clinical diagnosis. *J. Am. Acad. Child Adolesc. Psychiatry 26*:389-394.
30. Shulman, K. I., MacKenzie, S., and Hardy, B. (1987). The clinical use of lithium carbonate in old age: A review. *Prog. Neuropsychopharmacol. Biol. Psychiatry 11*:159-164.
31. Johnson, F. N. (1987). *Lithium Combination Treatment*. Basel, New York, Karger, pp. 1-273.
32. Rudorfer, M. V. and Linnoila, M. (1987). Electroconvulsive therapy. In *Lithium Combination Treatment*. Lithium Therapy Monographs, Vol. 1. Edited by F. N. Johnson. Basel, New York, Karger, pp. 164-178.
33. Jefferson, J. W. and Greist, J. H. (1987). Lithium carbonate and carbamazepine side effects. In *Psychiatry Update*. American Psychiatric Association Annual Review. Vol. 6. Edited by R. E. Hales and A. J. Frances, Washington, D. C., American Psychiatric Press, pp. 746-780.
34. Anonymous (1987). Thyroid changes with lithium therapy. *Psychiatry Drug Alerts 1*:64.
35. Maarbjerg, K., Vestergaard, P., and Schou, M. (1987). Changes in serum thyroxine (T_4) and serum thyroid stimulating hormone (TSH) during prolonged lithium treatment. *Acta Psychiatr. Scand. 75*:217-221.
36. Hetmar, O., Brun, C., Clemmesen, L., Ladefoged, J., Larsen, S., and Rafaelsen, O. J. (1987). Lithium: Long-term effects on the kidney. 2. Structural changes. *J. Psychiatr. Res. 21*:279-288.
37. Lassen, E., Vestergaard, P., and Thomsen, K. (1986). Renal function of patients in long-term treatment with lithium citrate alone or in combination with neuroleptics and antidepressant drugs. *Arch. Gen. Psychiatry 43*:481-482.
38. Greist, J. H., Jefferson, J. W., Ackerman, D. L., Baudhuin, M. G., Erdman, H. P., and Carroll, J. A. (1985). Lithium Information Center: The Lithium Library revisited. *J. Clin. Psychiatry 46*:327-331.

8

Anticonvulsants for the Lithium-Resistant Bipolar Patient

ROBERT M. POST

Biological Psychiatry Branch, National Institute of Mental Health
Bethesda, Maryland

INTRODUCTION

Treatment of the bipolar depressed patient raises unique problems in comparison with the unipolar depressed patient. A much wider range of treatment modalities is available for the unipolar depressed patient because the primary and sole concern is alleviation of the depressive mood, whereas a secondary concern in the treatment of the bipolar patient is achieving this latter goal without the induction of a manic episode, continuous cycling, or rapid cycling. Clinical experience and a considerable literature (1,2) indicate that some bipolar patients are indeed susceptible to the induction of these antidepressant-related side effects—hypomania, conversion to continuous cycling, or rapid cycling.

Bunney and associates (3) noted a 9.6% incidence of hypomania during treatment with a variety of heterocyclic and monoamine oxidase inhibitor (MAOI) antidepressants. They indicated that the tricyclic- and L-dopa-induced switches among bipolar patients occurred with an incidence statistically greater than chance expectations. As noted in the review of Wehr and Goodwin (1,2), there is some controversy over the prevalence of this problem, but less

For presentation at Symposium for Treatment-Resistant Depression, Philadelphia, 1988 controversial are the data that patients who are already showing rapid cycling may increase the rapidity of cycling while treated with an antidepressant and then show a return to slower-cycling frequencies when the medication is removed. Such a patient is illustrated in Figure 1.

This 59-year-old woman showed a pattern of cycling between depression and mania for several decades. Upon treatment with lithium carbonate in conjunction with a variety of heterocyclic and MAOI antidepressants, her cycle frequency changed from several episodes each year to a much faster rate. This change, coincident with the use of medications, did not appear to be a spontaneous change in her course of illness, since placebo substitution at National Institutes of Health (NIH) was associated with a slowing down

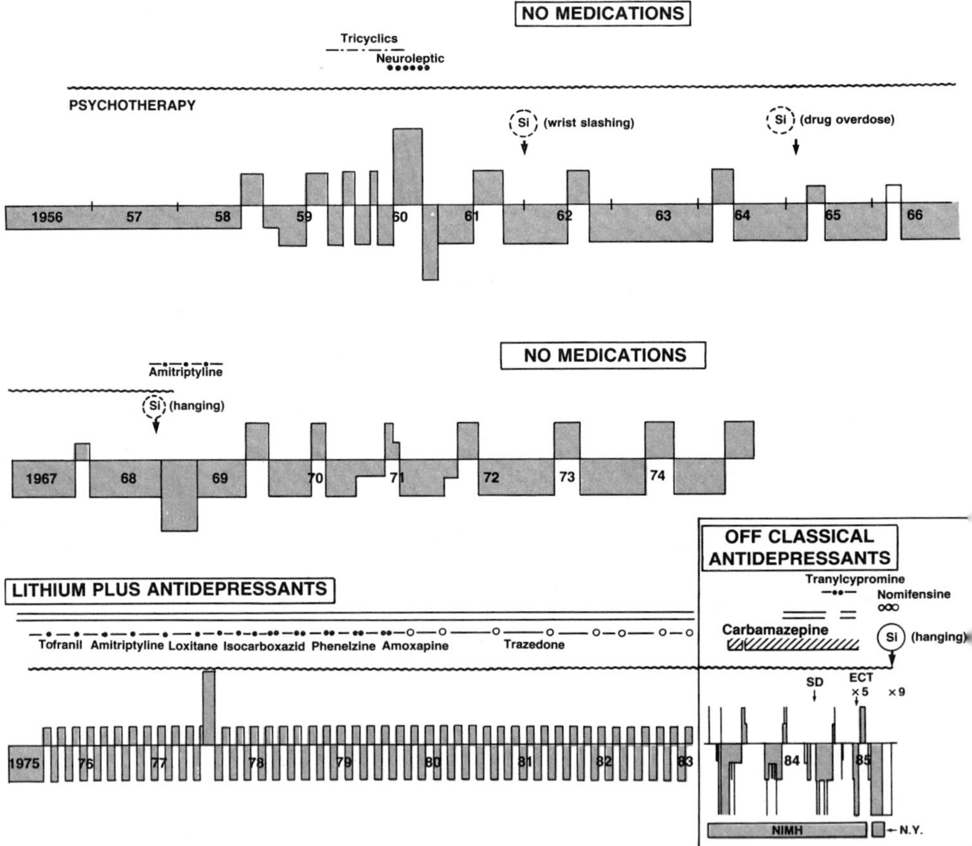

Figure 1 Rapid cycling associated with antidepressants.

of her cycling pattern. Treatment with lithium and carbamazepine in combination resulted in periods of euthymia lasting up to several months, but never adequately stopped her recurrent cycles of severe depression, functional incapacity, and suicidality. Following dramatic clinical improvement from depression after a single ECT treatment given at NIMH, the patient was discharged with a regimen of prophylactic ECT on a 2-week basis. Despite this treatment, the next depressive episode occurred "on schedule" and a new series of ECT treatments were begun. In contrast with the initial response at NIMH, little clinical improvement was observed with this treatment, and shortly after discharge the patient committed suicide. Thus, this patient demonstrated a lack of response to lithium and a proclivity to rapidly cycle during treatment with tricyclic or MAOI antidepressants, in spite of cotreatment with lithium. Furthermore, her failure to respond to ECT prophylaxis as well as a loss of acute effectiveness of ECT typifies the need for alternative treatment options for refractory bipolar depressed patients, and highlights the potential for very tragic consequences if this serious medical illness is not successfully treated.

Kukopulos and associates (4) suggested that tricyclic antidepressants may also be associated with a conversion from a pattern of intermittent episodes to continuous cycling. Although these observations are open to methodological criticisms, they do raise the concern that treatment with antidepressants in bipolar-prone patients could ultimately change the pattern of illness to a more malignant form that is relatively more resistant to intervention with lithium carbonate. Whether tricyclic and related antidepressants are, in fact, associated with this conversion, or whether these patients would have spontaneously changed their pattern at this time, deserves further prospective and randomized studies. Nonetheless, these three potential hazards associated with the traditional antidepressant modalities (mania and rapid or continuous cycling) serve as the backdrop for consideration of alternative modes of treatment for bipolar depression.

In this context, treatment of the depressive episode in a bipolar patient should be approached with two temporal perspectives: (1) immediate relief of the suffering associated with the acute episode and (2) consideration for the longer-term course of the illness and the potential for recurrence. Therefore, treatments associated with the potential for long-term prophylaxis of both manic and depressive episodes might be expected to have a higher priority in the treatment of bipolar patients than heretofore considered. Considerable evidence suggests the acute and prophylactic efficacy of carbamazepine in both manic and depressive episodes. Given this emerging spectrum of clinical efficacy, carbamazepine deserves special attention in the treatment of the acutely depressed patient. In the following discussion, other anticonvulsants will also be mentioned briefly, but little data exists on their short- and long-term effects on depression.

CARBAMAZEPINE IN THE TREATMENT OF ACUTE DEPRESSION

To date, we have entered 47 patients in a double-blind clinical trial of carbamazepine in depression. Thirty-five of these patients have been previously reported (5). In that study, 12 patients (34%) showed moderate to marked antidepressant response during treatment with carbamazepine, as illustrated in Figure 2. The percentage of moderate to marked responders has remained approximately the same, as 15 of the 47 patients (32%) have now shown this degree of improvement. Although this rate of response is no higher than that observed following placebo in other studies, the patients included in this sample had demonstrated substantial refractoriness, and each received an extensive period of medication-free evaluation before the active clinical trial, when carbamazepine was substituted for placebo. Several other noteworthy points are illustrated in Figure 2. In the responder group, there was little evidence of improvement in the first week of treatment, but they dem-

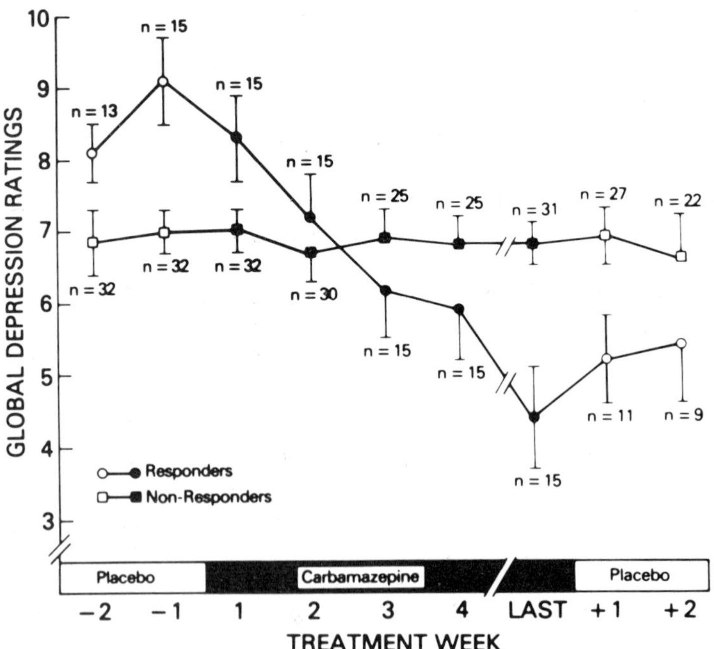

Figure 2 Antidepressant course in marked response to carbamazepine.

onstrated gradual improvement thereafter, with maximum benefit occurring by the 4th, 5th, or 6th week of treatment. This lag in response with carbamazepine parallels that observed with traditional tricyclic and MAOI drugs. Interestingly, the patients with more severe symptoms in the week before treatment with carbamazepine began were among those with the most substantial antidepressant response. Furthermore, in the nonresponder group, there was little evidence of any withdrawal symptoms when carbamazepine was discontinued. Moreover, in contrast with the many patients who show a rapid relapse into mania following carbamazepine discontinuation (6), depressed patients who respond to carbamazepine do not usually relapse when the drug is stopped.

In addition to the severity of the present episode of depression, other potential predictors of acute antidepressant response to carbamazepine include a history of less chronic depression and more discrete episodes in the past. Several factors have not been associated with acute antidepressant response to carbamazepine and include minor electroencephalogram abnormalities and a history of paraepileptic or psychosensory symptoms associated with psychomotor seizures. Finally, a negative family history of affective illness was not a predictor of antidepressant response. Although we initial observed an association between an immediate antidepressant response to one night of sleep deprivation and subsequent response to carbamazepine, this association has not held up in the larger series of patients. Nevertheless, this interesting observation deserves further investigation because this relationship could be of considerable clinical importance as a potential predictor of subsequent antidepressant response to carbamazepine.

The antidepressant efficacy of carbamazepine, compared with standard treatment modalities, deserves further clinical investigation using randomized, double-blind techniques. Because most of the patients who responded to carbamazepine in our series had previously been refractory to other agents (including lithium, tricyclic and MAOI drugs), the utilization of a crossover design would also delineate whether subgroups of patients respond selectively to some agents and not to others. Our initial observations of an antidepressant effect of carbamazepine were in accord with those of Neumann et al. (7) and Prasad (8), but still leaves open the question of antidepressant efficacy of carbamazepine. Despite several decades of clinical research on the acute antidepressant effects of lithium carbonate, it also remains a subject of some controversy. Thus, the clinical profile of lithium and carbamazepine, at this point, appears to indicate a substantial antimanic, but less consistent antidepressant efficacy for these compounds.

Carbamazepine Dose, Blood Levels, and Side Effects

Conventional dosages of carbamazepine in the treatment of epilepsy and trigeminal neuralgia range from 400 mg/day to 1600 mg/day. A similar dosage and blood level range appear indicated for the treatment of affective disorder. However, treatment of individual patients should be directed at attaining optimal dose and blood level in the absence of clinical side effects. Because there is a wide range of doses and blood levels at which side effects can occur, an individualized dose titration approach appears critical for optimum management with carbamazepine. We suggest very slow increases in doses starting at 100 or 200 mg/day at bedtime and holding or reducing doses if side effects occur. Most commonly, these include sedation, dizziness, ataxia, or diplopia. These usually occur several hours after an initial dose when peak blood levels are obtained. After 2-3 weeks of treatment, carbamazepine usually reduces hepatic microsomal enzymes that increase the metabolism of the drug. As a result, a dose that was initially poorly tolerated during the first several weeks of treatment may ultimately be easier to take after more extended administration. When the dose is titrated in this fashion, a benign side effects profile can often be achieved, as illustrated in Figure 3.

Interestingly, in our research studies, patients' self-rating of "side effects" during placebo showed a pattern similar to the observed during administration

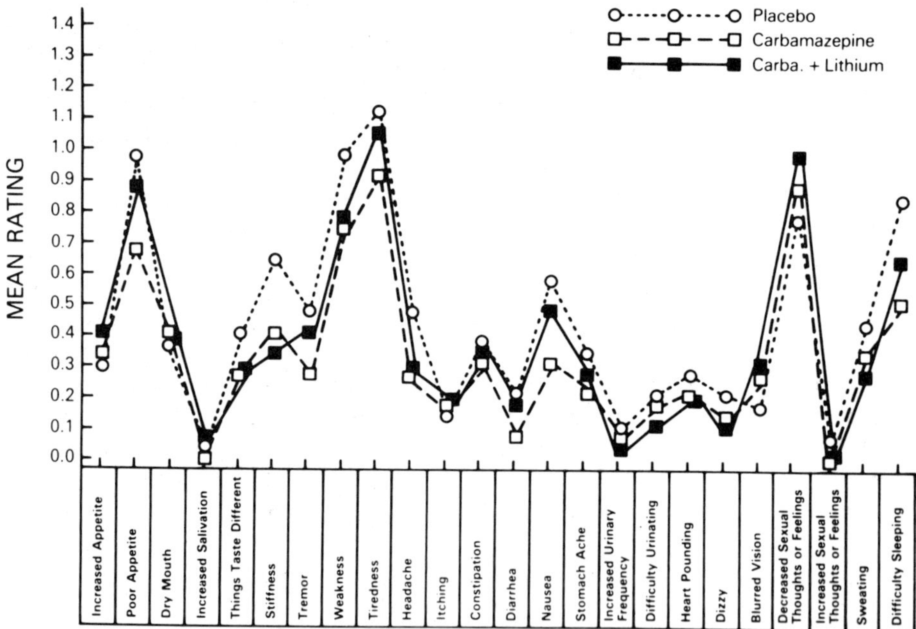

Figure 3 Side effects profile on carbamazepine and lithium combination: Open circles, placebo; open squares, carbamazepine; closed squares, carbamazepine-lithium combination.

of carbamazepine or the combination of carbamazepine plus lithium (discussed later). These data suggest that many reported "drug-related" side effects may, in fact, be symptoms of the underlying depressive illness. This perspective is particularly important in the management of side effects in patients who often experience a wide range of somatic concerns associated with their illness.

Within the dose range employed, we have observed no consistent relationship between carbamazepine blood levels and the degree of clinical response, as illustrated in Figure 4. This absence of a relationship further supports the appropriateness of dose titration, rather than a regimented approach of attempting to bring all patients within a poorly delineated "therapeutic window." As illustrated in Figure 5, many patients have different slopes as well as thresholds for side effects (9). Some patients will have a very steep slope and show severe side effects with small dose and blood level changes in carbamazepine, whereas other patients will demonstrate a very subtle slope and mild increases in side effects, despite rather substantial increases in dose and blood levels. This factor can be altered by the concomitant use of other drugs that could substantially increase carbamazepine blood levels and result in acute carbamazepine toxicity.

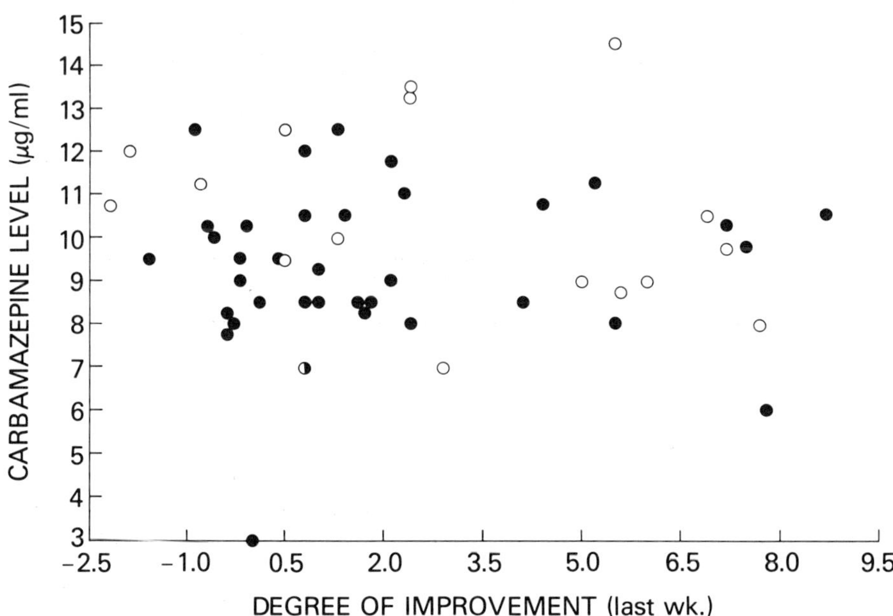

Figure 4 Lack of relationship between carbamazepine levels and degree of clinical response.

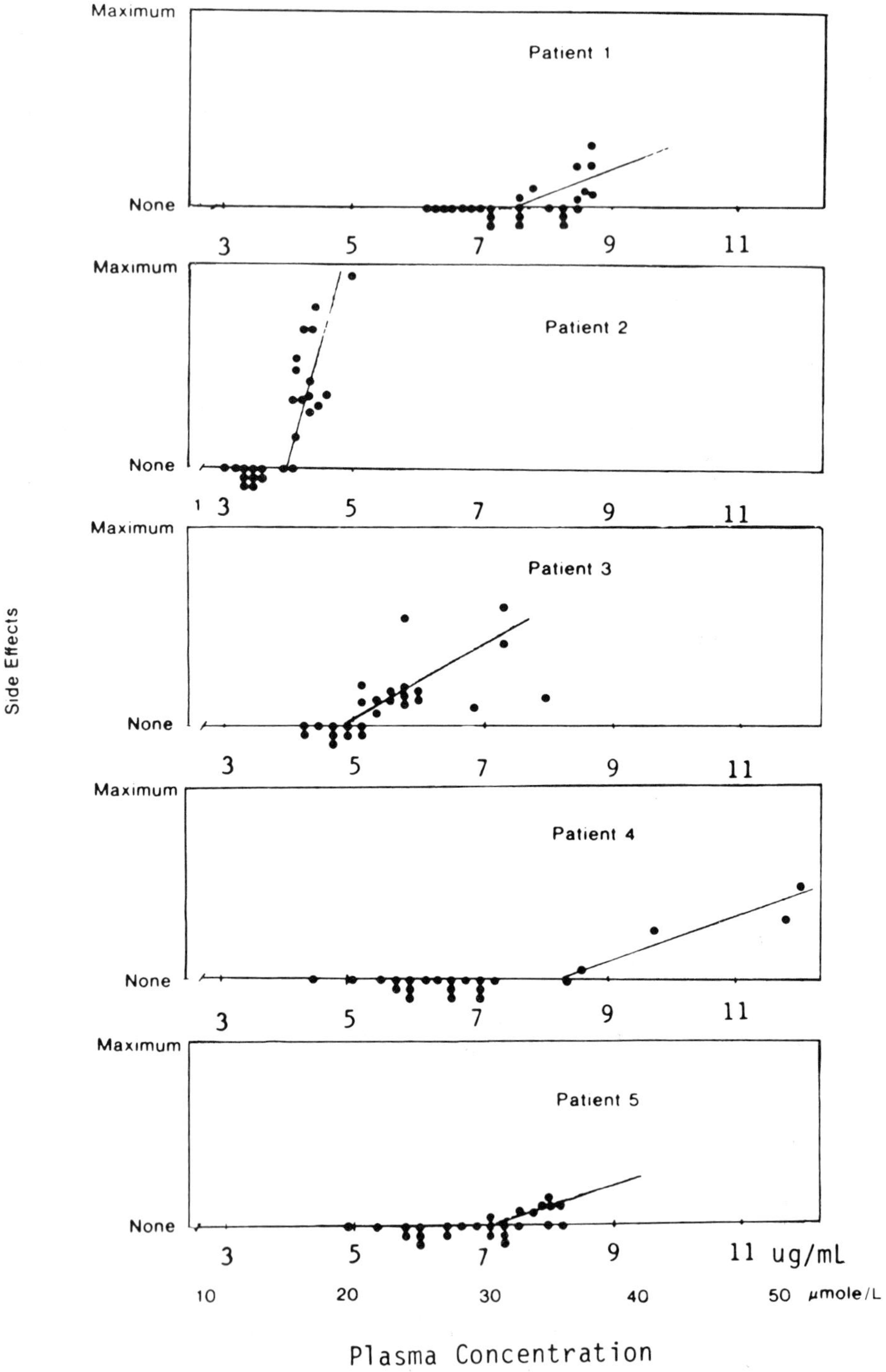

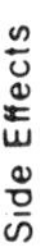

Figure 5 Comparison of side effects thresholds and slopes as a function of plasma drug concentration. (Adapted from Ref. 9.)

As summarized in Table 1, a variety of commonly used drugs may increase carbamazepine blood levels. These include erythromycin, the calcium channel blockers verapamil and diltiazem (but not apparently nifedipine), isoniazid (but not other MAOIs such as tranylcypromine), and several other agents. Thus, patients should be warned about the use of these drugs in combination with carbamazepine. Cimetidine may cause mild transient increases in carbamazepine blood levels which are usually of little clinical concern. Sodium valproate may increase the amount of carbamazepine epoxide in the blood, but usually without clinical consequence (10).

We initially observed a better relationship between the degree of elevation in carbamazepine epoxide levels and clinical response (11), but further analysis suggested that this relationship was not particularly robust, although the relationship of cerebrospinal fluid (CSF) levels of carbamazepine-10,11-epoxide to the degree of clinical response needs further study. Therefore, it would not now appear necessary to consistently monitor carbamazepine or its epoxide blood levels in patients who are showing good clinical response with an absence

Table 1 Interactions Between Carbamazepine and Other Drugs

A. Influence of other drugs on carbamazepine levels

Increased levels associated with toxicity	Increased levels without toxicity
Erythromycin	Valproate and progabide
Josamycin	(carbamazepine-10,11-epoxide only)
Triacetyloleandomycin	Nicotinamide
Verapamil	Nicotinamide
Diltiazem	Cimetidine
(not nifedipine)	(mild acute increases, none after 1 week)
Isoniazid	
(not tranylcypromine)	Decreased levels
Viloxazine	Phenobarbital
Nafimidone	Phenytoin
Danazol	Primidone
Propoxyphene (Darvon)	Theophylline

B. Influence of carbamazepine on other drugs

Carbamazepine increases	Carbamazepine decreases
Escape from dexamethasone suppression	Clonazepam
	Dicumarol
Desmethylclomipramine	Doxycycline
Clomipramine	Valproate
Phenytoin	Theophylline
	Ethosuximide
	Warfarin
	Haloperidol
	Birth control pills and pregnancy tests

of side effects. That is, most patients can be titrated to their optimum dosage by using efficacy and side effects as the main determinants. In the presence of side effects or the absence of clinical efficacy, assessment of carbamazepine (and epoxide) blood levels may be of help in appropriately determining dose increases or decreases.

LITHIUM AND CARBAMAZEPINE COMBINATION TREATMENT: EFFICACY AND SIDE EFFECTS

We have found that approximately 50% of patients who are inadequate responders to the acute antidepressant effects of carbamazepine will show a substantial improvement after the addition of lithium carbonate. This rapid onset of antidepressant response to lithium potentiation is illustrated in Figure 6 from Kramlinger and Post (12). This rapid response onset appears to represent a true potentiation by lithium, as the response is more rapid than that observed with lithium alone. The lithium dosages used in this study were 300-1500 mg/day, with a mean ($\pm$SEM) blood level of 0.7 $\pm$ 0.03 mEq/L and a range between 0.2 and 1.0 mEq/L. These data on lithium potentiation of carbamazepine are consistent with similar literature (summarized in Table 2) regarding lithium potentiation of other antidepressant medication. The rapid onset of effect is more consistent with the reports of de Montigny et al. (13,14), although slower onsets of action have also been observed by Price et al. (15).

Thus, lithium potentiation of a variety of antidepressants appears capable of inducing rapid clinical improvement in more than 50% of refractory depressed patients. This is of considerable clinical import for the bipolar patient who is being treated with carbamazepine or another antidepressant drug. It remains to be seen if patients treated with lithium will show a similar potentiation effect if carbamazepine is added to the treatment program. Potentiating lithium and carbamazepine with tricyclics and MAOIs, although commonly attempted, remains to be systematically explored, and data regarding efficacy are limited.

Overall, we have found that lithium potentiation is well tolerated (see Fig. 3), and no patient had to be discontinued from the clinical trial because of side effects. The comparative clinical and side effects profile of lithium, carbamazepine, and the combination reveals an interesting differential pattern (Table 3). For example, the most problematic side effects of lithium therapy are not often of concern with carbamazepine, including symptoms of polydipsia, polyuria, diabetes insipidus, tremor, diarrhea, cognitive slowing, the subjective sense of cognitive impairment, psoriasis, and hypothyroidism. In contrast, side effects typically encountered with carbamazepine include pruritic rash in 10-15% of patients, dizziness, ataxia, sedation, diplopia, mild white

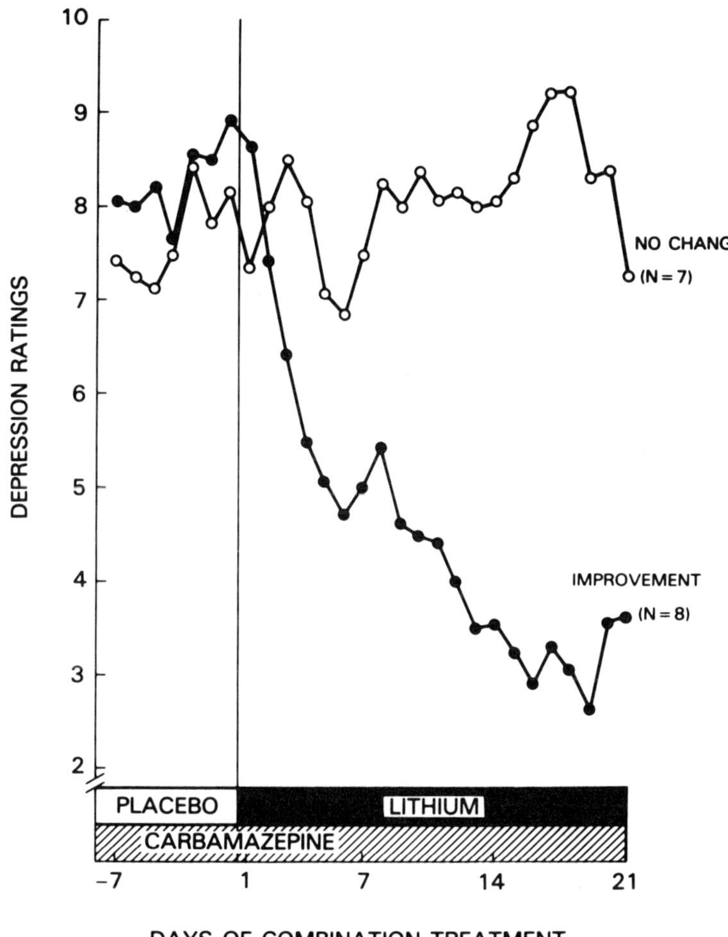

Figure 6 Lithium potentiation in nonresponders to carbamazepine. (From Ref. 12.)

blood cell (WBC) count suppression, hyponatremia, hypocalcemia, and rarely, atrial-ventricular (AV) block. These side effects are usually dose related and diminish with dose adjustment. Very rare side effects of serious medical concern, include idiosyncratic agranulocytosis, aplastic anemia, hepatitis, water intoxication, and an allergic syndrome with lymphadenopathy.

The effect of lithium plus carbamazepine on the WBC is illustrated in Figure 7. Although mild to moderate suppression of the total WBC occurs with carbamazepine, when lithium is introduced WBC values begin to rise and can even exceed the initial medication-free values. This observation, in

Table 2 Antidepressants Potentiated by Lithium Carbonate

Drug	Total no. responders/ total no. reported	Study
Tricyclic		
Amitriptyline	32/40	de Montigny et al. [3/3] (14); [12/16; 5/5] (66); Joyce et al. [2/2] (67); Heninger et al. [5/5] (68); Price et al. [1/1] (69); Garbutt et al. [2/2] (70); Pai et al. [2/2] (71); Madakasira [2/2] (72); Kantor et al. [0/2] (73)
Nortriptyline	2/5	Louie and Meltzer [1/3] (74); Price et al. [1/2] (75)
Imipramine	15/21	(de Montigny et al. [1/1] (14), [8/12] (66); Louie and Meltzer [1/1] (74); Garbutt et al. [2/2] (70); Roy and Pickar [3/3] (76); Kantor et al. [0/2] (73)
Desipramine	42/63	Price et al. [5/6] (75), [1/1] (69); de Montigny et al. [4/4] (66); Heninger et al. [3/6] (68); Nelson and Mazure [11/21] (77); Kushnir [3/3] (78); Price et al. [15[a]/22] (15)
Trimipramine	4/6	de Montigny et al. [4/6] (66)
Clomipramine	1/1	Schrader and Levien [1/1] (79)
Doxepin	7/9	de Montigny et al. [2/2] (14), [3/4] (66); Louie and Meltzer [1/1] (74); Kantor et al. [1/2] (73)
Dothiepin	2/2	Pai et al. [2/2] (71)

Tetracyclic		
Mianserin	13/15	Joyce et al. [2/2] (67); Heninger et al. [4/4] (68); Pai et al. [1/1] (71); Price et al. [6/8] (75)
Maprotiline	2/2	Weaver [1/1] (80); Kushnir [1/1] (78)
MAOI		
Phenelzine	6/7	Nelson and Byck [3/3] (81); Louie and Meltzer [2/3] (74); Madakasira [1/1] (72)
Tranylcypromine	3/3	Joyce et al. [2/2] (67); Tariot et al. [1/1] (82)
Other		
Iprindole	9/9	de Montigny et al. [2/2] (14); [7/7] (13)
Zimelidine	4/4	Joyce [4/4] (83)
Trazodone	4/11	Birkhimer et al. [1/1] (84); Kushnir [1/1] (78); Price et al. [2/9] (75)
Amoxapine	1/2	Louie and Meltzer [1/1] (74); Kantor et al. [0/1] (73)
Bupropion	3/7	Price et al. [3/7] (75)
Alprazolam	1/1	Cerra et al. [1/1] (85)
Adinazolam	3/10	Price et al. [3/10] (75)
Fluvoxamine	5/11	Price et al. [5/11] (75)
Carbamazepine	8/15	Kramlinger and Post [8/15] (12)
	167/243[a] (68%)	

[a]Joyce et al.: One patient treated with amitriptyline (AMI) and tranylcypromine (TRP) included in both AMI and TRP.

Source: from Ref. 12

Table 3 Comparative Clinical and Side-Effect Profiles of Lithium and Carbamazepine

	Lithium	Carbamazepine	Lithium-Carbamazepine combination
Clinical profile			
Mania	+ +	+ +	+ + +
Dysphoric	+	+	+ +
Rapid cycling	+	+ +	+ +
Continuous cycling	+	+	+ +
Family history negative	+	+ +	+ + +
Depression	+	+	+ + +
Prophylaxis of mania and depression	+ +	+ +	+ + +
Epilepsy	0	+ +	?
Pain syndromes	0	+ +	?
Side effects			
White blood count	↑	↓	(↓), Li*
Diabetes insipidus	↑	↓	↑, Li*
Thyroid hormones: T_3, T_4	↓	↓	↓↓
TSH	↑	– – –	↑, Li*

Serum calcium	(↑)	↓
Weight gain	↑	– – –
Tremor	↑	– – –
Memory disturbances	(↑)	?
Diarrhea	(↑)	– – –
Teratogenesis	(↑)	(↑)
Psoriasis	↑	– – –
Pruritic rash (allergy)	– – –	↑
Agranulocytosis	– – –	(↑)
Hepatitis	– – –	(↑)
Hyponatremia, water intoxication	– – –	(↑)
Dizziness, ataxia, diplopia	– – –	↑
Hypercortisolism, escape from dexamethasone suppression	– – –	↑

Legend:

Clinical Efficacy	Side Effects
0, None	↑, Increase
+, Effective	↓, Decrease
+ +, Very Effective	( ), Inconsistent or rare
+ + +, Possible synergism	– – –, Absent
	↓↓, Potentiation
	Li*, Effect of lithium predominates

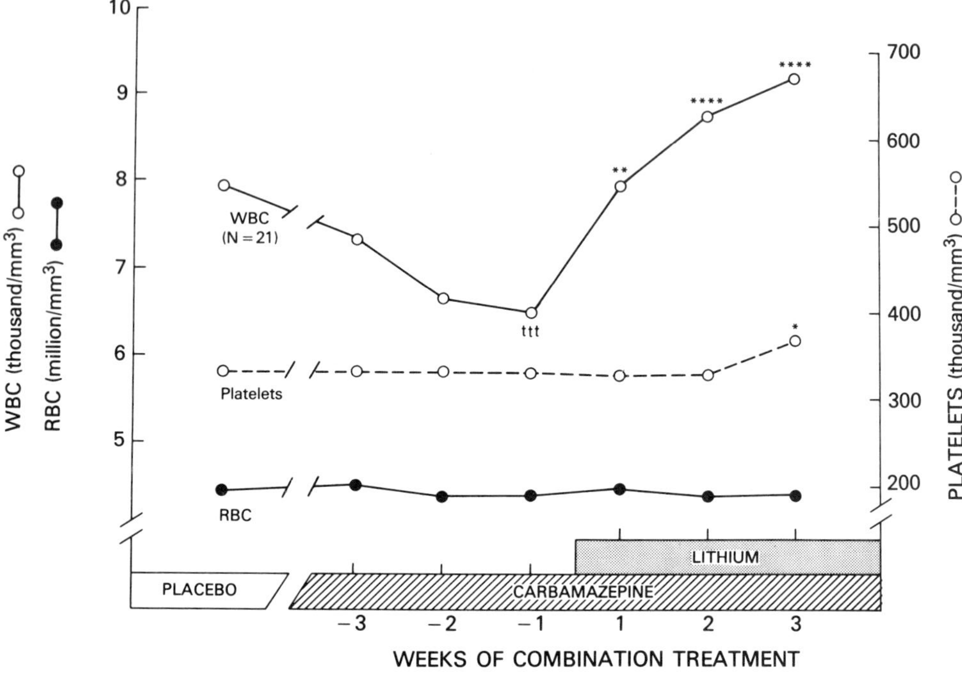

Figure 7 Hematological indices during lithium potentiation of carbamazepine. (From Ref. 122.)

conjunction with the reports by Brewerton et al. (16) and Joffe et al. (17), supports the notion that lithium potentiation is able to reverse the benign WBC suppression of carbamazepine. Whether lithium would have salutory effects against the more rare, idiosyncratic hematological reactions remains to be determined. Serious hematological effects are extraordinarily rare and are estimated to occur at a rate of 1:20,000 to 1:40,000 (18,19). More recent estimates by Pellock et al. (20) suggest that the incidence may be of the order of 8:1 million or 1:125,000 for either agranulocytosis or aplastic anemia. This extremely small occurrence rate appears to be similar to that of other psychotropic and anticonvulsant medications in inducing serious hematological problems.

The FDA-approved guidelines for monitoring hematological changes with carbamazepine have recently been changed from the recommendation of frequent hematological monitoring to that of a more flexible schedule based upon physician and patient need. We would suggest a middle-of-the-road approach whereby baseline complete blood counts would be obtained and followed on a regular basis until the patient and physician are convinced that only the benign WBC suppression is occurring and that overall hematological indices appear stable. Certainly, the patient should be instructed to call the physician should any signs of severe hematological suppression develop, including fever, rash, sore throat, petechiae, or bleeding.

The effect of the lithium-carbamazepine combination on thyroid hormones is also of interest (Fig. 8). Here, two potentially antithyroidal agents have an additive effect in reducing circulating levels of thyroxine (T_4), free T_4, and triiodothyronine (T_3). However, in spite of this suppression, the degree of thyrotropin (thyroid stimulating hormone; TSH) increase observed with this drug combination is similar, or even less, than that seen with lithium alone. This suggests that the antithyroid effects of carbamazepine, which are not usually associated with clinical hypothyroidism, might be occurring by a different mechanism than that observed with lithium and, when the combination is used, it is the lithium-induced increase in TSH that is observed. Therefore, if TSH should increase in the face of decreasing thyroid indices, then thyroid supplementation would appear indicated. Carbamazepine alone does not appear to produce clinically significant hypothyroidism, and to date only two cases have been reported in the literature.

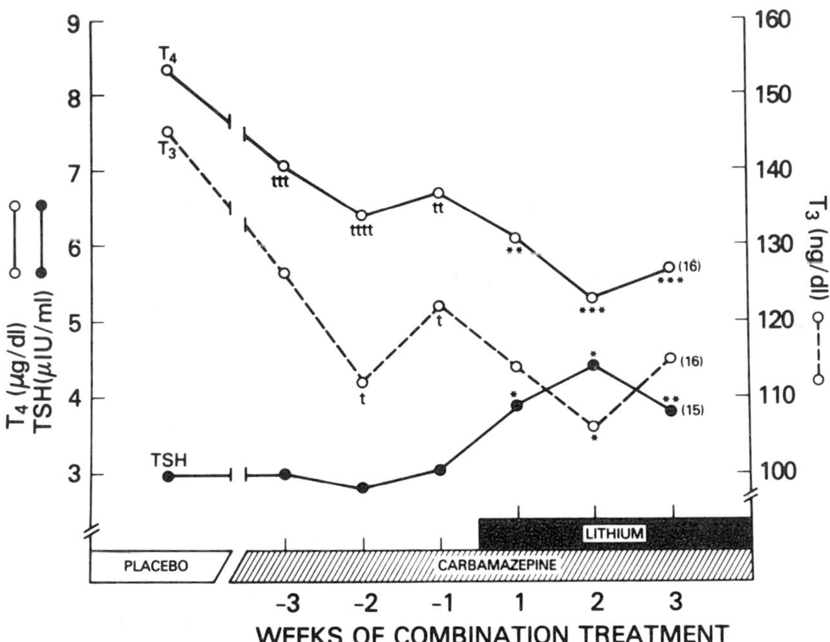

Figure 8 Thyroid indices during lithium potentiation of carbamazepine. (From Ref. 122.)

It is of considerable theoretical interest that the patients who show the most robust clinical antidepressant response to carbamazepine may also show the greatest reduction in circulating total T_4 and free T_4 (Fig. 9). These data complement those of Baumgartner et al. (21), who reported a similar relationship between T_4 levels and clinical response to clomipramine and maprotiline. However, a similar relationship was not observed following response to tranylcypromine (22). Nonetheless, these data with carbamazepine and the other antidepressants raise the interesting possibility that antidepressant response may be associated with a relative lowering of circulating thyroid hormone, or that the pharmacologic actions of these agents may be linked to a reduction in circulating thyroid hormone. These data may be consistent with the view that relative hyperthyroidism is associated with some types of recurrent affective illness. Cowdry et al. (23) reported that patients with rapid cycling had higher levels of TSH and a higher prevalence of clinical hypothyroidism compared with a group of less rapidly cycling patients. The degree that lithium accounted for this effect was uncertain. In contrast, Joffe et al. (24) found no relationship between thyroid indices and the rapidity

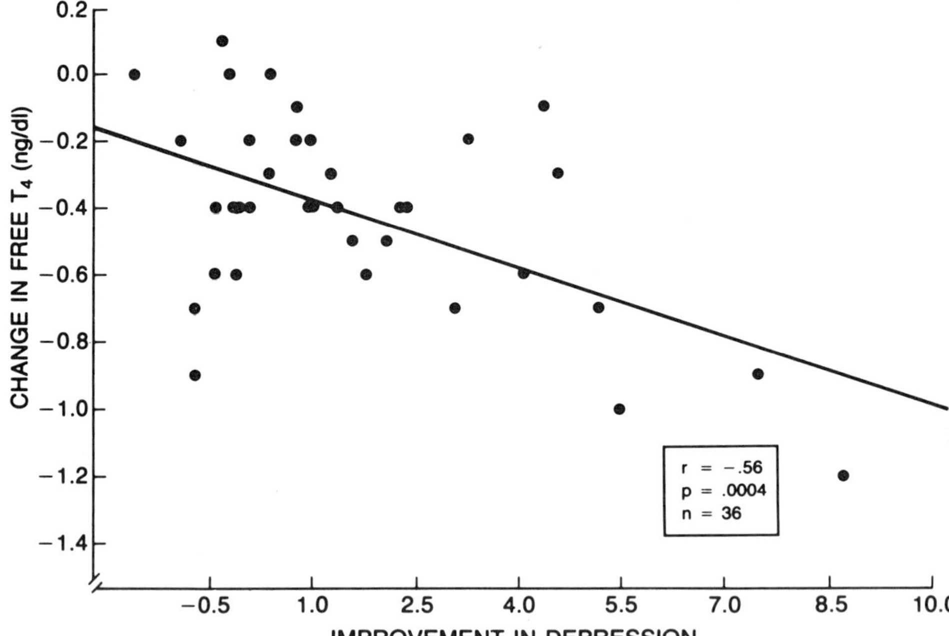

Figure 9 Antidepressant effects of carbamazepine: relationship to decreases in free T_4. (From Ref. 25.)

of cycling. In fact, when our group (25) examined thyroid indices before beginning pharmacotherapy, we observed a statistically significant relationship between higher levels of free T_4 and T_4 and degree of rapid cycling ($r = 0.22$, $N = 103$, $P < 0.05$). When groups were divided on the basis of rapid cycling (four or more episodes a year) and nonrapid cycling (less than four episodes a year), the rapid cyclers showed higher levels of T_4 and free T_4. There appeared to be a trend for T_4 and free T_4 values to increase during a period of medication-free evaluation, whereas T_3 values decreased, suggesting relatively less conversion of T_4 to T_3. Patients with more rapid cycling and those with higher levels of urinary free cortisol showed the greatest
cycling and those with higher levels of urinary free cortisol showed the greatest
changes in thyroid indices. Therefore, rather than rapid cycling per se being associated with relative hypothyroidism (23), our data would suggest the opposite. Viewed from this perspective, the clinical efficacy of lithium and carbamazepine could in some way be linked to the thyroid axis, and rather than relative hypothyroidism being an unwanted side effect, it is possible that the relative antithyroidal effects of these agents could be related to clinical effectiveness (26).

In a similar fashion, Joffe et al. (26) conceptualized the acute effects of T_3 potentiation in depression as providing a relatively antithyroidal effect. When T_3 is given, levels of T_4 are suppressed by a feedback mechanism. Because T_4 appears to be the main thyroid hormone in the brain, it is possible that T_3 potentiation (through its suppressive effect on T_4) could also be acting as a relative thyroid-suppressing mechanism for cerebral thyroid metabolism. This interesting proposition remains to be tested in animals, but deserves further clinical and basic investigation.

Nonetheless, initial data would suggest a possible clinical utility for T_3 potentiation of a variety of antidepressant treatment modalities [see review by Joffe and Post (27)]. T_3, rather than T_4, is suggested for the acute antidepressant potentiation for several reasons. Most clinical trials have utilized T_3 and an extensive data base has accumulated. Furthermore, recent data from Joffe et al. (28) suggest that T_3 was more effective than T_4 when the two drugs were given on a randomized basis to refractory depressed patients. Nine of 17 (53%) patients responded to T_3 potentiation, whereas only 4 of 21 (19%) responded to T_4. Although we have not observed the same frequency of antidepressant response to T_3 potentiation, we feel that it would be a useful clinical strategy to use thyroid potentiation with T_3, 25 or 50 μg in the morning, before switching antidepressant treatments or the addition of lithium carbonate.

The differential effects of lithium and carbamazepine on fluid and electrolyte function are noteworthy. Whereas lithium may produce diabetes insipidus, carbamazepine has been used to treat it. However, carbamazepine does not reverse lithium-induced diabetes insipidus. Carbamazepine seems to exert its effect at the level of the vasopressin receptor, whereas the antivasopressin effect of lithium probably occurs at a subreceptor level by interfering with adenylate cyclase function. Thus, although carbamazepine is an alternative to lithium for the patient with severe lithium-induced diabetes insipidus, it will not ameliorate this effect during combination treatment. Whether or not concurrent lithium administration will protect against carbamazepine-induced hypoatremia is controversial.

To the extent that lithium may impair learning and memory or produce a subjective sense of cognitive slowing because of its ability to impair vasopressin function, one would not expect a parallel effect from carbamazepine. Initial clinical and laboratory studies suggest that carbamazepine does produce less impairment in cognition when compared with other anticonvulsants; however, a direct comparison with lithium remains to be performed.

CARBAMAZEPINE PROPHYLAXIS FOR RECURRENT BIPOLAR DEPRESSION

As illustrated in Figure 10, a decreased frequency of depressive and manic episodes has been observed in bipolar patients taking prophylactic carbamazepine. Not only was there a diminished frequency of depressive episodes, but there was also a decrease in the total time each episode lasted. These patients were preselected on the basis of evidence of a good acute antimanic or antidepressant response to carbamazepine. In preliminary analysis of a larger

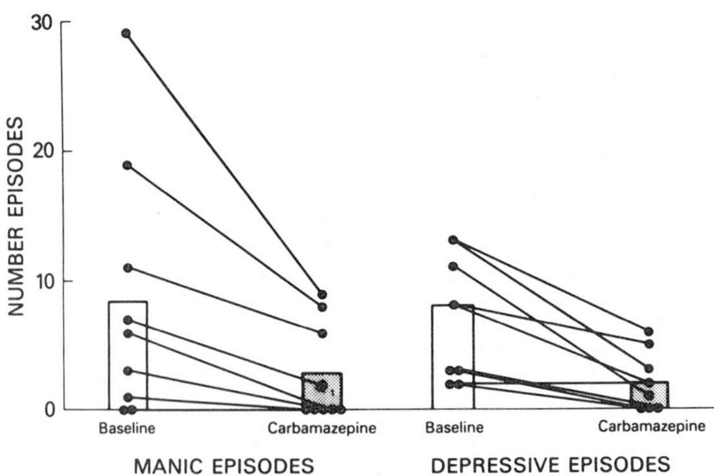

Figure 10 Significant reduction in number of manic and depressive episodes during carbamazepine prophylaxis. (Adapted from 28a.)

group of 22 patients, followed for an average of more than 4 years while on carbamazepine therapy, 50% showed a pattern of stable prophylaxis, and half the patients demonstrated a pattern of escape from carbamazepine prophylaxis during the later years of the study (28a).

These data on prophylaxis are consistent with the earlier data of Okuma et al. (29), who reported that a subgroup of patients will show moderate to excellent response when carbamazepine is used alone or in combination with another antidepressant, such as lithium. In a subsequent double-blind study (30) Okuma's group showed a modest benefit from carbamazepine in preventing depressive episodes when compared with placebo. These data are also consistent with a recent trial by Watkins et al. (31) and an open study by Kishimoto and Okuma (32). Further double-blind controlled trials of the relative efficacy of carbamazepine, lithium, and the combination appear indicated. Finally, Joffe et al. (33) suggested that more rapid-cycling patients may respond better to carbamazepine than to lithium and that patients with continuous cycling may require the combination of carbamazepine and lithium carbonate.

The clinical usefulness of adjunctive tricyclic and MAOI treatment with carbamazepine alone or in combination with lithium remains to be systematically explored in refractory bipolar patients. In particular, whether or not the combination of lithium and carbamazepine is able to block the propensity for increased cycling in some bipolar patients treated with tricyclic or MAOI antidepressants deserves further attention.

The role of adjunctive thyroid hormone in combination with carbamazepine and other antidepressants deserves further study. An early observation by Gjessing (34) and more recent reports by Stancer and Persad (35), Wehr et al. (36), and Bauer and Wybrow (37) suggest the utility of thyroid augmentation in some rapid-cycling, treatment-refractory patients. Although Wehr et al. (36) observed considerable toxicity with high-dose thyroid treatment, some of the patients in the study of Bauer and Wybrow (37) responded to more conventional T_4 dose supplementation. We observed a patient who had ultrarapid cycling for more than 20 years and did not respond to a combination of carbamazepine, lithium, and valproate until T_3 was added. This intervention converted the patient from a pattern of depressive cycles of several days to several weeks duration to a period of euthymia lasting up to nine months.

OTHER ANTICONVULSANTS FOR TREATMENT-REFRACTORY BIPOLAR PATIENTS

Although valproic acid (38) and clonazepam (39) have been reported to exert antimanic efficacy, their utility in the depressed phase of bipolar illness remains to be confirmed. Nonetheless, evidence suggests that some rapid-cycling patients who do not adequately respond to carbamazepine may respond to valproic acid (38,40,41). However, in the study of Puzynski and Klosiewicz (42), the depressed phase of the illness did not respond as well as the manic phase, and some patients experienced an increased frequency of depressive episodes. Although the number of manic episodes decreased by 57% with valproate, depressive episodes showed only a 19% reduction.

The usefulness of clonazepam in prophylaxis of bipolar patients also awaits further clinical confirmation, particularly in light of reports that some benzodiazepines may precipitate depression in patients with panic attacks (43, 44).

Although claims for the antidepressant efficacy of phenytoin have been expressed (45), systematic studies of this anticonvulsant in major affective disorders have not been performed.

Both the acute and long-term efficacy of γ-aminobutyric acid (GABA) active agents such as progabide and its congeners remains to be systematically explored (46,47).

Calcium channel blockers, with the exception of nimodipine and flunarizine, are not widely recognized for their anticonvulsant efficacy. Nonetheless, they remain of considerable interest as possible treatment options in refractory bipolar depression considering recent reports of acute antimanic effectiveness.

The anticonvulsant treatment with the clearest profile of clinical efficacy in resistant depression remains electroconvulsive therapy (ECT) (48). It has been frequently shown that electroconvulsive seizures (ECS) in patients, as well as in laboratory animals, exert potent anticonvulsant effects. Repetitive ECS often cause an increase in the threshold for seizures, with some patients becoming refractory, even at maximal settings (49-52). We have found that ECS in the rat can inhibit the development of amygdala-kindled seizures, as well as inhibit the seizures themselves, once they are fully developed (53). Others have demonstrated that a substance is released into CSF of animals given experimental seizures, and this factor exerts an anticonvulsant effect that is naloxone reversible when the CSF of one animal is given to a recipient. This observation suggests the possibility that this substance is an endogenous opiate (54). Regardless of the mechanism of the anticonvulsant effects of ECS, it is evident that this therapy is among the most potent in treating patients with refractory depression. Clearly, it remains a treatment for further investigation in the refractory bipolar patient. However, the long-term efficacy of this treatment and its suitability for prophylaxis remain to be confirmed (see Fig. 1).

LIFE-CHARTING LONGITUDINAL COURSE OF MANIC-DEPRESSIVE ILLNESS: A POSSIBLE DIFFERENTIAL PHARMACOTHERAPY AS A FUNCTION OF STAGE OF EVOLUTION OF ILLNESS

Elsewhere we have discussed the importance of considering the longitudinal course of the illness in the overall assessment and treatment of the bipolar patient with recurrent or refractory illness (55,56). We believe that this life-charting technique (57-59) has many practical clinical benefits.

In particular, there is considerable evidence that lithium is less efficacious in rapidly cycling bipolar patients compared with those with slower cycles (33,60-62) and that carbamazepine may be relatively more effective in rapid cycling (6,32,33). The clinical efficacy of carbamazepine when administered earlier in the course of illness and to patients who are not lithium refractory requires further clinical study. Although tricyclic and MAOI antidepressants have traditionally been used with some success early in the course of bipolar depression, these agents appear to be relatively contraindicated in the later stages of the illness, especially when characterized by rapid or continuous cycling (1,2).

A hypothetical schema for treatment is illustrated in Figure 11 and suggests the possibility that different agents may be effective at different stages of the illness. Although only limited data exist for this preliminary schema, the proposition deserves careful experimental evaluation.

In two nonhomologous animal models for the evolution of the course of a variety of neuropsychiatric syndromes (63), there is clear-cut evidence that the time frame of pharmacologic intervention may be associated with the presence or lack of efficacy for a given agent. For example, in cocaine-induced behavioral sensitization, neuroleptics given on day 1 will block its development. In contrast, when neuroleptics are given on day 2, after the initial sensitization effect has occurred, they will be insufficient to block the expression of cocaine-induced behavioral sensitization (64). Other pharmacologic agents do not show this dissociation, such that clonazepam and clonidine appear active on both the development and the expression of cocaine-induced behavioral sensitization. Conversely, carbamazepine is ineffective on this animal model in either the early or late phases of sensitization (55).

In contrast, carbamazepine is effective in some stages of kindling, but not in others, and this varies according to the type of kindling (56). For example, carbamazepine is ineffective in inhibiting the development of amygdala kindling in the rat, but it is highly effective on completed kindled seizures. Conversely, carbamazepine will block the development of cocaine- and lidocaine-

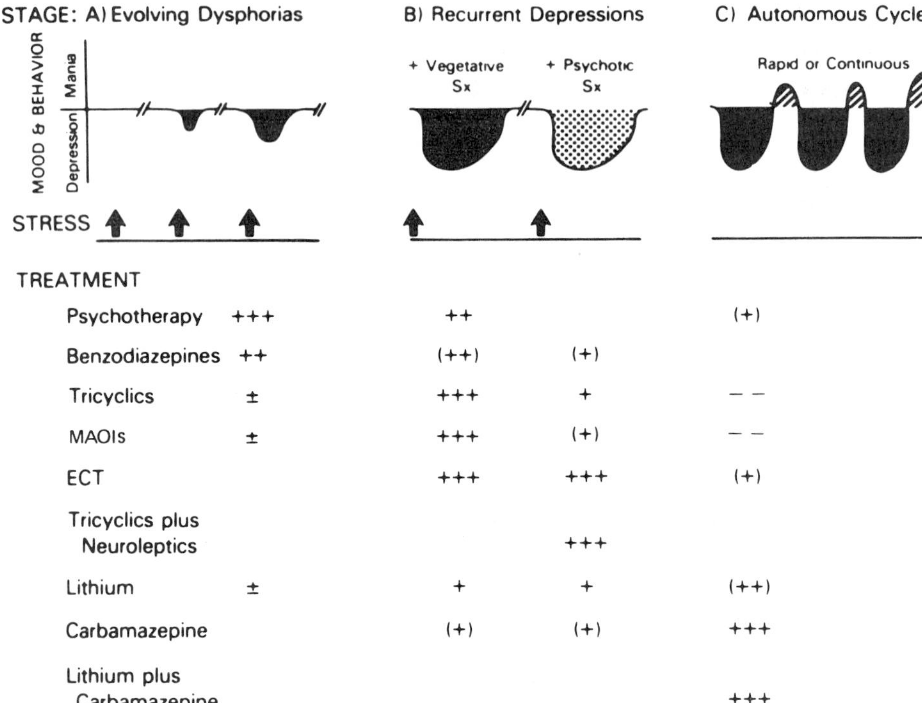

TREATMENT	A) Evolving Dysphorias	B) Recurrent Depressions + Vegetative Sx	B) Recurrent Depressions + Psychotic Sx	C) Autonomous Cycles
Psychotherapy	+++	++		(+)
Benzodiazepines	++	(++)	(+)	
Tricyclics	±	+++	+	−−
MAOIs	±	+++	(+)	−−
ECT		+++	+++	(+)
Tricyclics plus Neuroleptics			+++	
Lithium	±	+	+	(++)
Carbamazepine		(+)	(+)	+++
Lithium plus Carbamazepine				+++

Figure 11 Psychopharmacotherapy of affective illness as a function of type and stage of development. (From Ref. 56.)

induced kindled seizures, but it is ineffective at blocking these seizures once they are in the completed phase. Pinel (65) has demonstrated that, in the late spontaneous phases of kindling, there is a differential responsiveness to various pharmacologic agents. For example, animals responded to phenytoin, but not diazepam; although earlier in the development of the kindling the response was the opposite. Thus, it appears that in the development of amygdala kindling and in behavioral sensitization, pharmacotherapy may vary in its effect as a function of time in the evolution of the pathological process.

We have also elucidated a model of conditioned tolerance to the anticonvulsant effects of carbamazepine in amygdala-kindled seizures (65a). This tolerance can be reversed by a period of carbamazepine administration after kindled seizures are expressed, rather than before. We are currently investigating the possibility that conditioned tolerance could also develop in other neuropsychiatric syndromes, including trigeminal neuralgia and affective illness. Prevention or slowing the development of contingent tolerance could be relevant to patients with epilepsy and possibly with affective disorders. The preclinical findings on contingent tolerance suggest that discontinuing carbamazepine when it appears to be ineffective may induce renewed responsiveness when the drug is restarted.

CONCLUSIONS

A variety of treatment modalities are now available for the lithium-resistant bipolar depressed patient. Evaluation of the course of illness and the temporal relationship between symptom development and pharmacologic intervention may be relevant for determining the appropriate clinical management of patients with recurrent or resistant affective illness. New treatment modalities are obviously needed for the substantial percentage of patients with refractory illness. In particular, patients with bipolar depressions characterized by rapid or continuous cycling often appear to be the most refractory to traditional treatments.

It is hoped that through advances in basic neuroscience and clinical studies a new range of treatment modalities will emerge for this group of patients.

REFERENCES

1. Wehr, T. A. and Goodwin, F. K. (1987). Can antidepressants cause mania and worsen the course of affective illness? *Am. J. Psychiatry 144*:1403-1411.
2. Wehr, T. A. and Goodwin, F. K. (1987). Do antidepressants cause mania? *Psychopharmacol. Bull. 23*:61-65.
3. Bunney, W. E., Jr., Wehr, T. R., Gillin, J. C., Post, R. M., Goodwin, F. K., and van Kammen, D. P. (1977). The switch process in manic-depressive psychosis. *Ann. Intern. Med. 87*:319-335.
4. Kukopulos, A., Reginaldi, D., Laddomada, P., Floris, G., Serra, G., and Tondo, L. (1980). Course of the manic-depressive cycle and changes caused by treatments. *Pharmakopsychiatria 13*:156-167.
5. Post, R. M., Uhde, T. W., Roy-Byrne, P. P., and Joffe, R. T. (1986). Antidepressant effects of carbamazepine. *Am. J. Psychiatry 143*:29-34.
6. Post, R. M., Uhde, T. W., Roy-Byrne, P. P., and Joffe, R. T. (1987). Correlates of antimanic responses to carbamazepine. *Psychiatry Res. 21*:71-83.
7. Neumann, J., Seidel, K., and Wunderlich, H.-P. (1984). Comparative studies of the effect of carbamazepine and trimipramine in depression. In *Anticonvulsants in Affective Disorders*. Edited by H. M. Emrich, T. Okuma, and A. A. Muller. Amsterdam, Excerpta Medica, pp. 160-166.
8. Prasad, A. J. (1985). Efficacy of carbamazepine as an antidepressant in chronic resistant depressives. *J. Indian Med. Assoc. 83*:235-237.
9. Tomson, T. (1984). Interdosage fluctuations in plasma carbamazepine concentration determine intermittent side effects. *Arch. Neurol. 41*:830-834.

10. Post, R. M. and Uhde, T. W. (1986). The use of carbamazepine in mania. In *Drugs in Psychiatry,* Vol. 4, *Antimanics, Anticonvulsants, and Other Drugs.* Edited by G. D. Burrows, T. R. Norman, and D. Davies. Amsterdam, Elsevier/North-Holland Biomedical Press, pp. 49-79.
11. Post, R. M., Uhde, T. W., Ballenger, J. C., Chatterji, D. C., Greene, R. F., and Bunney, W. E., Jr. (1983). CSF carbamazepine and its -10,11-epoxide metabolite in manic-depressive patients: Relationship to clinical response. *Arch. Gen. Psychiatry 40*:673-676.
12. Kramlinger, K. G. and Post, R. M. (1989). The addition of lithium carbonate to carbamazepine: Antidepressant efficacy in treatment-resistant depression. *Arch. Gen. Psychiatry 46*:794-800.
12a. Kramlinger, K. G. and Post, R. M. (1990). Addition of lithium carbonate to carbamazepine: Hematological and thyroid effects. *Am. J. Psychiatry* (in press).
13. de Montigny, C., Elie, R., and Caille, G. (1985). Rapid response to the addition of lithium in iprindole-resistant unipolar depression: A pilot study. *Am. J. Psychiatry 142*:220-223.
14. de Montigny, C., Grunberg, F., Mayer, A., and Deschenes, J.-P. (1981). Lithium induces rapid relief of depression in tricyclic antidepressant drug non-responders. *Br. J. Psychiatry 138*:252-256.
15. Price, L. H., Charney, D. S., and Heninger, G. R. (1986). Variability of response to lithium augmentation in refractory depression. *Am. J. Psychiatry 143*:1387-1392.
16. Brewerton, T. D. (1986). Lithium counteracts carbamazepine-induced leukopenia while increasing its therapeutic effect: A case report. *Biol. Psychiatry 21*:677-685.
17. Joffe, R. T. (1988). Hematological effects of lithium potentiation of carbamazepine in patients with affective illness. *Int. Clin. Psychopharmacol. 3*:53-57.
18. Pisciotta, A. V. (1982). Carbamazepine: Hematologic toxicity. In *Antiepileptic Drugs.* Edited by D. M. Woodbury, J. K. Penry, and C. Pippenger. New York, Raven Press, pp. 533-541.
19. Pisciotta, A. V. (1975). Hematologic toxicity of carbamazepine. In *Complex Partial Seizures and Their Treatment: Advances in Neurology.* Vol. 11. New York, Raven Press, pp. 355-368.
20. Pellock, J. M. (1987). Carbamazepine side effects in children and adults. *Epilepsia 28*:64S-70S.
21. Baumgartner, A. (1987). Thyroid hormones and antidepressant therapies. In *Proceedings of the American Psychiatric Association 140th Annual Meeting.* (Chicago, May 9-11, 1987) Symposium 104.A, p. 142.
22. Joffe, R. T., Post, R. M., and Uhde, T. W. (1985). Lack of pharmacokinetic interaction of carbamazepine with tranylcypromine. *Arch. Gen. Psychiatry 42*:738.
23. Chowdry, R. W., Wehr, T. A., Zis, A. P., and Goodwin, F. K. (1983). Thyroid abnormalities associated with rapid-cycling bipolar illness. *Arch. Gen. Psychiatry 40*:414-420.
24. Joffe, R. T., Kutcher, S., and MacDonald, C. (1988). Thyroid function and bipolar affective disorder. *Psychiatry Res. 25*:117-121.
25. Post, R. M., Kramlinger, K. G., Joffe, R. T., Gold, P. W., and Uhde, T. W. (1987). Effects of carbamazepine on thyroid function. In *Abstracts, American Psychia-*

tric Association 140th Annual Meeting. (Chicago, May 9-14, 1987) Symposium 104-D, p. 142.

26. Joffe, R. T., Roy-Byrne, P. P., Uhde, T. W., and Post, R. M. (1984). Thyroid function and affective illness: A reappraisal. *Biol. Psychiatry 19*:1685-1691.
27. Joffe, R. T. and Post, R. M. (1986). Experimental treatment for affective disorder. In *American Handbook of Psychiatry,* Vol. 8. Edited by P. A. Berger and K. H. Brodie. New York, Basic Books, pp. 386-407.
28. Joffe, R. T. and Singer, W. (1988). Thyroid hormone potentiation of antidepressants. In *New Research Abstracts of the American Psychiatric Association 141st Annual Meeting.* (Montreal, May 7-12, 1988) NR126, p. 74.

28a. Post, R. M., Leverich, G., Rosoff, A., and Altschuler, L. L. (1990). Carbamazepine prophylaxis in refractory affective disorders. *J. Clin. Psychopharmacology* in press.

29. Okuma, T., Kishimoto, A., Inoue, K., Matsumoto, H., Ogura, A., Matsushita, T., Naklao, T., and Ogura, C. (1973). Antimanic prophylactic effects of carbamazepine on manic-depressive psychosis. *Folia Psychiatr. Neurol. Jpn. 27*:283-297.
30. Okuma, T., Inanaga, K., Otsuki, S., Sarai, K., Takahashi, R., Hazama, H., Mori, A., and Watanabe, M. (1981). A preliminary double-blind study of the efficacy of carbamazepine in prophylaxis of manic-depressive illness. *Psychopharmacology 73*:95-96.
31. Watkins, S. E., Callender, K., Thomas, D. R., Tidmarsh, S. F., and Shaw, D. M. (1987). The effect of carbamazepine and lithium on remission from affective illness. *Br. J. Psychiatry 150*:180-182.
32. Kishimoto, A. and Okuma, T. (1985). Antimanic and prophylactic effects of carbamazepine in affective disorders. In *Abstracts of the Fourth World Congress of Biological Psychiatry.* (Philadelphia, Sept. 8-13, 1985) p. 363, Abstr. 506.4.
33. Joffe, R. T. (1990). Lithium and carbamazepine in manic-depressive illness: A clinical evaluation. Unpubl. manuscript.
34. Gjessing, L. R. (1975). A review of periodic catatonia (Academic Address). *Biol. Psychiatry 8*:23-45.
35. Stancer, H. C. and Persad, E. (1982). Treatment of intractable rapid-cycling manic-depressive disorder with levothyroxine. *Arch. Gen. Psychiatry 39*:311-312.
36. Wehr, T. A., Sack, D. A., Cowdry, R. W., and Rosenthal, N. E. (1985). Thyroid-axis abnormalities in bipolar depression. In *Abstracts, Fourth World Congress of Biological Psychiatry.* (Philadelphia, Sept. 8-13, 1985) p. 326, Abstr. 414.6.
37. Bauer, M. S. and Whybrow, P. C. (1986). The effect of changing thyroid function on cyclic affective illness in a human subject. *Am. J. Psychiatry 143*:633-636.
38. Emrich, H. M., Dose, M., and von Zerssen, D. (1984). Action of sodium-valproate and of oxcarbazepine in patients with affective disorders. In *Anticonvulsants in Affective Disorders.* Edited by H. M. Emrich, T. Okuma, and A. A. Muller. Amsterdam, Excerpta Medica, pp. 45-55.
39. Chouinard, G., Young, S. N., and Annable, L. (1983). Antimanic effect of clonazepam. *Biol. Psychiatry 18*:451-466.

40. Post, R. M. and Uhde, T. W. (1986). Anticonvulsants in non-epileptic psychosis. In *Aspects of Epilepsy and Psychiatry*. Edited by M. R. Trimble and T. G. Bolwig. Chichester, John Wiley & Sons, pp. 177-212.
41. McElroy, S. L., Keck, P. E., Jr., and Pope, H. G., Jr. (1987). Sodium valproate: Its use in primary psychiatric disorders. *J. Clin. Psychopharmacol. 7*:16-24.
42. Puzynski, S. and Klosiewicz, L. (1984). Valproic acid amide as a prophylactic agent in affective and schizoaffective disorders. In *Anticonvulsants in Affective Disorders*. Edited by H. M. Emrich, T. Okuma, and A. A. Muller. Amsterdam, Excerpta Medica, pp. 68-75.
43. Pollack, M. H., Tesar, G. R., Rosenbaum, J. F., and Spier, S. A. (1986). Clonazepam in the treatment of panic disorder and agoraphobia: A one-year follow-up. *J. Clin. Psychopharmacol. 6*:302-304.
44. Lydiard, R. B., Laraia, M. T., Ballenger, J. C., and Howell, E. F. (1987). Emergence of depressive symptoms in patients receiving alprazolam for panic disorder. *Am. J. Psychiatry 144*:664-665.
45. Dreyfus, J. (1981). *A Remarkable Medicine Has Been Overlooked*. New York Simon & Schuster.
46. Morselli, P. L., Fournier, V., Macher, J. P., Orofiamma, B., Bottin, P., and Huber, P. (1986). Therapeutic action of progabide in depressive illness: A controlled clinical trial. In *GABA and Mood Disorders*. [Laboratoires d'Etudes et de Recherches Synthelabo (L.E.R.S.) Monograph Series, Vol. 4]. Edited by G. Bartholini, K. G. Lloyd, and P. L. Morselli, New York, Raven Press, pp. 119-126.
47. De Maio, D. (1984). Progabide in mania: Preliminary observations. In *Proceedings of the Ninth International Union of Pharmacology (IUPHAR) Congress*. (Paris, Aug. 6-7) 1984.
48. Fink, M. (1984). Theories of the antidepressant efficacy of convulsive therapy (ECT). In *Neurobiology of Mood Disorders*. Edited by R. M. Post and J. C. Ballenger. Baltimore, Williams & Wilkins, pp. 721-730.
49. Hinkle, P. E., Coffey, C. W., Weiner, R. D., Cress, M., and Christison, C. (1987). Use of caffeine to lengthen seizures in ECT. *Am. J. Psychiatry 144*:1143-1148.
50. Coffey, C. E., Weiner, R. D., Hinkle, P. E., Cress, M., Daughtry, G., and Wilson, W. H. (1987). Augmentation of ECT seizures with caffeine. *Biol. Psychiatry 22*:637-649. [published erratum appears in *Biol. Psychiatry 22*:1299, 1987]
51. Shapira, B., Lerer, B., Gilboa, D., Drexler, H., Kugelmass, S., and Calev, A. (1987). Facilitation of ECT by caffeine pretreatment. *Am. J. Psychiatry 144*: 1199-1202.
52. Sackeim, H. A., Decina, P., Portnoy, S., Neeley, P., and Malitz, S. (1987). Studies of dosage, seizure threshold, and seizure duration in ECT. *Biol. Psychiatry 22*:249-268.
53. Post, R. M., Putnam, F., Uhde, T. W., and Weiss, S. R. B. (1986). ECT as an anticonvulsant: Implications for its mechanism of action in affective illness. In *Electroconvulsive Therapy: Clinical and Basic Research Issues*. Edited by S. Malitz and H. A. Sackeim. *Ann. N. Y. Acad. Sci. 462*:376-388.

54. Holaday, J. W., Tortella, F. C., Long, J. B., Belenky, G. L., and Hitzeman, R. J. (1986). Endogenous opioids and their receptors: Evidence for involvement in the postictal effects of electroconvulsive shock. *Ann. N. Y. Acad. Sci. 462*:124-139.
55. Post, R. M., Rubinow, D. R., and Ballenger, J. C. (1984). Conditioning, sensitization, and kindling: Implications for the course of affective illness. In *Neurobiology of Mood Disorders*. Edited by R. M. Post and J. C. Ballenger. Baltimore, Williams & Wilkins, pp. 432-466.
56. Post, R. M., Rubinow, D. R., and Ballenger, J. C. (1986). Conditioning and sensitization in the longitudinal course of affective illness. *Br. J. Psychiatry 149*: 191-201.
57. Squillace, K. M., Post, R. M., Savard, R., and Erwin, M. (1984). Life charting of the longitudinal course of affective illness. In *Neurobiology of Mood Disorders*. Edited by R. M. Post and J. C. Ballenger. Baltimore, Williams & Wilkins, pp. 38-59.
58. Roy-Byrne, P. P., Post, R. M., Uhde, T. W., Porcu, T., and Davis, D. (1985). The longitudinal course of recurrent affective illness: Life chart data from research patients at the NIMH. *Acta. Psychiatr. Scand. Suppl. 317*:3-34.
59. Post, R. M., Roy-Byrne, P. P., and Uhde, T. W. (1988). Graphic representation of the life course of illness in patients with affective disorder. *Am. J. Psychiatry 145*:844-848.
60. Goodnick, P. J., Fieve, R. R., Schlegel, A., and Baxter, N. (1987). Predictors of interepisode symptoms and relapse in affective disorder patients treated with lithium carbonate. *Am. J. Psychiatry 144*:367-369.
61. Bouman, T. K., Niemantsverdriet-van Kampen, J. G., Ormel, J., and Slooff, C. J. (1986). The effectiveness of lithium prophylaxis in bipolar and unipolar depressions and schizo-affective disorders. *J. Affect. Disord. 11*:275-280.
62. Hanus, H. and Zapletalek, M. (1984). the prophylactic lithium treatment in affective disorders and the possibilities of the outcome prediction. *Sb. Ved. Pr. Lek. Fak. Univ. Karlovy 27*:5-75.
63. Post, R. M. (1988). Non-homologous animal models of affective illness: Clinical relevance of sensitization and kindling. In *Animal Models of Depression*. Edited by G. F. Koob, C. L. Ehlers, and D. Kupfer. Boston, Berkhauser (in press).
64. Weiss, S. R. B., Post, R. M., Pert, A., Woodward, R., and Murman, D. (1989). Context-dependent cocaine-sensitization: Differential effect of haloperidol on development versus expression. *Pharmac. Bio. & Behavior 34*:655-661.
65a. Weiss, S. R. B. and Post, R. M. (1990). Development and reversal of conditioned inefficacy and tolerance to the anticonvulsant effects of carbamazepine. *Epilepsia*, in press.
65. Pinel, J. P. (1983). Effects of diazepam and diphenylhydantoin on elicited and spontaneous seizures in kindled rats: A double dissociation. *Pharmacol. Biochem. Behav. 18*:61-63.
66. de Montigny, C., Cournoyer, G., Morissette, R., Langlois, R., and Caille, G. (1983). Lithium carbonate addition in tricyclic antidepressant-resistant unipolar depression. *Arch. Gen. Psychiatry 40*:1327-1334.
67. Joyce, P. R., Hewland, H. R., and Jones, A. V. (1983). Rapid response to lithium in treatment-resistant depression. *Br. J. Psychiatry 142*:204-214.

68. Heninger, G. R., Charney, D. S., and Sternberg, D. R. (1983). Lithium carbonate augmentation of antidepressant treatment. *Arch. Gen. Psychiatry 40*:1335-1342.
69. Price, L. H., Charney, D. S., and Heninger, G. R. (1984). Manic symptoms following addition of lithium to antidepressant treatment. *J. Clin. Psychopharmacol. 4*:361-362.
70. Garbutt, J. C., Mayo, J. P., Jr., Gillette, G. M., Little, K. Y., and Mason, G. A. (1986). Lithium potentiation of tricyclic antidepressants following lack of T_3 potentiation. *Am. J. Psychiatry 143*:1038-1039.
71. Pai, M., White, A. C., and Deane, A. G. (1986). Lithium augmentation in the treatment of delusional depression. *Br. J. Psychiatry 148*:736-738.
72. Madaksira, S. (1986). Low dose potency of lithium in antidepressant augmentation. *Psychiatr. J. Univ. Ottawa 11*:107-109.
73. Kantor, D., McNevin, S., Leichner, P., Harper, D., and Krenn, M. (1986). The benefit of lithium carbonate adjunct in refractory depression—fact or fiction? *Can. J. Psychiatry 31*:416-418.
74. Louie, A. K. and Meltzer, H. Y. (1984). Lithium potentiation of antidepressant treatment. *J. Clin. Psychopharmacol. 4*:316-321.
75. Price, L. H., Conwell, Y., and Nelson, J. C. (1983). Lithium augmentation of combined neuroleptic-tricyclic treatment in delusional depression. *Am. J. Psychiatry 140*:318-322.
76. Roy, A. and Pickar, D. (1986). Lithium potentiation of imipramine in treatment resistant depression. *Br. J. Psychiatry 148*:582-583.
77. Nelson, J. C. and Mazure, C. M. (1986). Lithium augmentation in psychotic depression refractory to combined drug treatment. *Am. J. Psychiatry 143*:363-366.
78. Kushnir, S. L. (1986). Lithium-antidepressant combinations in the treatment of depressed, physically ill geriatric patients. *Am. J. Psychiatry 143*:378-379.
79. Schrader, G. D. and Levien, H. E. M. (1985). Response to sequential administration of clomipramine and lithium carbonate in treatment-resistant depression. *Br. J. Psychiatry 147*:573-575.
80. Weaver, K. E. C. (1983). Lithium for delusional depression [Letter]. *Am. J. Psychiatry 140*:962-963.
81. Nelson, J. C. and Byck, R. (1982). Rapid response to lithium in phenelzine nonresponders. *Br. J. Psychiatry 141*:85-86.
82. Tariot, P. N., Murphy, D. L., Sunderland, T., Mueller, E. A., and Cohen, R. M. (1986). Rapid antidepressant effect of addition of lithium to tranylcypromine. *J. Clin. Psychopharmacol. 6*:165-167.
83. Joyce, P. R. (1985). Mood response to methylphenidate and the dexamethasone suppression test as predictors of treatment response to zimelidine and lithium in major depression. *Biol. Psychiatry 20*:598-604.
84. Birkhimer, L. J., Alderman, A. A., Schmitt, C. E., and Ednie, K. J. (1983). Combined trazodone-lithium therapy for refractory depression [Letter]. *Am. J. Psychiatry 140*:1382-1383.
85. Cerra, D., Meacham, T., and Coleman, J. (1986). A possible synergistic effect of alprazolam and lithium carbonate [Letter]. *Am. J. Psychiatry 143*:552.

9

Use of Psychostimulants in Affective Disorders

MICHAEL GARVEY, RUSSELL NOYES, JR., and BRIAN COOK

University of Iowa College of Medicine and VA Medical Center, Iowa City, Iowa

INTRODUCTION

Are psychostimulants useful in the treatment of affective disorders? A typical response to this question is that, at best, these medications produce transient improvement in some depressed patients. However, because of their significant abuse potential, they have no place in the treatment of affective disorders.

How well does the literature support these ideas? Many articles about treatment of depression with psychostimulants were published more than 20 years ago. This chapter will review these older studies, as well as more recent reports that have examined psychostimulant treatment in elderly and medically ill depressed patients. We will also review side effects and abuse potential of the stimulants, the use of stimulants to predict responses to tricyclic antidepressants, the use of stimulants as a challenge test for certain neuroendocrine substances, and, finally, the use of stimulants in mania.

BRIEF HISTORY OF AMPHETAMINE

Amphetamine was first synthesized in 1877. The pressor effects of this drug were initially described in 1930 by Piness and colleagues (1). Amphetamine

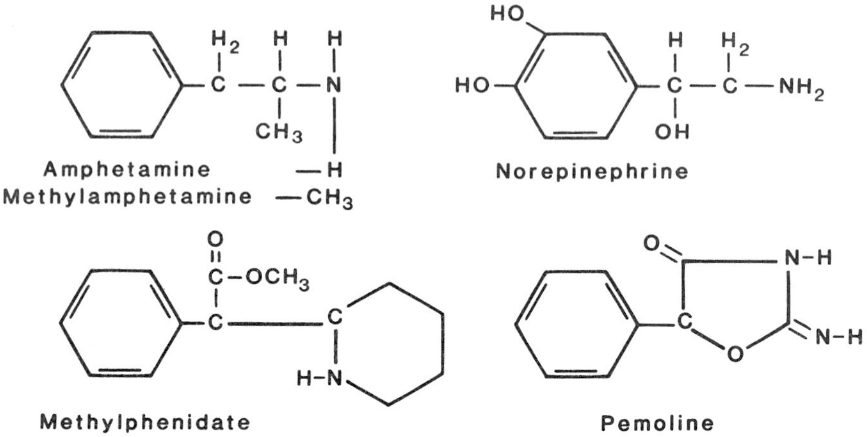

Figure 1 Chemical structures of stimulants.

was used as a bronchodilator by 1933 (2), and the psychostimulant properties were utilized to treat narcolepsy in 1935 by Prinzmetal and Bloomberg (3).

Amphetamine was initially an over-the-counter drug (4), and it was not until 1938 that the Food and Drug Administration (FDA) classified it as a prescription drug (5). However, the law was not vigorously enforced, and amphetamine continued to be available as an over-the-counter and mail order drug until the passage of federal laws in 1951 to restrict its use (6). Today, the only approved indications for its use are attention deficit disorder with hyperactivity, narcolepsy, and as a short-term adjunct in the treatment of endogenous obesity (7).

Amphetamine (Benzedrine) is a racemic mixture of *d* and *l* isomers with the *d* isomer (Dexedrine) possessing fewer cardiac effects and more central nervous system (CNS) stimulation than the *l* isomer. The CNS stimulant properties of methamphetamine (Methedrine) may be the same or slightly more potent than *d*-amphetamine. The chemical structures of these and other stimulants are illustrated in Figure 1.

USE OF PSYCHOSTIMULANTS IN THE TREATMENT OF DEPRESSION

This section reviews studies that have examined the efficacy of stimulants in the treatment of depression, including those examining treatment outcome in (1) "general" depression, (2) geriatric patients, and (3) medically ill depressed patients. Studies are also categorized and reviewed by the medications used (e.g., amphetamine, methamphetamine, methylphenidate, pemoline). Some of these categories overlap.

Treatment of Depression with Amphetamine

It became apparent by the early 1930s that amphetamine stimulated the CNS and could be used to treat depression (Table 1; 8-12). However, there were many problems with these early investigations. For example, only one of these studies used a placebo control group, but it was apparently a single-blind study (8). Treatment schedules and dosages were quite variable and patient assessments were open to rater bias. None of the authors detailed what criteria were used to diagnose depression. The diagnosis included not only patients with depression, but also those with other primary diagnoses, if they appeared to have depressionlike symptoms. Several studies included schizophrenic patients who appeared to be depressed. This lack of diagnostic precision certainly could produce a distorted picture of amphetamine's usefulness in the treatment of depression. The lack of controls in most of these projects produced results that are difficult to interpret. The only placebo-controlled investigation found amphetamine to be noticeably superior to placebo (85% improvement versus 9% improvement, respectively; 8). These pioneer investigations produced relatively mixed and noninformative results.

During the next three decades, several more trials examined the efficacy of amphetamine for the treatment of depression (Table 2; 13-18). Most of these "second-generation" studies used a placebo control or a comparison antidepressant drug. Several employed a crossover design, such that patients served as their own controls. However, here again, the diagnostic criteria were not stated, and the types of "depressed" patients being treated are unclear. For example, Wheatley (13) observed an 88% response for placebo in patients with acute depression, whereas for chronic depression, it was nearly 60%. Such a finding would suggest that the depressed patients included in these early trials would not be similar to those treated in present-day depression studies with an average placebo response less than 35%. In spite of this notable deficiency, some authors have cited the Wheatley study as evidence that *d*-amphetamine is no more effective than placebo. Given these rates of placebo response, it would be very hard to demonstrate the superiority of any antidepressant medication!

Four other depression-stimulant studies that employed controls (see Table 2) did not give data for individual treatment outcomes (14-17), but rather, they report the results of statistical comparisons between the groups. All of these studies had control groups who were given a monoamine oxidase inhibitor or tricyclic antidepressant, and in all but one study a second control group

Table 1 Early Studies of Amphetamine-Treated Depressions

Author (Ref.)	Diagnosis	Design	Medication	Patients improved (%)
Dub and Lurie (8)	Mixed diagnoses all had depressive-like symptoms (N = 48)	Single-blind multiple crossovers	Benzedrine	85
			placebo	9
Davidoff and Reinfenstein (9)	Depression (N = 20)	Open-label: 3 d-3 mo	Benzedrine	30
Anderson (10)	Depression (N = 28)	Open-label 1 d-1 yr	Benzedrine (50% of sample dropped out)	32
Wilbur et al. (11)	Depression (N = 30)	Open-label 1 d-6 mo	Benzedrine	
			1-wk trial	50
			3-mo trial	20
Meyerson (12)	Neurosis (N = 9)	Case series	Benzedrine	78

Table 2 Amphetamine Treatment for Depression

Author (Ref.)	Diagnosis	Design	Medication	Patients improved[a] (%)
Wheatley (13)	Acute depression (N = 70)	Random double-blind, 3-wk trial	d-Amphetamine	86 partial improvement 52 complete improvement
			Placebo	88 partial improvement 72 complete improvement
Wheatley (13)	Chronic depression (N = 40)	Random double-blind multiple crossover, 8-wk trial	d-Amphetamine	66 partial improvement 26 complete improvement
			Placebo	58 partial improvement 25 complete improvement
Hare et al. (14)	Primary depression (N = 78)	Random double-blind crossover, 6-wk trial	Imipramine Drinamyl (d-amphetamine + amylobarbitone)	Group I Assessors: Imipramine more effective Group II Assessors: NS
Hare et al. (15)	Primary depression (N = 43)	Random double-blind multiple crossover, 2 wk each medication	d-Amphetamine, phenelzine, placebo	NS
Overall et al. (16)	Depression (N = 113)	Random double-blind, 12-wk trial	d-Amphetamine, amobarbitone, imipramine, isocarboxazide, placebo	Imipramine better at week 3 NS at week 12
Doust et al. (17)	Depression (N = 24)	Double-blind multiple crossover	d-Amphetamine, imipramine, placebo	NS
Rudolf (18)	Depression (N = 117)	Open-label	Methamphetamine	73 Improved

[a]NS, no significant difference.

was given a placebo. Two of the four studies found imipramine superior to *d*-amphetamine and placebo; but the results were less convincing because these differences were present at 3 weeks, but not at 12 weeks in one study (16), whereas in the other study (14), the differences reported by one group of raters conflicted with those by another group for the same patients. No differences were found among treatment outcomes for patients given *d*-amphetamine, imipramine, phenelzine, or placebo in the other two studies (15, 17). One can have little confidence in studies that were unable to demonstrate differences in outcome between placebo versus imipramine or phenelzine. Even so, certain reviews on the efficacy of stimulants for the treatment of depression have cited one or more of these studies (see Table 2) to illustrate the lack of efficacy of *d*-amphetamine for treatment of depression. The methylphenidate studies repeat this theme.

Other methodological problems are present for the studies listed in Table 2. Many employed crossover designs. Patients often received a relatively short course of a particular medication, thereby making it difficult to show drug-placebo differences. Furthermore, after a crossover, it is difficult to tell whether a patient who improves is responding to the new treatment or to delayed effects from the discontinued old treatment. Another methodological problem was the lack of information on the most appropriate dose range for *d*-amphetamine treatment. A range of 5-40 mg/day was usually chosen because previous work indicated that such dosages might provide activating effects. However, dose-ranging studies were not systematically performed, and it is unknown whether this same dosage range, or a larger or smaller range, would provide for optimal therapeutic benefit.

Even though, these latter studies were relatively uninformative, no large-scale placebo-controlled trial examining the efficacy of *d*-amphetamine in major depression has been undertaken in the past 20 years. This lack of research has, in part, been due to the proven efficacy of tricyclic antidepressants, which were devoid of the problem of drug dependence.

Comparison of Methamphetamine and Electroconvulsive Therapy

A handful of studies published between 1945 and 1955 compared methamphetamine and electroconvulsive therapy (ECT) (Table 3) (19-21). The most serious flaw in all of these studies was the apparent lack of random assignment to each treatment, which raised the question of whether the more seriously ill patients were preferentially given ECT. One study showed ECT to be superior, whereas another found methamphetamine to be slightly better, and the third reported that both treatments were equivalent.

A review (19) of the pre-1956 literature concluded that both methamphetamine and ECT were effective in treating depression (Table 4), although these

Table 3 Comparisons of Methamphetamine and ECT

Author (Ref.)	Diagnosis	Design	Medication	Patients improved (%)
Rudolf (19)	Depression (58 separate episodes) (N = 20)	Naturalistic	M-AMPH (22 episodes)	86
			ECT (36 episodes)	69
Monro and Conitzer (20)	Depression (N = 234)	Naturalistic	M-AMPH (N = 34)	33
			ECT (N = 200)	78
Rudolf (21)	Depression (N = 72)	Naturalistic	M-AMPH (N = 42)	83
			ECT (N = 30)	83

[a]M-AMPH, methamphetamine.

Table 4 Review of Pre-1956 Literature Examining Efficacy of ECT and Methamphetamine

Diagnosis	Publications reviewed	Number patients	Treatment[a]	Patients improved[a] (%)
Manic-depression	9	938	ECT	91
	2	54	M-AMPH	78
Reactive depression	3	101	ECT	78
	2	45	M-AMPH	86
Involutional depression	18	1255	ECT	88
	1	33	M-AMPH	91

Numbers reported are approximations (see Ref. 19).
[a]M-AMPH, methamphetamine.

studies apparently lacked random treatment assignment. Consequently, although it is difficult to draw meaningful conclusions about the efficacy of methamphetamine, these data suggest that stimulants might be useful in the treatment of some depressions.

Use of Newer Stimulants in the Treatment of Depression

The nonamphetamine stimulants methylphenidate and, to lesser extent, pemoline (see Fig. 1), have gained a wider acceptance in medical practice than has *d*-amphetamine, probably because it is thought that these medications have less abuse potential. Since the 1950s, methylphenidate has been tested as an antidepressant, and studies on the antidepressant effects of pemoline began in 1970 (Table 5).

Seven studies examined the antidepressant effects of methylphenidate or pemoline (22-28) and found the stimulant medication superior to placebo in four of six studies (Table 5). In one os the positive studies (24), the patient ratings showed beneficial effects, whereas general practice physician ratings did not. All six of the placebo-controlled studies were methodological improved over the earlier *d*-amphetamine studies, but they still had substantial flaws. Only two of the studies (23,27) described a selection criteria that suggested the patients had major depressive disorder. Most studies chose patients who were "mildly depressed" or were suffering from fatigue or apathy. Some studies had the advantage of using previously tested rating scales.

Perhaps the most soundly designed study was that of Elizur et al. (23), who found that 60% of the methylphenidate patients responded, compared with 30% on placebo. However, this study involved only 20 patients. Similarly, Rickels et al. performed two sizeable studies in the early 1970s (24,25). Mildly depressed patients were selected from general medical practice or psychiatric outpatient settings. In one study, the patients judged methylphenidate to be superior to placebo, but their physicians did not (24), whereas in the other study, only in two of the three clinical settings were methylphenidate and pemoline more effective than placebo (25). Landman found that methylphenidate was more effective than placebo in patients with depressive symptoms (28), although it is unclear how many patients had major depression. In an open-label study, Kerenyi found methylphenidate to be effective in 76% of 121 depressed patients (26).

Of the two negative studies listed in Table 5, one appeared to be methodologically sound (27), but the raw data suggest that, although there were no drug-placebo differences, the 60% improvement response would not be typical of depressed patients involved in modern-day treatment studies. The second

Table 5 Treatment of Depression with Methylphenidate or Pemoline

Author (Ref.)	Diagnosis	Design	Medication	Patients improved (%)
Mattes (22)	Mixed diagnoses with depressive symptoms and adult ADD symptoms (N = 20)	Random double-blind crossover	M-PHEN vs placebo	NS
Elizur et al. (23)	Depression (N = 20)	Random double-blind 3-wk trial	Pemoline vs Placebo	60 30
Rickels et al. (24)	Depression (N = 101)	Random double-blind 4-wk trial	MD rating M-PHEN vs placebo	NS
			Patient rating (M-PHEN better)	$p < 0.5$
Rickels et al. (25)	Depression (N = 120)	Random double-blind 4-wk trial	M-PHEN vs pemoline vs placebo	For most comparisons both drugs better than placebo
Kerenyi et al. (26)	Depression (N = 121)	Open-label	M-PHEN	76
Robin and Wiseberg (27)	Depression (N = 40)	Random double-blind 4-wk trial	M-PHEN vs placebo	NS
Landman et al. (28)	Depression (N = 89)	Random double-blind 4-day trial	M-PHEN vs placebo	Drug superior to placebo

[a]NS, no significant difference; M-PHEN, methylphenidate.

negative study (22) found no difference between methylphenidate and placebo in a group of 20 patients with mixed diagnoses, only seven of whom had major depressive disorder. Additionally, all patients had to have adult attention deficit disorder-like symptoms.

Taken together, these studies offered some design improvements and suggested that methylphenidate and pemoline might be useful in the treatment of some depressive disorders.

USE OF PSYCHOSTIMULANTS FOR DEPRESSION IN THE ELDERLY AND MEDICALLY ILL PATIENT

During the past decade, several articles have indicated that stimulants may be useful in treating depressed geriatric patients or for the treatment of depression in patients with medical illness. To some extent, stimulant use for depression in those groups has been recommended because of the frequent side effects with conventional antidepressants, and because symptoms of fatigue and apathy, which seem to respond to stimulants, are often present.

Table 6 describes studies of stimulants for depression in the elderly. At a glance, it appears that methylphenidate (the stimulant used in all of these studies) is an effective antidepressant, although closer inspection reveals a number of methodological problems. For example, one study was a retrospective review (29), whereas another was a small series of case reports (30). A third study (31) employed a randomized double-blind design, but examined patients who were apathetic and not necessarily depressed. The fourth study (32) appeared to have been single-blind and, therefore, was open to rater bias.

Four studies examined the use of stimulants in a total of 44 medically ill patients (Table 7) (33-36). Overall, the reported effectiveness of stimulants was good, but all of the studies were case series with no controls. Obviously, studies with random assignment and a double-blind, placebo-controlled design are needed.

Use of Stimulants for Treatment-Resistant Depression

There are case reports suggesting that stimulant medications may be useful in treatment-resistant depression, either as a primary therapy or as an adjunct to antidepressants. Treatment resistance may arise from either nonresponse to conventional antidepressants or from an inability to achieve an adequate trial of therapy because of side effects. A recent report examined the efficacy of adding stimulant medications to monoamine oxidase inhibitors (MAOIs) or to a combination of MAOIs and tricyclic antidepressants (37). Of the 11 patients treated and followed for 6 months or more, 1 patient worsened, 1 patient had no change, 4 showed slight improvement, and 5 experienced

Table 6 Psychostimulant Treatment of Depression in the Elderly

Author (Ref.)	Diagnosis	Design	Medication[a]	Patients improved (%)
Askinazi et al. (29)	Depression (N = 13)	Retrospective review	M-PHEN	54
Kanton and Raskind (30)	Depression (N = 3)	Case series	M-PHEN	100
Clark and Mankikar (31)	Senile apathy ? depression (N = 44)	Random double-blind	M-PHEN	76
			vs placebo	16
Jacobson (32)	Unipolar depression (N = 54)	? Single-blind	M-PHEN	37
		alternate assignment	vs placebo	15

[a]M-PHEN, methylphenidate.

Table 7 Psychostimulant Treatment of Depression Secondary to Medical Illness

Author (Ref.)	Diagnosis	Design	Medication[a]	Patients improved (%)
Woods et al. (33)	Major depression (N = 21)	Case series	d-AMPH	52
	Major depression (N = 11)		M-PHEN	36
Frisch (34)	Depression (N = 3)	Case series	M-PHEN	100
Kaufmann et al. (35)	Depression (N = 4)	Case series	M-PHEN	100
Kaufmann et al. (36)	Depression (N = 5)	Case series	M-PHEN or d-AMPH	100

[a]d-AMPH, d-amphetamine, M-PHEN, methylphenidate.

moderate to marked improvement. Thus, approximately half of this treatment-resistant group responded favorably to the addition of stimulants. The possibility that all of these patients had spontaneous remissions can not be ruled out until appropriate treatment controls are employed. A recent case report also decribed a treatment-resistant patient who responded to the combination of methylphenidate and desipramine (38). Several participants of the studies reviewed here (Tables 1-7) had treatment resistant depressions that responded to stimulants. Although the data base for the use of stimulants for treatment-resistant depression is limited, the available information suggests that stimulants may be useful.

STIMULANT SIDE EFFECTS AND ABUSE POTENTIAL

The most commonly reported side effects of stimulants include insomnia, drowsiness, restlessness, sweating, dry mouth, tremor, palpitations, dizziness, feelings of "butterflies in the stomach," nausea, weight gain, weight loss, constipation, hypertension, and hypotension. However, these adverse side effects are relatively infrequent, and usually occur in only 1-9% of patients. Insomnia appears to be the exception and affects 5-25% of patients. These side effects are generally mild and clinically insignificant. When hypertension occurs, the increase in blood pressure is about 5-10-mm.

In many studies, 60-75% of patients experienced no side effects, but effects did necessitate discontinuation of stimulant medication in 0-7%. Importantly, discontinuation rates for geriatric and medically ill depressed patients were below 10% (29-36), which compare favorably with the 32% for medically ill depressed patients who discontinued tricyclic antidepressants for this reason (39).

The issue of stimulant abuse potential is serious. There is ample evidence that these drugs lead to psychological and physical dependence in some individuals; however, the extent of this problem in patients taking these drugs for therapeutic reasons is not known. Probably a combination of genetic and environmental factors are necessary for drug abuse to occur.

In contrast, the use of stimulants by individuals not predisposed to drug abuse may not be a problem. In fact, we were unable to locate a single case of drug abuse in the various affective disorder studies previously reviewed. However, only a few studies specifically commented on this issue, and certainly this should not be construed to mean that depressed patients would never abuse stimulants, but rather, it should place this potential probelm in context.

Clinical Perspectives in the Use of Psychostimulants for Depression

There appears to be increasing interest in the use of stimulants for the treatment of depression in the geriatric and medically ill patient. Methylphenidate and *d*-amphetamine have been used to treat such depressed patients, with a typical starting dosage for methylphenidate of 5-10 mg in the morning. If no response occurred within 1 to several days, the dosage was gradually increased to 20-30 mg in divided doses, given in the morning and early afternoon. Slightly smaller dosages were used for *d*-amphetamine. If the therapy was beneficial, improvement appeared within hours to days of treatment initiation or a dose increase. The stimulant medication was discontinued, in some patients, after a few weeks of treatment, with an apparent low rate of immediate relapse (29-36); others were maintained on stimulant therapy for many months. Possibly, patients who continued with stimulants were those with mild, but persistent, symptomatology or those who had a chronic course of affective disorder.

USE OF THE STIMULANT CHALLENGE TEST TO PREDICT TRICYCLIC ANTIDEPRESSANT RESPONSE

Fawcett and Siomopoulos (40) initially used a *d*-amphetamine challenge test to predict treatment response to imipramine, and subsequent studies have confirmed these initial observations (41-44). The stimulant challenge test commonly involves the morning administration of *d*-amphetamine, 10-30 mg (or an equivalent amount of methylphenidate). Many challenge tests last for several days and employ placebos in a crossover design. A positive test result is based on rating improvement for depression, mood, motor activity, or combinations of various symptoms. Table 8 summarizes the various studies employing a stimulant challenge to predict antidepressant response (41-49).

Table 8 Use of Stimulant Activation Response to Predict Tricyclic Antidepressant Response

Author (Ref.)	Test Drug[a]	Treatment Drug[a]	Outcome
Fawcett et al. (41)	d-AMPH (N = 12)	IMI or DMI	Six of 6 positive d-AMPH activation improved One of 6 with no d-AMPH activation improved
van Kamman and Murphy (42)	d-AMPH (N = 13)	IMI	Significant positive correlation between d-AMPH activation and IMI response
van Kamman and Murphy (43)	d-AMPH (N = 18)	$LiCO_3$	Significant positive correlation between d-AMPH activation and $LiCO_3$ response; for unipolar women only
Ward and Lampe (44)	d-AMPH (N = 1)	DMI	Positive d-AMPH response predicted positive DMI response
Brown and Brawley (45)	M-PHEN (N = 41)	IMI or AMI	94% (of 17) positive M-PHEN activation improved with IMI 96% (of 24) with no M-PHEN activation improved with AMI
Ettigi et al. (46)	d-AMPH (N = 18)	DMI	77% (of 13) positive d-AMPH activation improved with DMI 60% (of 5) with no d-AMPH activation improved with DMI
Sabelli et al. (47)	M-PHEN (N = 43)	IMI DMI AMI NOR	26 patients with positive M-PHEN activation: IMI (5) 100% improved DMI (21) 100% improved AMI (5) 0% improved 17 patients with no M-PHEN activation AMI (5) 100% improved NOR (12) 100% improved DMI (4) 0% improved
Joyce (48)	M-PHEN (N = 11)	Zimelidine	2 of 5 positive d-AMPH activation improved 4 of 6 with no d-AMPH activation improved
Spar and LaRue (49)	M-PHEN (N = 71)	DMI AMI	Significant positive correlation between M-PHEN activation and DMI improvement no correlation between M-PHEN and AMI improvement

[a]d-AMPH, *d*-amphetamine; M-PHEN, methylphenidate; IMI, imipramine; DMI, desipramine; AMI, amitriptyline; NOR, nortriptyline.

Seven studies used imipramine or desipramine as the treatment medication (41,42,44-47,49), and six of these (41,42,44,45,47,49) found a positive relationship between stimulant-induced activation and treatment outcome. In the seventh study (46), regardless of whether or not the patients showed stimulant-induced improvement, they responded well to desipramine. However, only a few (N = 5) patients showed no stimulant-induced improvement in that study.

Three studies looked at the relationship between stimulant-induced improvement and response to amitriptyline (45,47,49). Two of these trials (45, 47) found that a lack of stimulant-induced activation was related to a positive amitriptyline outcome, whereas the third study (49) found no relationship between the stimulant challenge and treatment outcome.

Three other medications have been examined in this paradigm. A positive stimulant test result predicted a response to lithium (43), whereas in another, a lack of stimulant response predicted a good nortriptyline outcome (47). The response to zimelidine was unrelated to the outcome of a stimulant challenge (48).

These studies suggest that acute stimulant-induced activation may be a predictor of positive response to imipramine, desipramine, and possibly lithium. A lack of stimulant activation may predict a positive outcome with amitriptyline and, possibly, nortriptyline.

STIMULANT CHALLENGE AS A NEUROENDOCRINE PROBE IN DEPRESSION

The noradrenergic, serotoninergic, and cholinergic neurotransmitter systems are believed to be involved in some depressions (50). Certain endocrine substances, such as cortisol and growth hormone, are controlled, in part, by these same neurotransmitters (51-54). Stimulant medications such as *d*-amphetamine and methylphenidate have effects on these neurotransmitter systems (55). These various factors led investigators during the past 15 years to explore if depressed patients differed from other patients or healthy controls in their output of certain endocrine substances in response to a stimulant challenge. Investigations have focused on three general areas: cortisol response to stimulant challenge, growth hormone response to such a challenge, and the relationship between postdexamethasone cortisol levels and the activation produced by stimulant challenge.

Stimulant-Induced Growth Hormone Release

Growth hormone (GH) release is thought to be partially under control of central noradrenergic mechanisms, and several investigators have hypothesized that a reduced GH response to a stimulant challenge test would be evident in patients with endogenous depression. To this end, there have been four studies examining GH release after a stimulant challenge test (Table 9; 56-59). Three studies compared depressed patients and healthy controls. They reported that "endogenous," but not "reactive," depressive patients had a blunted GH response (56); a modest nonsignificant blunting of GH (59); and no differences between controls and depressed patients (58). A fourth study, which did not utilize a healthy control group, found no difference in GH response between depressed patients and other psychiatric patients (57). These investigations provide no clear evidence of whether or not the GH response to stimulant challenge is blunted in depressed patients. The few studies and their conflicting results indicate the need for additional research.

Stimulant-Induced Cortisol Release

Cortisol response to a stimulant challenge has also been examined (Table 10) (57,59-63). Unlike GH release, there is more consistency in the cortisol stimulation studies. In four studies (59-61,63), which compared depressed patients with healthy controls, either blunting of the cortisol response or an actual decrease in cortisol output was found in depressed patients during the 30-90 min following stimulant challenge. In comparisons of endogenous depressive patients with those who had nonendogenous depression, one study found that patients with endogenous depression had a decreased cortisol output, compared with the nonendogenous depressive patients (57), whereas another study found no difference between these two groups (62).

Table 9 Stimulant-Induced Serum Growth Hormone Changes

Author (Ref.)	Challenge medication[a]	Outcome
Langer et al. (56)	d-AMPH (N = 16)	Peak GH release: 9 endogenous depressives < 21 normal subjects < 7 reactive depressives
Checkley (57)	Methamphetamine (N = 26)	No differences between depressives and other psychiatric patients
Halbreich et al. (58)	d-AMPH (N = 19)	No significant within-sex differences between normals and depressives
Joyce et al. (59)	M-PHEN (N = 20)	Nonsignificant trend for controls to have larger rise than depressives

[a]d-AMPH, d-amphetamine; M-PHEN, methylphenidate.

Table 10 Stimulant-Induced Serum Cortisol Changes

Author (Ref.)	Challenge medication[a]	Outcome
Checkley (57)	M-AMPH (N = 16)	Total 1-hr output Endogenous depressives Reactive depressives Other psychiatric patients
Sachar et al. (60)	d-AMPH (N = 16)	AM cortisol: 30-90 min after challenge increased in 5 normals decreased in 11 depressives
Sachar et al. (61)	d-AMPH (N = 40)	PM cortisol: 30-60 min. after challenge increased in 18 normals decreased in 22 depressives
Feinberg et al. (62)	d-AMPH (N = 64)	NS between 14 endogenous and 7 nonendogenous depressives ? decrease 60 min after challenge
Stewart et al. (63)	d-AMPH	Blunted cortisol in depressives compared with controls

[a]NS, no significant difference; M-AMPH, methamphetamine; d-AMPH, d-amphetamine.

Relationship of Stimulant-Induced Psychomotor Activation to Postdexamethasone Cortisol Concentrations

Three studies examined the relationship between stimulant-induced activation and postdexamethasone cortisol levels (Table 11) (45,64,65). One study involved only eight patients and is difficult to interpret (65). The other two studies both found significant associations between dexamethasone suppression test (DST) escape and a lack of activation to a stimulant challenge (45,64).

The results from these studies of stimulants as neuroendocrine probes suggest that some neurotransmitters (such as norepinephrine) may be involved in some of the neuroendocrine abnormalities in depression (50,51). However, more research will be needed to clarify the relationships between depression and the specific stimulant-induced neuroendocrine abnormalities.

Table 11 Relationship Between DST-Cortisol and Stimulant Activation Response

Author (Ref.)	Challenge medication[a]	Substance examined	Outcome
Sternbach et al. (64)	M-PHEN (N = 19)	DST-cortisol, mood-activation	Significant association DST escape and mood nonresponse to M-PHEN
Roy-Byrne et al. (65)	M-PHEN (N = 8)	DST-cortisol, mood-activation	Small numbers, difficult to interpret
Brown and Brawley (45)	M-PHEN (N = 30)	DST-cortisol, mood-activation	Significant association between DST escape and mood nonresponse to M-PHEN

[a]M-PHEN, Methylphenidate.

Table 12 Stimulant Treatment of Mania

Author (Ref.)	Medication[a]	Design	Outcome
Janowsky et al. (66)	M-PHEN (N = 10)	Open-label	2 of 10 improved
Beckmann and Heinemann (67)	d-AMPH (N = 6) IV 30-50 mg	Open-label single-dose	All 6 patients showed short-term improvement
Brown and Mueller (68)	d-AMPH (N = 2) oral, 15 mg	Open-label single-dose	Short-term improvement in both patients
Garvey et al. (69)	d-AMPH (N = 6) oral, 60 mg/d	Ratings and medications were blinded: 3-day trial	50% improvement in 5 of 6 patients

[a]d-AMPH, d-amphetamine; M-PHEN, methylphenidate.

USE OF STIMULANTS IN THE TREATMENT OF MANIA

The treatment of mania with stimulants may seem counterintuitive. Can a medication that causes insomnia, restlessness, irritability, anxiety, increased energy, and mood elevation, be effective in mania? Four separate studies have examined the response of manic patients to stimulants (Table 12; 66-69). Although the total patient numbers are small, three studies showed improvement in most of the manic patients (67-69), whereas one study found that only two of ten patients were benefited (66).

In several of these studies, manic patients were sedated for several hours following a *d*-amphetamine dose. Interestingly, 13 of 20 healthy adults also experienced drowsiness after receiving 10 mg of *d*-amphetamine (70).

The following strategies may help clarify the usefulness of *d*-amphetamine in the treatment of mania: (1) double-blind placebo comparisons; (2) larger doses of *d*-amphetamine; (3) longer treatment times, if the attrition rate can be decreased; (4) examination of possible predictors of response; and (5) combining *d*-amphetamine with other antimanic agents, such as lithium.

If future research shows that *d*-amphetamine is useful in the treatment of mania, then a possible mechanism of action could be the enhancement of the neurotransmitters serotonin and acetylcholine. L-Tryptophan, a precursor of serotonin, has been reported to be effective in the treatment of some manic patients (71-73), and indirect evidence in animal studies suggests that *d*-amphetamine may serve as a serotonin receptor agonist (52) and a releaser and reuptake blocker of serotonin (53). *d*-Amphetamine also increases the rate of firing of midbrain raphe cells, which are a primary source of brain serotonin (74). Similarly, an increase in brain levels of acetylcholine has been therapeutic in some manic patients. Two studies (75,76) have demonstrated the effectiveness of the acetylcholine precursor, lecithin, in mania. Physostigmine, an anticholinesterase inhibitor that increases brain levels of acetylcholine, has been effective in reducing manic symptoms (77,78). Animal studies suggest that *d*-amphetamine stimulates the release of brain acetylcholine (54).

COMMENT

Are stimulant medications useful in the treatment of major depressive disorders? Prior reviews have provided a negative answer (79,80). However, one recent review has suggested that the studies examining the efficacy of stimulants in the treatment of depression often are methodologically flawed and insufficient to warrant firm conclusions (81). We agree that the data do not firmly signify whether stimulants are efficacious. The early studies employing amphetamine (see Tables 1 through 4) for the treatment of depression have substantial problems in methodology and, therefore, are uninformative. The methamphetamine-ECT comparisons suggest that stimulant treatment of depression may be of some value. The methylphenidate-pemoline studies (see Table 5) are more supportive of efficacy in the treatment of depression. In particular, there may be clinical utility for psychostimulants in treating depression in the elderly, the medically ill, and patients suffering from treatment-resistant depression.

REFERENCES

1. Piness, G., Miller, H., and Alles, G. A. (1930). Clinical observations on phenylaminoethanol sulphate. *JAMA 94*:790-791.
2. Alles, G. A. and Prinzmetal, M. (1930). The comparative physiological actions of dl-^{3}-phenylisopropylamines: II. Brochial effect. *J. Pharmacol. Exp. Ther. 48*:161-174.
3. Prinzmetal, M. and Bloomberg, W. (1935). The use of Benzedrine for the treatment of narcolepsy. *JAMA 105*:2051-2054.
4. Lake, C. R. and Quirk, R. S. (1984). CNS stimulants and the look-alike drugs. *Psychiatr. Clin. North Am. 7*:689-701.
5. Anderson, R. J. (1983). Nasal inhaler abuse. *Pharm. Chem. Newslett. 12*:106.
6. Grinspoon, L. and Hedbloom, P. (1975). *The Speed Culture: Amphetamine Use and Abuse in America.* Cambridge, London, Harvard University Press.
7. *Physicians' Desk Reference* (1988). Oradell, N. J., Medical Economics, pp. 2016.
8. Dub, L. A. and Lurie, L. A. (1939). Use of Benzedrine in the depressed phase of the psychotic state. *Ohio State Med. J. 35*:39-45.
9. Davidoff, E. and Reinfenstein, E. C. (1939). The results of eighteen months of Benzedrine Sulfate therapy in psychiatry. *Am. J. Psychiatry 95*:945-969.
10. Anderson, E. W. (1938). Further observations on Benzedrine. *Br. Med. J. 1*:60-64.
11. Wilber, D. L., MacLean, A. R., and Allen, E. U. (1937). Clinical observations on the effect of Benzedrine Sulfate. *JAMA 109*:549-554.
12. Myerson, A. (1936). Effect of Benzedrine Sulfate on mood and fatigue in normal and in neurotic persons. *Arch. Neurol. Psychiatry 36*:816-822.
13. Wheatley, D. (1969). Amphetamines in general practice: Their use in depression and anxiety. *Semin. Psychiatry 1*:163-173.
14. Hare, E. H., McCance, C., and McCormick, W. O. (1964). Imipramine and "Drinamyl" in depressive illness: A comparative trial. *Br. Med. J. 1*:818-820.
15. Hare, E. H., Dominian, J., and Sharpe, L. (1962). Phenelzine and dexamphetamine in depressive illness. *Br. Med. J. 1*:9-12.
16. Overall, J. E., Hollister, L. E., Pokorny, A. D., Casey, J. F., and Katz, G. (1961). Drug therapy in depressions: Controlled evaluation of imipramine, isocarboxazide, dextroamphetamine-amobarbitol, and placebo. *Clin. Pharmacol. Ther. 3*:16-22.
17. Doust, J. W. L., Lewis, D. J., Miller, A., Spratt, D., and Wright, R. L. D. (1959). Controlled assessment of antidepressant drugs, including Tofranil. *Can. Psychiatr. Assoc. J. 4*(suppl.):S190-S194.

18. Rudolf, G. D. (1955). Treatment of depression with sympathomimetic preparations. *Practitioner 174*:180-183.
19. Rudolf, G. D. (1956). The treatment of depression with methylamphetamine. *J. Ment. Sci. 102*:358-363.
20. Monro, A. B. and Conitzer, H. (1950). A comparison of desoxyephedrine (Methedrine), and electroshock in the treatment of depression. *J. Ment. Sci. 96*:1037-1042.
21. Rudolf, G. D. (1949). The treatment of depression with desoxyephedrine (Methedrine). *J. Ment. Sci. 95*:920-929.
22. Mattes, J. A. (1985). Methylphenidate in mild depression: A double-blind controlled trial. *J. Clin. Psychiatry 46*:525-527.
23. Elizur, A., Wirtner, I., and Davidson, S. (1979). The clinical and psychological effects of pemoline in depressed patients: A controlled study. *Int. Pharmacopsychiatry 14*:127-134.
24. Rickels, K., Gingrich, R. L., McLaughlin, F. W., Morris, R. J., Sabloskey, L., Silverman, H., and Wentz, H. S. (1972). Methylphenidate in mildly depressed outpatients. *Clin. Pharmacol. Ther. 13*:595-601.
25. Rickels, K., Gordon, P. E., Gransman, D. H., Weise, C. C., Pereira-Ogan, J. A., and Hesbacher, P. T. (1970). Pemoline and methylphenidate in mildly depressed outpatients. *Clin. Pharmacol. Ther. 11*:698-710.
26. Kerenyi, A. B., Koranyi, E. K., and Sarwer-Foner, G. J. (1960). Depressive states and drugs. III. Use of methylphenidate (Ritalin) in open psychiatric settings and in office practice. *Can. Med. Assoc. J. 83*:1249-1254.
27. Robin, A. A. and Wiseberg, S. (1958). A controlled trial of methylphenidate (Ritalin) in the treatment of depressive states. *J. Neurol. Neurosurg. Psychiatry 21*:55-57.
28. Landman, M. E., Preisig, R., and Perlman, M. (1958). A practical mood stimulant. *J. Med. Soc. N. J. 55*:55-58.
29. Askinarzi, C., Weintraub, R. J., and Karamouz, N. (1986). Elderly depressed females as a possible subgroup of patients responsive to methylphenidate. *J. Clin. Psychiatry 47*:467-469.
30. Katon, W. and Raskind, M. (1980). Treatment of depression in the medically ill elderly with methylphenidate. *Am. J. Psychiatry 137*:963-965.
31. Clark, A. N. G. and Mankikar, G. D. (1979). *d*-amphetamine in elderly patients refractory to rehabilitation procedures. *J. Am. Geriatr. Soc. 27*:174-177.
32. Jacobson, A. (1958). The use of Ritalin in psychotherapy of depressions of the aged. *Psychiatr. Q. 32*:474-483.
33. Woods, S. W., Tesar, G. E., Murray, G. B., and Cassen, N. H. (1986). Psychostimulant treatment of depressive disorders secondary to medical illness. *J. Clin. Psychiatry 47*:12-15.
34. Fisch, R. Z. (1985). Methylphenidate for medical inpatients. *Int. J. Psychiatry Med. 15*:75-79.
35. Kaufmann, M. W., Cassen, N., Murray, G., and MacDonald, D. (1984). The use of methylphenidate in depressed patients after cardiac surgery. *J. Clin. Psychiatry 45*:82-84.
36. Kaufmann, M. W., Murray, G. B., and Cassem, N. H. (1982). Use of psychostimulants in medically ill depressed patients. *Psychosomatics 23*:817-819.

37. Feighner, J. P., Herbstein, J., and Damlouji, N. (1985). Combined MAOI, TCA, and direct stimulant therapy of treatment-resistant depression. *J. Clin. Psychiatry 46*:206-209.
38. Drimmer, E. J., Gitlin, M. J., and Gwirtsman, H. E. (1983). Desipramine and methylphenidate combination treatment for depression. *Am. J. Psychiatry 140*: 241-242.
39. Popkin, M. K., Callies, A. L., and MacKenzie, T. B. (1985). The outcome of antidepressant use in the medically ill. *Arch. Gen. Psychiatry 42*:1160-1163.
40. Fawcett, J. and Siomopoulos, V. (1971). Dextroamphetamine response as a possible predictor of improvement with tricyclic therapy in depression. *Arch. Gen. Psychiatry 25*:247-255.
41. Fawcett, J., Maas, J. W., and DeKirmenjian, H. (1972). Depression and MHPG excretion: Response to dextroamphetamine and tricyclic antidepressants. *Arch. Gen. Psychiatry 26*:246-251.
42. van Kammen, D. P. and Murphy, D. L. (1978). Prediction of imipramine antidepressant response by a one-day d-amphetamine trial. *Am. J. Psychiatry 135*: 1179-1184.
43. van Kammen, D. P. and Murphy, D. C. (1979). Prediction of antidepressant response to lithium carbonate by a 1-day administration of *d*-amphetamine in unipolar depressed women. *Neuropsychobiology 5*:266-273.
44. Ward, N. G. and Lampe, T. H. (1982). A challenge of dextroamphetamine in patients with involutional agitated depression. *J. Clin. Psychiatry 43*:35-36.
45. Brown, P. and Brawley, P. (1983). Dexamethasone suppression test and mood response to methylphenidate in primary depression. *Am. J. Psychiatry 140*:990-993.
46. Ettigi, P. G., Hayes, P. E., Narasimhachari, N., Hamek, R. M., Goldberg, S., and Secord, G. J. (1983). *d*-amphetamine response and dexamethasone suppression test as predictors of treatment outcome in unipolar depression. *Biol. Psychiatry 18*:499-504.
47. Sabelli, H. S., Fawcett, J., Javaid, J. I., and Bagri, S. (1983). *Am. J. Psychiatry 140*:212-214.
48. Joyce, P. R. (1985). Mood response to methylphenidate and the dexamethasone suppression test as predictors of treatment response to zimelidine and lithium in major depression. *Biol. Psychiatry 20*:598-604.
49. Spar, J. A. and LaRue, A. (1985). Acute response to methylphenidate as a predictor of outcome of treatment with TCAs in the elderly. *J. Clin. Psychiatry 46*:466-469.
50. Lipton, M. A., DiMascio, A., and Killam, K. (eds.) (1978). *Psychopharmacology: A Generation of Progress.* New York, Raven Press.
51. Ganong, W. F. and Weiner, R. I. (1978). Role of brain monoamines and histamine in regulation of anterior pituitary secretion. *Physiol. Rev. 58*:905-976.
52. Innes, I. R. (1963). Action of dexamphetamine on 5-hydroxytryptamine receptors. *Br. J. Pharmacol. 21*:427-435.
53. Wong, D. T., Horngg, J. J., and Fuller, R. W. (1973). Kinetics of serotonin accumulation into synaptosomes of rat brain: Effects of amphetamine and chloramphetamines. *Biochem. Pharmacol. 22*:311-322.

54. Cheney, D. L. and Costa, E. (1978). Biochemical pharmacology of cholinergic neurons. In *Psychopharamcology: A Generation of Progress.* Edited by M. A. Lipton, A. DiMascio, and K. F. Killam. New York, Raven Press, pp. 283-291.
55. Moore, K. E. (1977). The actions of amphetamine on neurotransmitters: A brief review. *Biol. Psychiatry 12*:451-462.
56. Langer, G., Heinze, G., Rein, B., and Matussek, N. (1976). Reduced growth hormone responses to amphetamine in "endogenous" depressive patients. *Arch. Gen. Psychiatry 33*:1471-1475.
57. Checkley, S. A. (1979). Corticosteroid and growth hormone responses to methylamphetamine in depressive illness. *Psychol. Med. 9*:107-115.
58. Halbreich, U., Sachar, E. J., Asnis, G. M., Quitkin, F., Nathan, R. S., Halpern, F. S., and Klein, D. F. (1982). Growth hormone response to dextroamphetamine in depressed patients and normal subjects. *Arch. Gen. Psychiatry 39*:189-192.
59. Joyce, P. R., Donald, R. A., Nicholls, M. G., Livesey, J. H., and Abbott, R. M. (1986). Endocrine and behavioral responses to methylphenidate in depression. *Psychol. Med. 16*:531-540.
60. Sachar, E. J., Asnis, G., Nathan, R. S., Halbreich, U., Tabrizi, M. A., and Halpern, F. S. (1980). Dextroamphetamine and cortisol in depression. *Arch. Gen. Psychiatry 37*:755-757.
61. Sachar, E. J., Halbreich, U., Asnis, G. M., Nathan, R. S., Halpern, F. S., and Ostrow, L. (1981). Paradoxical cortisol responses to dextroamphetamine in endogenous depression. *Arch. Gen. Psychiatry 38*:1113-1117.
62. Feinberg, M., Greden, J. F., and Carroll, B. J. (1981). The effect of amphetamine on plasma cortisol in patients with endogenous and non-endogenous depression. *Psychoneuroendocrinology 6*:355-357.
63. Stewart, J. W., Quitkin, F., McGrath, P. J., Liebowitz, M. R., Harrison, W., Rabkin, J. G., Novacenko, H., Puig-Antich, J., and Asnis, G. M. (1984). Cortisol response to dextroamphetamine stimulation in depressed outpatients. *Psychiatry Res. 12*:195-206.
64. Sternbach, H., Gwirtsman, H., and Gerner, R. H. (1981). The dexamethasone suppression test and response to methylphenidate in depression. *Am. J. Psychiatry 138*:1629-1631.
65. Roy-Byrne, P. P., Gwirtsman, H. E., Baxter, L., and Gerner, R. H. (1983). Endocrine correlates of mood response to methylphenidate in depression. *J. Clin. Psychopharmacol. 3*:266-268.
66. Janowsky, D. S., El-Yousef, K., and Davis, J. M. (1973). Provocation of schizophrenic symptoms by intravenous administration of methylphenidate. *Arch. Gen. Psychiatry 28*:185-191.
67. Beckman, V. A. and Heinemann, H. (1976). *d*-Amphetamin manischen beim Syndrom. *Arzneimittelforschung 26*:1185-1186.
68. Brown, W. A. and Mueller, B. (1979). Alleviation of manic symptoms with catecholamine agonists. *Am. J. Psychiatry 136*:230-231.
69. Garvey, M. J., Hwang, S., Teubner-Rhodes, D., Zander, J., and Rehm, C. (1987). Dextroamphetamine treatment of mania. *J. Clin. Psychiatry 48*:412-413.
70. Tecce, J. J. and Cole, J. O. (1974). Amphetamine effects in man: Paradoxical drowsiness and lowered electrical brain activity (CNV). *Science 185*:451-453.

71. Prangue, A. J., Wilson, K., and Lynn, C. W. (1974). L-Tryptophan in mania. *Arch. Gen. Psychiatry 30*:56-62.
72. Chouinard, G., Jones, B. D., and Young, S. N. (1979). Potentiation of lithium by tryptophan in a patient with bipolar illness. *Am. J. Psychiatry 136*:719-720.
73. Murphy, D. L., Baker, M., and Goodwin, F. K. (1972). L-Tryptophan in affective disorders: Indoleamine changes and differential clinical effects. *Psychopharmacologia 34*:11-20.
74. Foote, W. E., Sheard, M. H., and Aghajanian, G. K. (1969). Comparison of effects of LSD and amphetamine on midbrain raphe units. *Nature 222*:567-569.
75. Cohen, B. M., Lipinski, J. F., and Altesman, R. I. (1982). Lecithin in the treatment of mania: Double-blind placebo-controlled trials. *Am. J. Psychiatry 139*: 1162-1164.
76. Cohen, B. M., Miller, A. L., and Lipinski, J. F. (1980). Lecithin in mania: A preliminary report. *Am. J. Psychiatry 137*:242-243.
77. Janowsky, D. S., El-Yousef, M. K., and Davis, J. M. (1973). Parasympathetic suppression of manic symptoms by physostigmine. *Arch. Gen. Psychiatry 28*: 542-547.
78. Carroll, B. J., Frazer, A., and Schless, A. (1973). Cholinergic reversal of manic symptoms. *Lancet 1*:427-428.
79. Ban, T. A. (1969). The use of the amphetamines in adult psychiatry. *Semin. Psychiatry 1*:129-143.
80. Wittenborn, J. R. (1982). Antidepressant use of amphetamines and other psychostimulants. *Mod. Probl. Pharmacopsychiatry 18*:178-195.
81. Chiarello, R. J. and Cole, J. O. (1987). The use of psychostimulants in general psychiatry. *Arch. Gen. Psychiatry 44*:286-295.

10

The Use of Light Therapy in the Treatment of Depression

ALFRED J. LEWY and ROBERT L. SACK

Oregon Health Sciences University, Portland, Oregon

INTRODUCTION

Early Circadian Rhythm Theories for Affective Disorders

Some types of depression may be related to a disturbance of biological rhythms (1). We have proposed the hypothesis that there are two types of biological rhythm disturbances: the phase-advance type and the phase-delay type. The phase-advance type was noted first by Papousek (2), Kripke et al. (3), and Wehr et al. (4). They speculated that patients with affective disorders had biological circadian rhythms that were phase advanced relative to real time and to the sleep-wake cycle. For example, the body temperature rhythm in these patients (as assessed by its nighttime minimum) was thought to occur abnormally early. Wehr et al. (4) were able to show that scheduling sleep earlier in the evening might have a transiently antidepressant effect. This manipulation seemed to restore the "correct" phase relationship between sleep and other endogenous circadian rhythms. It is possible to hypothesize that an altered phase relationship between sleep rhythms and the other circadian rhythms might occur in depression because sleep is influenced by stress and social cues, as well as by light—whereas the other circadian rhythms (e.g., temperature) are cued mainly to the light-dark cycle.

Discovery of the Effect of Bright Light in Humans

The effects of bright light were first documented in humans when we discovered (Fig. 1) that humans require substantially brighter light than ordinary room light for suppression of melatonin (a light-sensitive pineal gland hormone) production (5). Apparently, human circadian rhythms rely on sunlight exposure for proper synchronization to the day-night cycle, and exposure to ordinary-intensity room light has less effect on these rhythms. We

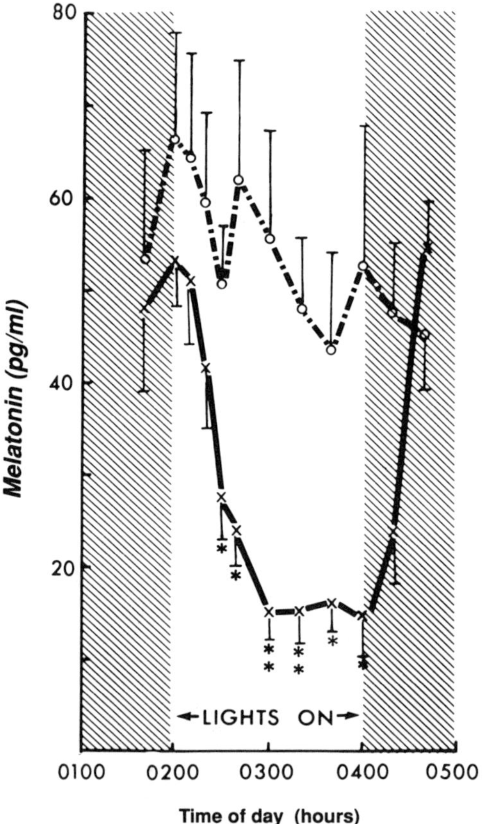

Figure 1 Effect of light on melatonin secretion. Each point represents the mean concentration of melatonin (± standard error) for six subjects. A paired *t*-test, comparing exposure to 500 lux with exposure to 2500 lux, was performed for each data point. A two-way analysis of variance with repeated measures and the Newman-Keuls statistic for the comparison of means showed significant differences between 2:30 AM and 4:00 AM (*, $p \leqslant 0.05$; **, $p \leqslant 0.01$). (From Ref. 5, with permission from AAAS.)

have subsequently shown that human circadian rhythms can be phase-shifted by artificial light exposure, providing it is sufficiently bright (1,6,7).

First Studies of Treating Winter Depression with Bright Light

Our first therapeutic use of bright light was in the treatment of a patient who had a recurrent pattern of depressions, which began when day length shortened in autumn and winter and spontaneously remitted when day length increased in the spring (8). Because we knew that seasonal rhythms in animals were regulated by day length (specifically, by the time interval between the twilight transitions), we extended the length of our patient's winter days by exposing him to 2000 lux light (about four times brighter than ordinary room light, but much less than the 10,000 to 100,000 lux sunlight commonly experienced outdoors) between 6:00 and 9:00 AM and between 4:00 and 7:00 PM. After 4 days on this treatment schedule, he began to switch out of his depression and was fully remitted after another 6 days of light therapy. Although this patient represented only an interesting case report, and a placebo response could not be ruled out, it did stimulate an additional study the next year in which treatment with bright was compared with dim light exposure in the morning and evening in 9 winter-depressive patients. Bright light exposure caused a statistically significant decrease in depression as rated by the Hamilton Depression Rating Scale, whereas dim light exposure did not (9). Consequently, evidence began to accumulate confirming our impression that winter depression had a biological basis.

THE PHASE-SHIFT HYPOTHESIS FOR THE ANTIDEPRESSANT EFFECT OF BRIGHT LIGHTS

The next step was to determine why patients with seasonal affective disorder became depressed in the winter and why they remitted with bright light exposure. A critical theoretical and practical question was whether or not these patients needed their day length extended both in the morning and in the evening. The knowledge that these patients did not like to wake up early in the morning led investigators at the National Institute of Mental Health to perform a study whereby they scheduled bright light exposure only in the evening, because most patients found this treatment time to be more convenient (10). In contrast, we interpreted the reluctance of these patients to awaken early in the morning in winter as possible evidence that they had abnormally delayed endogenous (biological) circadian rhythms during their winter depressions (11). Therefore, we speculated that bright light exposure in the morning (which would provide a corrective phase advance) would have more of an antidepressant effect than bright light exposure at other times of the day and would demonstrate greater antidepressant efficacy than bright light exposure scheduled in the late evening (which would exacerbate the phase delay). Furthermore, we had performed several studies comparing the circadian rhythm phase-shifting effects of morning versus evening bright light. In these studies, we found that the (bright) light-dark cycle could shift the circadian melatonin rhythms in healthy controls in the predicted direction, holding the light-dark cycle constant. Removal of bright light exposure in the evening caused a phase advance (shift to an earlier time), whereas removal of bright light exposure in the morning caused a phase delay (shift to a later time; 1,6).

TREATMENT OF CHRONOBIOLOGICAL SLEEP DISORDERS WITH BRIGHT LIGHT

We began to apply these findings to the treatment of winter depression and to the treatment of phase-advance and phase-delay type chronobiological sleep and mood disorders. The treatment of chronobiological sleep disorders was straightforward, and our preliminary results confirmed our initial predictions that delayed sleep phase syndrome (characterized by difficulty falling asleep before 1:00 to 3:00 AM) could be successfully treated with morning bright light exposure to provide a corrective phase advance in all circadian rhythms, including the sleep-wake cycle (11). Advanced sleep phase syndrome (characterized by difficulty staying awake until 11:00 PM) could also be successfully treated by using evening bright light exposure to provide a corrective phase delay in all circadian rhythms—including the sleep-wake cycle.

TREATMENT OF CHRONOBIOLOGICAL MOOD DISORDERS

The Internal-Phase Angle Disturbance

Treatment of chronobiological mood disorders appeared to be a more problematic, and therefore more interesting, research area. It is difficult to determine if and what type of biological rhythm disturbance is present during a depressive episode. Furthermore, there was no clear hypothesis for how a rhythm disturbance might cause a depressive episode.

As mentioned earlier, our thinking was influenced by the phase-advance hypothesis of Wehr et al. (4), which suggested that sleep is advanced in some patients with affective disorder, but not as advanced as are the other biological circadian rhythms. Wehr's sleep-manipulation studies suggested that there was an internal-phase angle disturbance between sleep and the other endogenous circadian rhythms, and the earlier scheduling of sleep produced a transient remission of depressive symptoms in at least one depressed bipolar patient. We thought that this hypothesis, if correct, was appropriate only for melancholic-type depressives (i.e., patients with early-morning awakening) and that these patients might also respond to bright light therapy applied in the evening while holding the sleep-wake cycle constant (11).

Thus, in this type of phase-shifted affective disorder, a variety of endogenous circadian rhythms are abnormally phase advanced relative to sleep and to real time. This means that in a phase-advance type disorder, sleep is abnormally delayed relative to the other circadian rhythms. Therefore, to avoid confusion, we phase type a disorder by conventionally describing the phase of the other endogenous circadian rhythms relative to sleep (and not the other way around).

Phase-Advance and Phase-Delay Types of Mood Disorders

Although we were intrigued by the possibility that winter-depressive patients might have a circadian rhythm mood disorder, these patients were obviously clinically different from depressed patients with melancholic features: whereas most melancholic patients awaken early, most seasonal depressives have difficulty awakening early during the autumn and winter. We thought that seasonal depressive patients might have a phase-delay type of chronobiological disorder (1), and to the best of our knowledge, this represented the first attempt to view the phase-advance hypothesis of depression as just one of two types of phase shift disorders. [Although phase-delay types have been described in the literature (3), they appear to have been considered anomalies (13).] We further hypothesized that winter depressive patients had circadian rhythms that were phase delayed relative to real time and to sleep (7).

Morning Versus Evening Bright Light for Winter Depression

Therefore, when we tested this hypothesis, we held sleep times constant (between 10:00 PM and 6:00 AM) for a baseline week, as well as for the subsequent light treatment weeks (14). Subjects were also instructed to avoid bright light between 5:00 PM and 8:00 AM (except when specifically scheduled for bright light treatment). During weeks 2 and 3 of the procedure, subjects were randomly assigned to a week of morning (6:00-8:00 AM) bright (2500 lux) light exposure and to a week of evening (8:00-10:00 PM) bright light exposure. During the fourth week they were exposed to both morning and evening bright light. Unlike the treatment pardigm for our first patient in which evening light was scheduled between 4:00 and 7:00 PM, evening light in this study was scheduled sufficiently late to cause a phase delay.

Circadian phase was assessed using the dim light melatonin onset measurement (DLMO), which is a highly useful marker for circadian phase. By avoiding bright light in the evening, we eliminate masking of the melatonin onset.

Evening light caused a phase delay in the DLMO in patients with winter depression and control subjects (Fig. 2), although the controls appeared to

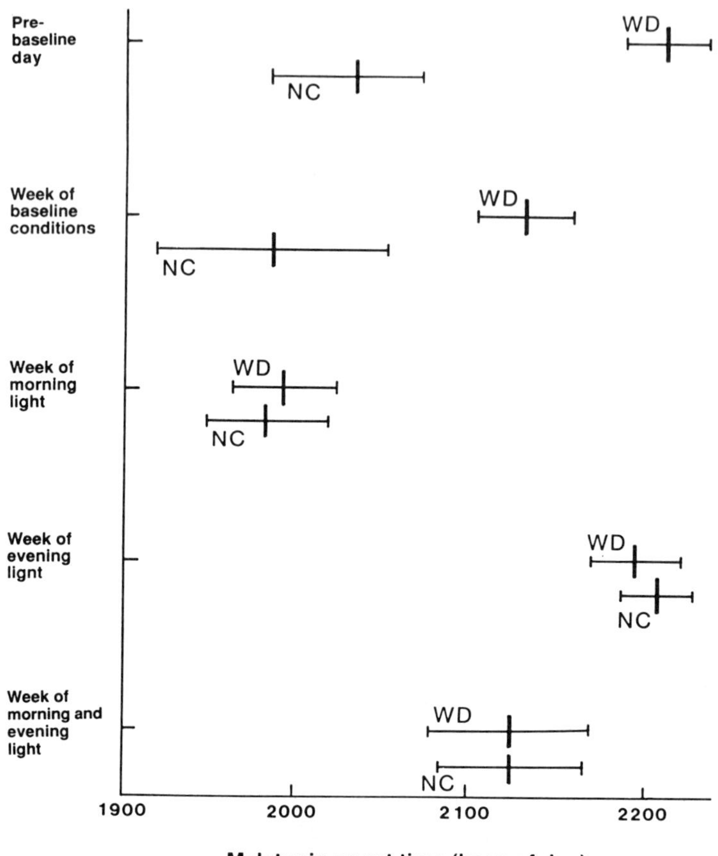

Figure 2 Average melatonin onset times (± SEM) for normal controls (NC) and patients with winter depression (WD) ($N = 6$ to 8, except $N = 4$ for the prebaseline melatonin values). An analysis of variance for repeated measures indicated a significant difference between treatments for both patients ($p \leq 0.001$) and normal controls ($p \leq 0.009$). Significant paired *t*-tests for the patients were baseline versus AM ($p \leq 0.001$), baseline versus PM ($p \leq 0.012$), and AM versus PM ($p \leq 0.001$). Significant paired *t*-tests for the normal controls were baseline versus AM + PM ($p \leq 0.039$), AM versus PM ($p \leq 0.004$), and AM versus AM + PM ($p \leq 0.003$). Melatonin onset times of the patients were compared with those of the normal controls at both prebaseline ($p \leq 0.02$) and baseline ($p \leq 0.05$) (Student's *t*-test). (From Ref. 15, with permission from AAAS.)

delay more than the patients (14). Morning light advanced the DLMO, although more so in the patients than in the control subjects. The relative phase-shift differences in magnitude between patients and controls suggested that the phase response curves (PRCs) of the patients were more phase delayed. Moreover, the prebaseline and baseline DLMO values were significantly phase delayed in the patients compared with control subjects.

Morning light had a significantly more antidepressant effect than evening light (14), and depression ratings after the week of morning light were significantly ($P \leqslant 0.004$) lower than those after the baseline week or after the week of evening light ($P \leqslant 0.045$) (Fig. 3). There were no other statistically significant differences observed. Therefore, morning light clearly had a greater

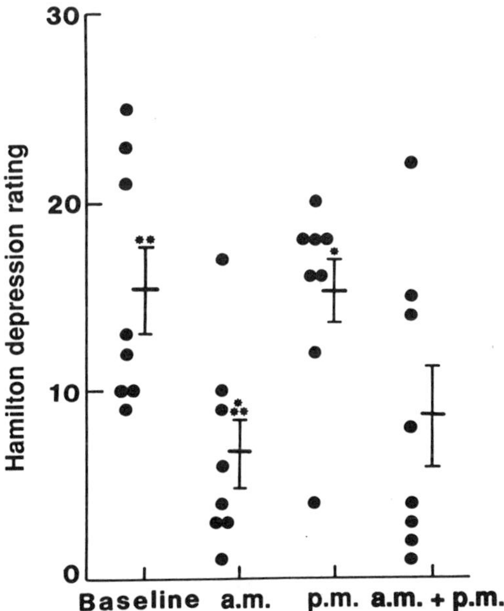

Figure 3 Individual and average 21-item Hamilton depression ratings (± SEM) for eight patients with winter depression for each of the 4 weeks of the study. An analysis of variance for repeated measures indicated a significant ($p \leqslant 0.026$) difference between treatments. Only the paired *t*-tests comparing the week of morning (AM) light and the baseline week (** $p \leqslant 0.004$) and comparing the week of AM light and the week of evening (PM) light (*$p \leqslant 0.045$) were significant. Average depression ratings (± SEM) for the seven normal control subjects were 3.0 ± 0.9 at baseline, 2.4 ± 0.3 (AM light), 6.1 ± 1.6 (PM light), and 4.3 ± 0.9 (AM + PM light). From Ref. 15, with permission from AAAS.)

antidepressant effect than evening light, whereas the combination of morning plus evening light had an intermediate antidepressant effect. Similarly, the DLMO values after the combination of morning plus evening light were at an intermediate phase between that of morning or evening light alone.

During the winter of 1987, this study was repeated with bright light being administered between 7:00 and 9:00 PM (Sack et al., in preparation). Results of this trial were similar to those of the first study. Although evening light produced a slight, but significant, antidepressant effect when compared with the baseline week, morning light still had a significantly greater antidepressant effect than evening light. These results were not unexpected, because the earlier-scheduled evening light caused less of a phase delay. Thus, the (modest) clinical response observed after evening light was probably due to some effect other than phase-shifting. Whether or not this is a placebo effect (patients are always aware of when they are being exposed to light) or is due to some other physiological mechanism is unknown at present.

Correlation Between Antidepressant and Phase-Shifting Effects

In another study (Fig. 4), we found that the antidepressant effect of bright light correlated with its ability to phase advance the DLMO (16). These data, although not conclusive, are consistent with our hypothesis that the antidepressant effect of bright light may be related to a corrective phase advance in the DLMO (and other circadian rhythms). Whether or not we can demonstrate significant phase delays at baseline in affectively ill patients, compared with normal controls, remains to be determined because patients may be delayed when ill and not during remission, and they may not necessarily be delayed relative to normal persons (17).

Phase Typing With the Baseline Dim Light Melatonin Onset

The baseline DLMO measurement may turn out to be a useful way to phase type patients. If this is true, a delayed baseline DLMO would suggest that patients initially be treated with morning light (to provide a corrective phase advance); whereas an advanced baseline DLMO value would suggest the use of evening light (to provide a corrective phase delay). However, the baseline DLMO may not be as good a marker for circadian rhythm changes as the phase-shift responses to light (16).

Phase Typing with the Advance-Delay Differential

In our studies, we measure the DLMO after a week of baseline conditions, a week of morning light, and a week of evening light. The phase-shift responses we observed were the DLMO's phase-advance response to morning light, and its phase-delay response to evening light. By subtracting the latter

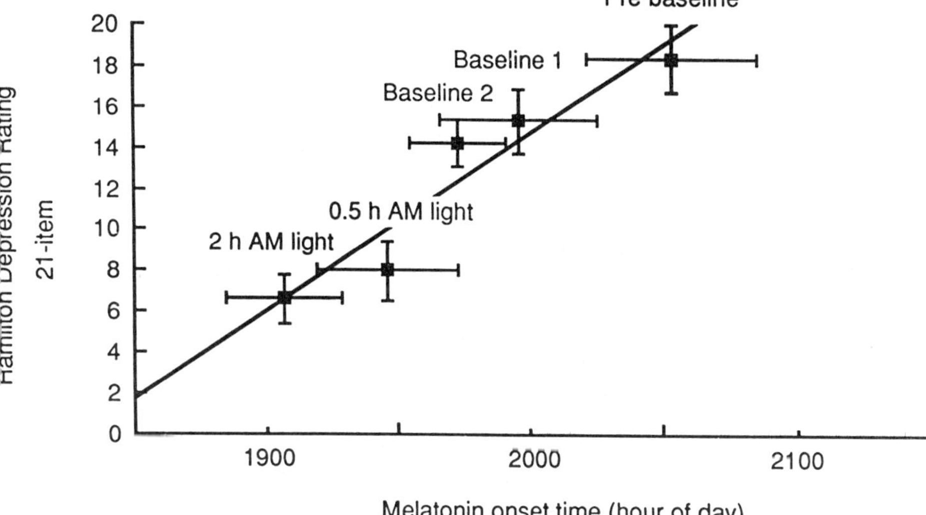

Figure 4 Correlation between melatonin onset and Hamilton Depression Rating in the study of 0.5 hr versus 2 hr of light. Patients received either 0.5 hr or 2 hr of morning light immediately upon awakening at 6 AM or awoke into dim light during the baseline weeks in a randomized crossover design. The average melatonin onsets are plotted on the abscissa, and the average Hamilton depression ratings are plotted on the ordinate. The five plotted points are as follows (from right to left): first day of the study, first baseline week, second baseline week, week of 0.5 hr of morning light and week of 2 hr of morning light. A linear regression, fitted for the five data points obtained for each of the 12 subjects for whom we had complete data, had a significant correlation coefficient ($r = 0.95$, $df = 4$, $p \leqslant 0.01$). When the slopes were calculated for each subject individually, the mean was also significantly different from zero ($p \leqslant 0.006$, $df = 11$, Student's *t*-test). These data indicate that clinical improvement is highly correlated with a phase advance in the melatonin onset. (From Ref. 16.)

response from the former, it is possible to calculate an advance-delay (A-D) differential value. The A-D differential takes into account interindividual differences in melatonin physiology and, ultimately, may represent a more useful way to phase type patients than the baseline DLMO measurement. However, the A-D differential is significantly correlated with the baseline DLMO (Fig. 5; 16). Therefore, it is not surprising that the later the baseline DLMO value, the greater (or more positive) the A-D differential, and the earlier the baseline DLMO, the smaller (or more negative) the A-D differential. Thus, seasonal depressive patients have greater A-D differentials than do normal controls.

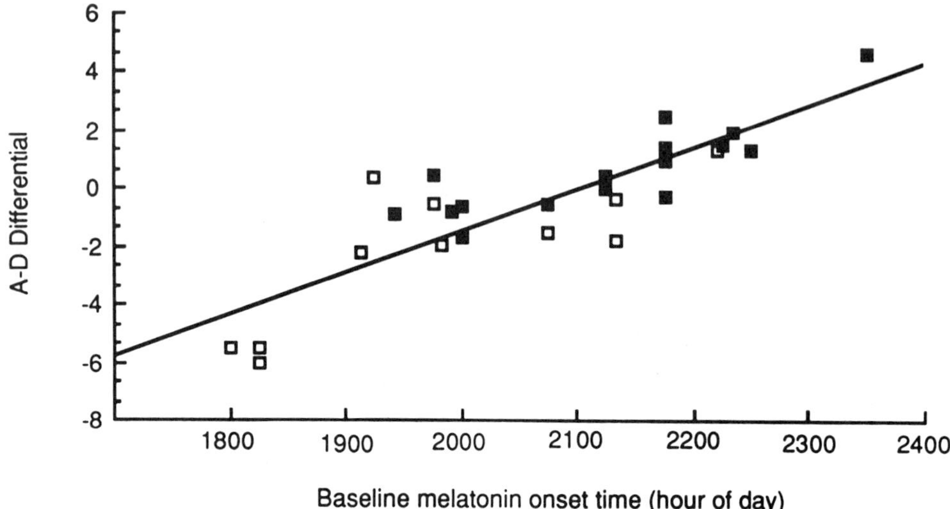

Figure 5 Data from the two studies of morning versus evening light were combined. The A-D differential was calculated for both patients (N = 16) and controls (N = 11). The A-D differential is calculated by subtracting the evening light delay shift relative to baseline from the morning light advance shift relative to baseline. The A-D differential may possibly indicate that phase of the PRC, in that a greater (more positive) A-D differential would be consistent with a relatively phase-advanced PRC and a lesser (more negative) A-D differential would be consistent with a relatively phase-delayed PRC. The good correlation shown here ($r = 0.86$, $df = 25$, $p \leqslant 0.0001$) indicates that the baseline melatonin onset (dim light melatonin onset) predicts the A-D differential, as if the baseline melatonin onset were marking the phase of its PRC. (From Ref. 16.)

THE USE OF BRIGHT LIGHT IN THE TREATMENT OF NONSEASONAL DEPRESSION

The use of bright light therapy in other types of depression is currently under investigation; however, it is not yet known just how beneficial light therapy will be for patients with endogenous (nonseasonal) major depression. This is not surprising, because major depression probably represents a heterogeneous group of illnesses. Winter depression, on the other hand, seems causally related to seasonal change in environmental light. However, if a patient with major depression also has a sleep-phase disorder, then appropriately timed bright light should be of benefit in correcting the sleep disorder (11). The effect of bright light on the other symptoms of depression is, in our experience, more variable.

Kripke initially began treating major depressed patients with morning light, with only modest success (13). In contrast, we (11) initially hypothesized that since these patients had phase-advanced circadian rhythms (17) the most appropriate time for bright light exposure should be in the evening. Switching to evening light has not produced dramatic reductions in depression ratings (13), and Kripke has now begun a protocol whereby patients receive evening light for several weeks. The results of this study are as yet not known.

The existence of a group of depressed patients with phase-advance type circadian rhythm disturbance is, in our opinion, controversial, and conclusive evidence for phase advance in depression has not been forthcoming. Therefore, advancing sleep has not become a common treatment, and evening light has not produced a robust antidepressant effect.

In summary, the efficacy of bright light in the treatment of depression, other than seasonal affective disorder, remains unknown. In contrast, bright light has been effective in treating advanced (12) and delayed (11) sleep-phase syndromes, and it may also be useful in the treatment of jet lag (18) and in problems associated with shift work (19). Furthermore, although bright light is very effective in the treatment of winter depression, there is still some controversy over whether or not the timing of the light is critical.

ALTERNATIVE HYPOTHESES FOR THE ANTIDEPRESSANT EFFECT OF LIGHT

The "Photon-Counting" Hypothesis

Most investigators agree that clinically effective light has to be of sufficient brightness and duration. However, some investigators have proposed a "photon-counting" hypothesis that states that the timing of the light is not critical for its antidepressant effect (10,20,21). According to this hypothesis, patients can have a satisfactory response to light by exposure to a sufficient number of photons at any time of day. Unfortunately, this hypothesis does not specify what physiological changes occur in the winter that might trigger recurrent depression, nor does it specify what physiological effect is produced by exposure to bright light.

This hypothesis had its genesis in the finding that evening bright light was effective in treating winter depression (10,20), and that extending the day length did not produce more antidepressant effect than bright light exposure in the middle of the day (21). We have critiqued these and other studies supportive of the photon-counting hypothesis (22,23). In general, most of these studies have failed to hold sleep time constant or to control for ambient bright light exposure around the critical times of dawn and dusk. Similarly, other studies have failed to maximize the effectiveness of scheduling morning light immediately upon awakening (24) or have utilized insufficient sample sizes or study design, all of which could contribute to the possibility of a type II error (failure to show a difference between treatment groups) (25). Nonetheless, at least one group has consistently maintained that patients can be treated with bright light at any time of the day (10,20,21,24). It is hoped that this controversy will be resolved as soon as possible, because more and more winter depressive patients are currently requesting light treatment.

There are several other possible ways for evening light (which is not capable of causing a phase advance) to have an antidepressant effect. For example, because the effect is usually modest and has been observed only after 1 week of treatment, a placebo effect cannot be ruled out, since patients are always aware of the light exposure conditions. Additionally, it is possible that some patients may be responding because they have a phase-advance type of disturbance. A third explanation for the antidepressant effect of evening light may be its ability to delay sleep (through some kind of energizing effect), thus causing patients to wake up later and into bright morning (sun)light. We have performed two pilot studies in which we have successfully treated winter depressives by delaying their sleep (26). In fact, we have frequently suggested to patients that they try to delay their sleep and go outside immediately upon awakening (but not look directly at the sun or they might suffer eye damage) if their schedule permits, before going to the expense of obtaining an artificial bright light fixture.

Midday light has also been claimed to have an antidepressant effect (24, 25), but unfortunately, circadian phase was not measured in these studies. It is, however, possible that the midday light, if given sufficiently early in the day, could produce a phase advance with antidepressant effect.

This controversy may soon be resolved, as a recent analysis of the pooled data from all research groups studying winter depression has shown that morning light is more effective than midday or evening light (27). Therefore, it is argued that evening light is probably working through nothing more than a placebo effect. In their attempt to find an alternative to the phase-shift hypothesis, the Bethesda group has found a number of summer versus winter physiological changes in seasonal depressive patients, as well as several patient versus control differences (28). However, a specific physiological hypothesis has not yet been proposed, other than the phase-shift hypothesis.

The Circadian Amplitude Hypothesis

A specific circadian amplitude hypothesis has also been proposed (29); however, it is not clear if this hypothesis is substantially different from the phase-shift hypothesis, because a change in circadian phase often causes a change in circadian amplitude and vice versa.

SUMMARY

In summary, our research of the phase-shift hypothesis has enabled us to develop some practical guidelines for the treatment of winter depression and other chronobiological disorders (30).

1. If patients are thought to have a phase-delay type disturbance, then the physician should schedule 1-2 hr of 2500 lux light immediately upon awakening.
2. The response should begin to be apparent within 2-4 days.
3. If patients have to advance their sleep to accommodate the morning light exposure schedule, their response may be somewhat delayed until their sleep has become readapted.
4. Incidental bright light exposure in the evening should be avoided.
5. If the response is not satisfactory after a few days of morning light exposure, a longer duration or increased light intensity may be necessary (beginning the exposure immediately upon awakening).
6. Once the antidepressant response has been established, the duration, or intensity, or both, of light therapy can be reduced.
7. If patients do not respond, have only a transient response, or show signs of becoming phase advanced, the duration or intensity of morning light should be reduced.
8. Patients with phase-advanced circadian rhythms should be treated with evening (7:00-9:00 PM) light and should avoid bright light in the morning. In addition, they should minimize delaying their sleep.
9. Bright artificial light should not be administered using an unapproved light source, such as a sun lamp or heat lamp.
10. Although outdoor sunlight is often effective (because of its brightness), patients should be instructed never to stare directly at the sun.

ACKNOWLEDGMENTS

We thank C. Simonton, M. Blood, and V. Bauer for their help in preparing this manuscript. We thank G. Clarke, M. MacReynolds, J. Peterson, and J. Gauthier for technical assistance. This research was supported by grants MH40161 and MH 00703.

REFERENCES

1. Lewy, A. J., Sack, R. L., and Singer, C. M. (1984). Assessment and treatment of chronobiologic disorders using plasma melatonin levels and bright light exposure: The clock-gate model and the phase response curve. *Psychopharmacol. Bull. 20*: 566-568.

2. Papousek, M. (1975). Chronobiological aspects of cyclothymia. *Fortschr. Neurol. Psychiatr. 43*:381-440.
3. Kripke, D. F., Mullaney, D. J., Atkinson, M., and Wolf, S. (1978). Circadian rhythm disorders in manic-depressives. *Biol. Psychiatry 13*:335-350.
4. Wehr, T. A., Wirz-Justice, A., Goodwin, F. K., Duncan, W., and Gillin, J. C. (1979). Phase advance of the circadian sleep-wake cycle as an antidepressant. *Science 20*:710-713.
5. Lewy, A. J., Wehr, T. A., Goodwin, F. K., Newsome, D. A., and Markey, S. (1980). Light suppresses melatonin secretion in humans. *Science 210*:1267-1269.
6. Lewy, A. J., Sack, R. L., and Singer, C. M. (1985). Immediate and delayed effects of bright light on human melatonin production: Shifting "dawn" and "dusk" shifts the dim light melatonin onset (DLMO). *Ann. N.Y. Acad. Sci. 453*:253-259.
7. Lewy, A. J., Sack, R. L., and Singer, C. M. (1985). Treating phase typed chronobiologic sleep and mood disorders using appropriately timed bright artificial light. *Psychopharmacol. Bull. 21*:368-372.
8. Lewy, A. J., Kern, H. E., Rosenthal, N. E., and Wehr, T. A. (1982). Bright artificial light treatment of a manic-depressive patient with a seasonal mood cycle. *Am. J. Psychiatry 139*:1496-1498.
9. Rosenthal, N. E., Sack, D. A., Gillin, J. C., Lewy, A. J., Goodwin, F. K., Davenport, Y., Mueller, P. S., Newsome, D. A., and Wehr, T. A. (1984). Seasonal affective disorder: A description of the syndrome and preliminary findings with light therapy. *Arch. Gen. Psychiatry 41*:72,80.
10. Rosenthal, N. E., Sack, D. A., Carpenter, C. J., Parry, B. L., Mendelson, W. B., and Wehr, T. A. (1985). Antidepressant effects of light in seasonal affective disorder. *Am. J. Psychiatry 142*:163-170.
11. Lewy, A. J., Sack, R. L., Frederickson, R. H., Reaves, M., Denney, D. D., and Zielske, D. R. (1983). The use of bright light in the treatment of chronobiologic sleep and mood disorders: The phase-response curve. *Psychopharmacol. Bull. 19*:523-535.
12. Lewy, A. J., Sack, R. L., and Singer, C. M. (1985). Melatonin, light and chronbiological disorders. In *Photoperiodism, Melatonin and the Pineal.* Edited by D. Evered and S. Clark. London, Pitman, pp. 231-252.
13. Kripke, D. F. (1985). Therapeutic effects of bright light in depressed patients. *Ann. N.Y. Acad. Sci. 453*:270-281.
14. Kripke, D. F. (1984). Critical hypotheses for depression. *Chronobiol. Int. 1*: 73-80.
15. Lewy, A. J., Sack, R. L., Miller, L. S., and Hoban, T. M. (1987). Antidepressant and circadian phase-shifting effects of light. *Science 235*:352-354.
16. Lewy, A. J., Sack, R. L., Singer, C. M., White, D. M., and Hoban, T. M. (1988). Winter depression and the phase shift hypothesis for bright light's therapeutic effects: History, theory and experimental evidence. *J. Biol. Rhythms 3*: 121-134.
17. Lewy, A. J., Sack, R. L., Singer, C. M., and White, D. M. (1987). The phase shift hypothesis for bright light's therapeutic mechanism of action: Theoretical considerations and experimental evidence. *Psychopharmacol. Bull. 23*:349-353.

18. Daan, S. and Lewy, A. J. (1984). Scheduled exposure to daylight: A potential strategy to reduce "jet lag" following transmeridian flight. *Psychopharmacol. Bull. 20*:566-568.
19. Eastman, C. I. (1987). Bright light in work-sleep schedules for shift workers: Application of circadian rhythm principles. In *Temporal Disorder in Human Oscillatory Systems.* Edited by L. Rensing, U. van der Heiden, and M. C. Mackey. Berlin, Springer-Verlag, pp. 176-185.
20. James, S. P., Wehr, T. A., Sack, D. A., Parry, B. L., and Rosenthal, N. E. (1985). Treatment of seasonal affective disorder with evening light. *Br. J. Psychiatry 147*:424-428.
21. Wehr, T.A., Jacobsen, F. M., Sack, D. A., Arendt, J., Tamarkin, L., and Rosenthal, N. E. (1986). Phototherapy of seasonal affective disorder. *Arch. Gen. Psychiatry 43*:870-875.
22. Lewy, A. J. and Sack, R. L. (1986). Minireview: Light therapy and psychiatry. *Proc. Soc. Exp. Biol. Med. 183*:11-18.
23. Lewy, A. J. and Sack, R. L. (1988). Letter to the Editor. *Am. J. Psychiatry 145*:1041-1042.
24. Jacobsen, G. M., Wehr, T. A., Skewer, R. A., Sack, D. A., and Rosenthal, N. E. (1987). Morning versus midday phototherapy of seasonal affective disorder. *Am. J. Psychiatry 144*:424-428.
25. Isaacs, G., Stainer, D. S., Sensky, T. E., Moor, S., and Thompson, C. (1988). Phototherapy and its mechanism of action in seasonal affective disorder. *J. Affect. Disord. 14*:13-19.
26. Lewy, A. J., Sack, R. L., and Singer, C. M. (1990). Bright light, melatonin and biological rhythms in humans. In *Sleep and Biological Rhythms*, Edited by J. Montplaisir and R. Godbout. New York, Oxford University Press.
27. Terman, M., Terman, J. S., Quitkin, F. M., McGrath, P. J., Steward, J. W., and Rafferty, B. (1989). Light therapy for seasonal affective disorder: A review of efficacy. *Neuropsychopharmacology 2*:1-22.
28. Skewer, R. G., Jacobsen, F. M., Duncan, C. C., Kelly, K. A., Sack, D. A., Tamarkin, L., Gaist, P. A., Kasper, S., and Rosenthal, N. E. (1988). Neurobiology of seasonal affective disorder and phototherapy. *J. Biol. Rhythms 3*: 135-154.
29. Czeisler, C. A., Kronauer, R. E., Mooney, J. J., Anderson, J. L., and Allan, J. S. (1987). Biologic rhythm disorders, depression, and phototherapy: A new hypothesis. *Psychiatr. Clin. North Am. 10*:687-709.
30. Lewy, A. J. (1988). Treating chronobiologic sleep and mood disorders with bright light. *Psychiatr. Ann. 17*:664-669.

11

Electroconvulsive Therapy

RICHARD D. WEINER and C. EDWARD COFFEY

Duke University Medical Center, Durham, North Carolina

INTRODUCTION

Overview

This chapter considers the practice of electroconvulsive therapy (ECT) and its role in contemporary psychiatric practice. We will begin with a definition of ECT, followed by a review of its historical evolution and present utilization and a discussion of its indications, contraindications, and adverse effects. A description of modern ECT technique will also be provided. We will conclude with a review of what is known about the mechanism of action of ECT, and we will offer recommendations for education and training in this treatment modality. Several general references are available to readers desiring a more comprehensive review of this topic (1-3).

Care has been taken to make sure that the material provided in this chapter is both up-to-date and consistent with available data, including new ECT clinical practice guidelines developed by the American Psychiatric Association (3a). Still, the reader must be aware that many issues regarding ECT have yet to be resolved, and, as new data become available, our knowledge base for ECT, along with the manner in which the practice of this treatment modality is carried out, will need to be revised.

What is Electroconvulsive Therapy?

Electroconvulsive therapy is the electrical induction of modified grand mal seizures for the purpose of inducing therapeutic change in patients suffering from distinct episodes of susceptible mental disorders. Electrical stimulation was chosen for this purpose because it represents the simplest, most reliable means of eliciting such seizures, not because there is anything "therapeutic" per se in the electricity itself.

History of Electroconvulsive Therapy

The historical roots of ECT lie in the misconception by early 20th century neuropsychiatrists that schizophrenia and epilepsy were incompatible (4). During this era, no effective means of inducing a remission in severe mental disorders was available, although with Wagner-Jauregg's discovery that induction of malaria produced a marked beneficial effect in patients with neurosyphilis (5), the time was ripe for a breakthrough.

In 1935, Lazlo Meduna, a Hungarian neuropsychiatrist, reported a series of schizophrenic patients whose psychosis showed a marked improvement after a series of epileptic seizures elicited by intramuscular injections of oil of camphor (6). Initially greeted with disbelief, Meduna's findings, once corroborated, led to an almost immediate acceptance of "convulsive therapy," as it was called, across the world. Within a very short space of time, this treatment modality was being applied to a wide variety of mental disorders, as psychiatrists of the day endeavored to determine its spectrum of action.

Unfortunately, camphor was an extremely unreliable means of inducing seizures. One could not be altogether sure whether an injection would lead to one seizure, several seizures, or, for that matter, any seizure activity at all. When seizures did occur, they were often ushered in by a series of painful myoclonic jerks. Because of such difficulties, patient acceptability of convulsive therapy in these early days was not high. The implementation of a purer, synthetic epileptogenic compound, pentylenetetrazol (Metrazol), was helpful, but only partially so.

Both the benefits and the liabilities associated with pharmacoconvulsive therapy were quite apparent to the Italian neuropsychiatrist, Ugo Cerletti, who, like many others, began to use this treatment modality in the mid-1930s. What distinguished Cerletti from his colleagues, however, was that he was also a well-known expert in the field of experimental epileptology, in which for some time, he had been involved in the study of various effects of seizures produced in animals by electricity.

Although it took little effort for Cerletti and his co-workers to conceptualize the possibility of using an electrical, rather than a pharmacologic, stimulus to elicit therapeutic seizures, the act of doing so was approached with considerable fear and trepidation, particularly coming at a time when the use of the "electric chair" in penal institutions was becoming commonplace. After much careful animal study of issues related to the safety of the electrical stimulus at intensity levels compatible with seizure generation, Cerletti and his assistant, Luciano Bini, performed the first application of "electroshock therapy," as they called it, in 1937, reporting the case in the psychiatric literature a year later (7). By 1940, the reliability of the electrical stimulus and the subsequent salutary effects upon patient acceptability led ECT to largely supplant pharmacoconvulsive therapy in most clinical settings.

Marked by an even more extensive utilization than pharmacoconvulsive therapy, ECT rapidly became the dominant form of somatic therapy for major mental disorders. During the 1940s, clinical investigations showed that the benefits of ECT were particularly great in severe depressive disorders and mania, and its use gradually became more diagnostically selective. Eventually, with the development of effective pharmacologic antidepressant and antipsychotic agents, beginning in the mid-1950s, the use of ECT began to wane. Over the last several decades, ECT utilization rates have continued to decline (8,9), although in recent years this process may have begun to level out, as the psychiatric profession comes to grips with the limitations of available psychopharmacologic alternatives.

What is the Contemporary Practice of Electroconvulsive Therapy?

At present, ECT remains an accepted form of treatment in most countries, with numerous national psychiatric and medical societies endorsing its continued use. Recently, a special NIH/NIMH Consensus Panel on ECT in the United States reached similar conclusions (10). Each year, approximately 30,000 patients in the United States receive ECT (8,9), primarily for major depressive disorder, with schizophrenia and mania making up nearly all of the remaining cases. Electroconvulsive therapy in the United States is mainly administered in general, university, and private psychiatric hospitals, where it is typically given to not more than several percent of the inpatient psychiatric population. This therapy appears to be relatively underutilized in public, state, and Veterans Administration hospitals, where utilization rates are often below 1%.

INDICATIONS

Depression

The main current diagnostic indication for ECT is major depression, which probably accounts for 80-90% of ECT referrals in the United States. Scientific data supporting the efficacy of ECT in major depression are quite compelling. Over the past three decades, in particular, a number of carefully controlled studies have firmly established that ECT represents an extremely potent means of establishing a therapeutic remission (11). Such studies have included double-blind placebo-controlled investigations, in which periods of anesthesia induction without an electrically induced seizure (i.e., "sham-ECT") were used for the control condition (12). Comparisons between ECT and a variety of antidepressant pharmacologic agents have also been carried out, largely demonstrating a significant therapeutic advantage for ECT, both in the degree and rate of response.

Areas that remain to be investigated adequately on a prospective basis include ECT versus combination antidepressant-neuroleptic pharmacotherapy in delusional depression and the combination of ECT and psychotropic agents in nonresponders to both treatment modalities. Overall, in carefully selected patient populations, response rates as high as 80-90% have been reported. Still, in some situations (e.g., largely treatment-refractory groups referred to tertiary care facilities) response rates may be as low as 60-70%.

Although traditionally it has been believed that the presence of melancholic (i.e., "endogenous") symptomatology represents a highly favorable prognostic sign, this belief has recently been questioned, and it now appears that both endogenous and nonendogenous types of major depression may respond equally well to ECT (13). A similar situation holds for unipolar versus bipolar forms of major depression. The indicators of therapeutic outcome for ECT are more related to the symptomatologic profile, treatment history, presence of concurrent chronic mental or physical disorders, and degree and manageability of ongoing stress factors than to the diagnostic subtype. The existence of delusions, for example, is considered a good prognostic sign, as is a history of a favorable ECT response. Unfortunately, the clinical usefulness of such indicators is marginal, and attempts to define meaningful prognostic indices on the basis of such factors have been unsuccessful. The ECT Prediction Scale designed by the Newcastle group in England has been most widely used for this purpose (14).

The existence of an indicated diagnosis represents only one factor in the determination of when to refer a patient for ECT. This decision should also be made on the basis of a comprehensive assessment of the risk/benefit ratio for all other viable treatment options. Situations that are compatible with an immediate referral for ECT might include an overriding necessity, on either psychiatric or medical grounds, for a rapid remission; a history of poor antidepressant drug response or good ECT response; patient preference; and the presence of lower overall risks with ECT. An actively suicidal individual, with electrocardiographic (ECG) evidence of heart block, for example, represents a case for whom a preference for ECT as the primary treatment modality would be supported.

In most situations, a trial of antidepressant medication, supplemented with a neuroleptic agent if the patient is psychotic, is attempted before ECT. If this trial is unsuccessful, or cannot be completed because of toxic effects, the use of ECT should then be considered. The decision for ECT referral versus switching to alternative psychotropic agents should be tempered by the diminished likelihood of pharmacologic response, as well as the present severity of symptomatology. The occurrence of substantial clinical deterioration during a drug trial is often a strong rationale for the initiation of ECT.

Mania

Until recently, data concerning the efficacy of ECT in mania consisted of retrospective series and case reports (15). Such data did, however, suggest that ECT was effective in inducing a remission in approximately 60-80% of cases, depending upon the series. Because of the rapid acceptance of lithium carbonate as an effective antimanic agent, however, little effort was expended in the demonstration of ECT's relative efficacy as a first-line treatment. Accordingly, the use of ECT in mania was largely relegated to lithium non-responders and those individuals for whom therapeutic levels of this agent could not be tolerated. Primary use of ECT was reserved for rare cases for whom the condition was too grave to allow waiting for a pharmacologic effect. A 1976 APA member survey estimated that only 3% of ECT patients were referred for treatment of mania (8).

Within the last few years, two controlled investigations of ECT versus lithium in mania have been carried out (16,17). For the first time, these studies suggest that the efficacy of ECT in mania may indeed be at least as great as that of lithium, and they provide further support of a role for ECT in the treatment of this disorder.

Schizophrenia

Electroconvulsive therapy was first used for treatment of schizophrenia. Over the intervening years, the many controlled and uncontrolled studies of ECT in schizophrenia have allowed several conclusions to be made (18). First, there is no apparent therapeutic advantage for ECT over neuroleptic agents, except for catatonia and also perhaps for schizoaffective disorder, in which a prominent affective component appears to be present. Second, ECT is roughly comparable with neuroleptics in the treatment of schizophreniform disorders and patients in whom an acute decompensation occurs without a history of preexisting residual symptomatology. However, such conditions may differ fundamentally from the classic chronic, or "process," schizophrenia.

Patients with chronic schizophrenia rarely show a beneficial response to ECT, which is unfortunate because the drug response in such patients is also often limited. Still, the presence of affective or catatonic features should at least suggest ECT as a treatment option. Conversely, the existence of prominent "negative" symptomatology (e.g., apathy, flattened affect, and alogia) should be considered a poor prognostic sign. The use of a long series of daily ECT, termed "regressive ECT," was thought to have a specific efficacy in cases of otherwise unresponsive chronic schizophrenia. However, because there was no adequate replication, and the severe organic deterioration, which was a hallmark of this technique, was invariable present, regressive ECT is no longer used.

Generally, neuroleptic agents are now considered the first-line treatment for schizophrenia, with ECT being relegated, as with mania, to a secondary role. Still, increasing concern about potentially irreversible neurologic effects associated with neuroleptic agents (i.e., tardive dyskinesia) may promote ECT as a primary therapy in some cases. Recent reports that the combination of ECT plus concomitant neuroleptic agents may be efficacious in drug nonresponders (19) has also renewed the general level of interest in ECT in the management of schizophrenia.

Other Conditions

Although ECT has been tried in many types of functional disorders other than major depression, mania, and schizophrenia, there is little evidence of true efficacy (11). However, multiple diagnoses may be present simultaneously; therefore, the occurrence of a major depressive episode, in an individual with dysthymia, generalized anxiety disorder, or personality disorder, should still lead to consideration of ECT as a viable treatment alternative, even though a favorable prognosis may be somewhat less likely.

Because ECT produces a wide range of neurochemical, neuroendocrine, and neurophysiological changes, most of which are probably not related to therapeutic action (see Mechanism of Action section), its use has been proposed for the management of several medical conditions for which, in theory, these ECT-induced changes might be therapeutic (20). In several of these situations, particularly Parkinson's disease, neuroleptic malignant syndrome, hypopituitary syndrome, and epilepsy, beneficial effects have, in fact, been reported. Although such effects have been only transient and should be considered experimental, further work in this area should be continued, for example, potential maintenance ECT in drug-refractory Parkinson's disease.

Occasionally, ECT has been used for treatment of a few other medical conditions for which its mechanism of action is less clear, namely organic delusional syndromes (including alcohol and drug withdrawal states), for which it is believed that ECT has a specific antidelusional action, and catatonia. Again, such uses are experimental and, because viable treatment alternatives are usually present, ECT should be reserved for the rare situation for which standard pharmacologic management has proved ineffective.

CONTRAINDICATIONS

Although there are no conditions under which one would "never" administer ECT (i.e., no "absolute" contraindications) several circumstances exist, which are associated with a sufficiently high risk of mortality or serious morbidity, to make one reluctant to institute ECT under what our surgical colleagues would term an "elective" basis. Examples of such conditions include space-occupying intracerebral lesions, other causes of increased intracranial pressure, recent myocardial infarction (particularly with unstable cardiac function), unstable vascular aneurysm or malformation, retinal detachment, pheochromocytoma, and other situations where there is markedly elevated anesthetic risk.

Practitioners must ask themselves several questions when confronted with these types of situations: What is the actual level of risk with ECT in this case? Are there means of lowering the risk of ECT by modifying treatment technique? How do the anticipated benefits and likely risks with ECT compare with those associated with alternative courses of action, including no active treatment at all? The answers to these questions will serve to determine whether or not a referral for ECT is indicated in a given case. It should also be recognized that such risk-benefit considerations represent an integral part of the informed consent process with ECT and, therefore, it is important that the patients themselves be appraised of this information.

ADVERSE EFFECTS

Mortality

The mortality of ECT is quite low. Figures quoted from large series tend to be around 1:10,000 patients (1), although the level of risk varies as a function of baseline medical status. Most deaths associated with ECT are usually related to either cardiac arrest or myocardial infarction. The next most likely causes of death appear to be cerebral herniation (typically in settings of unsuspected intracerebral mass lesions), and allergic or other toxic reactions to the anesthetic or relaxant agents used with the ECT procedure.

Cardiovascular

With the induction of the seizure with ECT, there are sudden marked elevations in both heart rate and blood pressure, both of which probably result from central sympathetic stimulation (21). These changes, which are typically transient and usually last no more than several minutes, are associated with increased cardiac output and myocardial oxygen demands. In addition to sympathetically mediated effects, parasympathetic discharges take place both at seizure onset and seizure termination. These latter changes are often manifested in the form of a transient bradycardia or, more rarely, as a brief period of asystole.

A variety of cardiac arrhythmias and other ECG alterations can occur secondary to these autonomic fluctuations, most commonly in the form of unifocal ventricular ectopic beats (22). These phenomena are particularly likely in patients with preexisting cardiac disease. In nearly all cases, such events are benign and disappear within several minutes. Only rarely is active treatment required, although personnel present in the treatment area should always be prepared to manage such occurrences. Risk of cardiac ischemia, as well as other sources of arrhythmias, can be greatly diminished by judicious use of preoxygenation, nitroglycerin, and, when indicated, antihypertensive or antiarrhythmic agents. However, routine use of antihypertensive agents with ECT is not indicated because this could unnecessarily diminish perfusion of cerebral tissue during the seizure (a time of high metabolic demands), and could potentially adversely impinge on the adequacy of seizure induction. Similarly, lidocaine (and probably newer related compounds as well) markedly diminishes seizure duration and compromises therapeutic response (23).

Cerebral

There is no evidence that either the brief electrical stimuli used with ECT or the seizure activity induced by this stimulation is associated with direct toxic effect upon the neural substrate (1,2,24). Metabolic effects of the induced seizures include a temporary increase in the permeability of the blood-brain barrier, resulting in related increases in extracellular fluid and both intracerebral and intraocular pressure (25). There is no evidence, however, that these changes typically produce cerebral anoxia or other aspects of cellular metabolic trauma. Recent primate studies, carried out on the basis of contemporary ECT technique, have failed to find evidence supporting irreversible pathophysiological alterations (26).

Despite the foregoing findings, the issue of "brain damage" with ECT has for many years remained at the forefront of the controversy that surrounds this treatment modality (24). In general, animal investigations, most of which were carried out 30-50 years ago, vary considerably for factors such as duration and intensity of stimulation, number and frequency of seizures, and use of oxygenation and muscle relaxation; and are far from consistent in their findings. Still, after controlling as much as possible for methodological inadequacies, the available data remain negative for the existence of irreversible structural alterations following induced seizures (24). In addition, recent noninvasive in vivo human studies, consisting of anatomical brain imaging [magnetic resonance imaging (MRI), computed tomography (CT)] as well as plasma assays for metabolic byproducts of neuronal degeneration, also have not demonstrated any such effects (27,28), although, by their nature, such measures are capable of reflecting changes only at the macroscopic level.

Electrophysiologically, varying amounts of electroencephalographic (EEG) slowing develop over the ECT course (29). This abnormality is typically nonspecific, generalized, and maximal frontally, although it may occasionally be asymmetrical or even focal, depending upon ECT type and the presence of preexisting cerebral dysfunction. Regardless of severity, slowing typically disappears within days to weeks after completion of the ECT course. Only minimal amounts are generally present by 1 month post-ECT.

The extent of cumulative EEG slowing is greatest with bilateral stimulus electrode placement, sinewave stimulus waveform, maximally superthreshold stimulus intensity, and many ECT treatments (30). The EEG slowing is also roughly correlated with interictal confusion and amnesia. With unilateral stimulus electrode placement, EEG slowing is frequently slightly greater over the stimulated hemisphere. This latter observation is of particular interest given recent data suggesting that grossly asymmetric slowing with unilateral ECT may be associated with a diminished therapeutic response, presumably secondary to inadequately generalized seizures (31).

The most widely recognized types of adverse cerebral effects with ECT are confusion and amnesia. Some degree of interictal confusion may develop over the ECT course, with severity a function of the same factors indicated for EEG slowing (32). Rarely, a full-blown organic delirium may occur. If present, its effect can often be greatly diminished by increasing the time interval between ECT treatments or by switching to a less toxic ECT technique. In terms of duration, ECT-related confusion is a transient phenomena and always disappears within a period of days after completion of the ECT course.

Similarly to EEG slowing and confusion, amnesia produced by ECT also varies considerably across individuals and is heavily influenced by technical factors, such as ECT type and the number and frequency of treatments (33). These amnestic changes are similar to other forms of organically based memory disturbances, including those occurring with spontaneous epilepsy. Two specific types of amnesia occur: an *anterograde* amnesia, which is a difficulty in retaining newly learned information; and a *retrograde* amnesia, which is a difficulty in remembering material learned before ECT (34).

Anterograde amnestic effects rapidly diminish following completion of the ECT course. It is quite uncommon, for example, for more than minimal changes to persist longer than a month following completion of the ECT course. Retrograde amnestic losses, which are most prominent for material learned relatively close to the time of ECT (i.e., most recent memories), also begin to dissipate rather quickly after the ECT course has been completed, although probably more slowly than with anterograde amnesia. Still, with bilateral stimulus electrode placement, a modest degree of spotty recent memory loss, particularly for autobiographical material, may persist for months or even years following ECT, although it is uncommon for such effects to be perceived as problematic by patients (35).

Studies of self-ratings of memory changes after ECT have been quite interesting, in that they demonstrate a strong relationship between functional and organic influences upon self-perceived memory function (36). In effect, these data reveal that memory self-ratings are actually more highly correlated with therapeutic outcome measures than with objective results of cognitive performance. This finding should not be altogether surprising, since depressive illness, in particular, is commonly associated with cognitive impairment, occasionally even presenting as a full-blown "pseudodementia." After successful treatment with ECT, such patients may actually experience considerable improvement in cognitive function.

In spite of the paucity of objective data supporting the presence of persistent memory dysfunction following ECT, a few anecdotal reports of substantial long-lasting memory loss have been described, with several extreme cases being highly publicized in the lay media. The pattern of amnesia described in such cases is often nonphysiological and may relate to either residual functional symptomatology or other aspects of underlying psychopathology (24). Patients with hysterical symptomatology, particularly those with a history of questionable complaints associated with other forms of treatment, appear to be particularly prone to such effects. Yet another contributing factor to this phenomenon may be a heightened sensitivity to "normal forgetting" in ECT patients. The experience of a transient amnestic episode after completion of an ECT course, could lead an individual to dwell upon occurrences of normal everyday forgetting that would otherwise be ignored.

Other Adverse Effects

Headaches, muscle aches and soreness, and nausea occasionally occur with ECT, but usually respond to supportive managment. Rarely, injuries to teeth, gums, or tongue can take place if protection of the oral airway is not properly managed. More dangerous adverse effects (e.g., musculoskeletal injuries, bladder rupture, and skin burns) are extremely rare and should not occur in the presence of adequate ECT technique.

PRE-ELECTROCONVULSIVE THERAPY EVALUATION AND PREPARATION FOR TREATMENT

Pre-electroconvulsive Therapy Evaluation

The evaluation of a patient for ECT consists of the demonstration of an appropriate clinical indication and an assessment of pertinent risk factors. Accordingly, the most important component of the pre-ECT evaluation is often the medical and psychiatric history and examination, which although general in scope, should focus in depth on areas of particular relevance to anticipated beneficial or adverse effects with ECT. Opinions differ concerning which laboratory tests are routinely indicated as part of the pre-ECT workup. In fact, only serum electrolyte levels, hemoglobin or hematocrit determinations, and an ECG should be considered necessary. Further procedures, such as spine and chest x-rays, EEG, or brain MRI should be ordered when specifically indicated.

To help assure that potential benefits and risks have been adequately defined, each case should be reviewed, both by a psychiatrist involved in the administration of ECT and by an anesthesia provider. Additional consultations should be considered when clinically appropriate. Because the final decision on use of ECT is made jointly by the patient and the treatment team, it should be understood that the role of the consultant is one of providing information, rather than "clearance."

Use of Ongoing Medications During Electroconvulsive Therapy

In general, it is best to discontinue psychotropic agents before the institution of ECT. Except perhaps for neuroleptic agents (11,19), there is no evidence that the concurrent use of psychotropic medications augments the efficacy of ECT. In addition, some psychotropic drugs interfere with the ability to induce seizures, (e.g., benzodiazepines and lithium; 37,38).

All nonpsychotropic medications should also be reviewed before ECT, and those not clearly indicated should be discontinued. Anticonvulsant agents and lidocaine increase seizure threshold or decrease seizure duration, thereby potentially compromising therapeutic response (23). Theophylline, on the other hand, has been reported to trigger status epilepticus (39). Other agents may interfere with the metabolism of anesthetic or relaxant agents, for instance, long-acting anticholinesterase compounds sometimes used in the treatment of glaucoma.

Finally, as part of the assessment of ongoing medications, the practitioner should ascertain which ongoing medications, by the nature of the protective effect they may exert, should be administered before ECT on the day of each treatment. Examples of such compounds include most cardiac drugs and corticosteroids.

Consent

Electroconvulsive therapy is a procedure for which voluntary informed consent is required, including the signing of a formal consent document (40). Such consent is provided for a specified course of ECT treatments or a time-limited period of continuation-maintenance ECT (see Post-ECT Management section). The practitioner should be aware of state regulations outlining the manner in which consent for ECT should be applied and see that they are followed. However, mental health professionals should work for change of any such regulations that are not wholly in the best interest of ECT patients.

Unless otherwise prescribed by law, consent should be provided by the patient. One assumes that such individuals have the capacity to provide consent unless compelling data exist to the contrary. Patients who are capable of providing consent, but refuse ECT should not be given the treatments against their will.

In the absence of adequate information, there cannot be true informed consent. The use of standard information sheets written in lay terms is quite helpful. Both verbal and written information should include the reason(s) for the ECT referral, the nature and merits of any alternative treatment options, a brief overview of pertinent aspects of ECT technique, the probable number of ECT treatments, and a delineation of major potential risks. In addition, patients should be assured that consent for ECT is a voluntary procedure and that they have the right to ask questions or to withdraw consent any time. The treatment team should make ongoing efforts to ensure that the patient remains aware of such rights.

ELECTROCONVULSIVE THERAPY TECHNIQUE

Overview of Procedure

Electroconvulsive therapy involves a series of electrically induced seizures, usually three per week. The plateau in therapeutic response determines the endpoint of the treatment course in responders. In contemporary practice, ECT treatments are modified by oxygenation, ultrabrief general anesthesia, and muscular relaxation. Physiological monitoring of seizure activity assures therapeutic potency and detects the occurrence of prolonged seizures. Similarly, monitoring the cardiovascular response helps minimize adverse systemic effects. The seizures themselves are induced by the application of a controlled electrical stimulus to the scalp after the patient has been oxygenated, anesthetized, and relaxed. Stimulus dosage levels, as well as the location of stimulus electrodes, are chosen on the basis of both beneficial and adverse effects.

Treatment Team and Setting

The ECT treatment team consists of a psychiatrist experienced in administering ECT, an anesthesia provider, an ECT nurse, and recovery nurse(s). The anesthesia provider is typically either an anesthesiologist or a nurse anesthetist. Regardless of discipline, this person needs to be capable of airway management, of providing anesthesia and muscular relaxation, and of handling the acute management of foreseeable medical emergencies.

The ECT treatment suite typically comprises areas for waiting, treatment, and recovery, all of which should be in close proximity. For outpatients, there should be an additional waiting area for family and patients. Although considerable variation exists in the location of the ECT treatment suite, optimally, it should be either on or adjacent to psychiatric inpatient units, but this is not always possible.

Anesthesia

Before anesthesia, the presence of an adequate airway is ascertained. Positive-pressure ventilation with 100% oxygen is provided from before anesthesia induction until return of spontaneous breathing. The ventilatory rate and volume should be consistent with mild hyperventilation, to maximize adequacy of seizure duration (41).

Many practitioners believe that anticholinergic premedication is routinely indicated to prevent bradycardia or asystole, although there is no consensus (1). When used, such agents are administered either intravenously (IV) 2 min before anesthesia induction, or intramuscularly (IM) or subcutaneously (SC) 30 min before entering the treatment area. The drugs typically used are either atropine—0.3-0.6 mg IM or SC or 0.4-1.0 mg IV—or glycopyrrolate (Robinul)—0.2-0.4 mg IM,SC, or IV. Recent data suggest that glycopyrrolate may be preferred because it does not cross the blood-brain barrier, and thereby is less likely to aggravate postictal confusion. However, there is evidence that glycopyrrolate may have less powerful cardiovascular effects than does atropine.

The anesthetic dose should be sufficient to provide amnesia for the treatment, but not so high that it adversely affects the seizure threshold. The usually preferred agent is methoxhexital (Brevital), 0.75—1.0 mg/kg IV, although some practitioners continue to report the use of thiopental (1).

For muscular relaxation, succinylcholine is usually used, with a typical dose range of 0.5-1.0 mg/kg IV. After the proper anesthetic dose has been established for a given patient, many anesthetists will administer the relaxant agent immediately after injection of the anesthetic drug (rapid sequence), rather than wait for the full anesthetic effect. Dosages of anticholinergic, anesthetic, and relaxant agents are adjusted at successive treatments to achieve the goal of light anesthesia and moderate muscular relaxation.

Stimulus Electrode Placement

Because of the nature of current flow, two stimulus electrodes are used with ECT. Traditionally, they have been applied bilaterally in frontotemporal regions (BL ECT), with the midpoint of each electrode located approximately 1 in. above the midpoint of a line between the tragus of the ear and the external canthus of the eye. In the 1940s, there were claims that unilateral stimulation might be associated with diminished cognitive side effects (42). However, this variation in ECT technique did not begin to catch on until after the late 1950s, when it was demonstrated that stimulation over the nondominant cerebral hemisphere was associated with much lower verbal memory impairment by ECT (43). More recent data suggest an advantage for unilateral nondominant electrode placement (ULND ECT), even with nonverbal memory function (44). In addition, electrode placement-related differences in retrograde amnesia for recent autobiographical events have been observed as long as 6 months post-ECT (35).

Because of its lesser effects upon memory function, there has been considerable movement within the psychiatric profession to make ULND electrode placement the preferred choice, at least for routine use. Unfortunately, reports continue to appear, including some based upon prospective controlled comparisons, that therapeutic response to ULND ECT may not be as potent, rapid, or enduring as that achieved with BL ECT (45), although other studies report a therapeutic equivalence (46). Because as yet, there is no consensus on this issue, various clinical practices abound, including switching ULND nonresponders to BL ECT, and switching BL ECT patients who develop substantial cognitive deficits to ULND ECT.

There is evidence that at least some of the reported efficacy differences between ULND and BL ECT may be secondary to technical factors (47). The ability to induce an adequate seizure with ULND electrode placement is a function of the precise location of the stimulus electrodes and (as discussed later) of stimulus intensity. The preferred location for right ULND ECT involves placing one electrode just to the right of the scalp vertex and the second electrode in the standard frontotemporal position (the "d'Elia" technique; 48).

Regardless of the type of electrode placement chosen, it is crucial to ensure adequate electrode contact. Several contemporary ECT devices offer a "self-test" feature, which provides a test of the adequacy of the coupling between the stimulus electrode and the scalp. This is accomplished by use of a very small electrical current that is substantially below the sensory threshold.

THE ELECTRICAL STIMULUS AND STIMULUS DOSING

The nature of the stimulus waveform has changed over the history of ECT. Initially, largely because of convenience, ECT devices incorporated the use of sinewave stimulus. In the 1940s, there began to be research interest in the use of interrupted patterns of electrical stimulation, such as the brief pulse, with which one could produce a seizure with much lower stimulus intensity (in terms of electrical charge or energy) (49). Claims were also made that such stimuli were associated with diminished cognitive impairment. Still, if the pulses were too brief, the treatments were not as therapeutic as those delivered using higher energy waveforms (50). The brief pulse stimulus did not catch on clinically, at least in the United States, until the mid-1970s when ECT devices of this type began to be available on a widespread basis. Since that time, data have established that the pulse stimulus is as therapeutically effective as the sinewave stimulus and, in addition, produces less confusion, amnesia, and EEG slowing (29,35). Hence, the pulse stimulus is now generally preferred for routine use.

Another issue pertinent to electrical parameters with ECT is stimulus dosing. A seizure threshold, below which a seizure cannot be elicited, exists for each patient. This threshold varies widely across individuals, covering more than a tenfold range, and is lower for females and with unilateral electrode placement (51). In addition, seizure threshold typically rises over the ECT course, reflecting this treatment modality's inherent anticonvulsant activity. Stimuli barely above seizure threshold may not be as therapeutic as more moderately suprathreshold stimulation, particularly with unilateral nondominant ECT (52). Grossly suprathreshold stimulation, on the other hand, may be associated with increased adverse cognitive effects.

Although it is as yet unclear about what type of stimulus dosing strategy is optimal to achieving a goal of "moderate" suprathreshold stimulation, two general approaches are presently in use. In the first, stimulus parameters for the initial ECT treatment are chosen empirically to reflect a relatively high probability of adequate seizure induction (e.g., 80% for a patient group with characteristics similar to the index case). Depending upon the ictal response, stimulus parameters are then adjusted up or down at successive treatments. The second type of stimulus dosing strategy involves an actual estimation of seizure threshold at the time of the first treatment. This determination is accomplished by starting at intensity levels that are likely to be subthreshold and increasing intensity in steps until an adequate ictal response takes place (51). Dosage levels for the second ECT treatment are then chosen to be a fixed level above this estimated seizure threshold (e.g., 100% greater with ULND electrode placement and 50% greater with BL placement).

Physiological Monitoring

Physiological monitoring with ECT includes measures of the ictal response as well as cardiovascular changes associated with treatment procedure. In terms of the ictal response, monitoring is carried out of both convulsive motor activity as well as the EEG. Because the motor aspects of the seizure are greatly suppressed by the muscle relaxant agent used with ECT, a special technique is used to assure that reliable monitoring of motor activity can be achieved. This technique consists of preventing the flow of this agent to a distal extremity by the use of a blood pressure cuff.

As ictal EEG activity persists longer than the motor convulsive response and, in addition, may be the only detectable evidence of a prolonged seizure, its use has been strongly encouraged. Such monitoring consists of one or more channels of EEG recording, each of which records the difference in scalp potential between two recording electrodes. Paper or auditory recording capabilities for EEG monitoring are now incorporated in several contemporary ECT devices in the United States. Because EEG tracings may sometimes be difficult to interpret, the use of EEG monitoring does not negate the need for concomitant monitoring of the motor response. Practitioners should also be aware of the nature of typical ictal EEG and postictal EEG patterns, the influence of anesthetic agents upon the EEG, and the appearance of various EEG artifacts (29).

Monitoring of heart rate, blood pressure, and ECG is indicated because of the pronounced transient, although usually benign, effects of ECT upon the cardiovascular system. Increases in heart rate and blood pressure typically occur within the first 30-60 sec of the seizure, with return to baseline by 3-5 min after stimulation. Relevant to cardiovascular function during ECT is the extent of oxygenation available to body tissues, and many anesthesiologists have recently implemented the use of noninvasive pulse oximetry.

Management of Missed, Inadequate, or Prolonged Seizures

The therapeutic potency of ECT is dependent upon the production of an adequate ictal response. However, the determination of seizure adequacy is now largely empiric. Most practitioners deal with this issue by restimulating at a higher stimulus intensity when the induced seizure is either totally absent or less than 25 sec by EEG criteria. Restimulation is carried out at 20-30 sec poststimulation for missed seizures and approximately 60 sec poststimulation for abortive seizures. In addition to the seizure duration cutoff criterion, some practitioners also use a higher stimulus intensity at the following treatment session if seizure duration is markedly decreased from that observed previously, or if the EEG seizure pattern is substantially lower in amplitude or regularity.

Prolonged seizures, defined here as longer than 180 sec by EEG criteria, are uncommon (29). As these events may be associated with increased toxicity, however, they should be aborted. Usually, this can be accomplished by the use of one or two repeated doses of anesthetic agent. Rarely, more powerful agents (e.g., diazepam or phenytoin) may be necessary.

Number and Frequency of Electroconvulsive Therapy

The number of ECT treatments administered should be tailored to therapeutic response. In an individual with an adequate response to ECT, the treatment course may be stopped after a therapeutic plateau has been achieved. This generally occurs by 6-12 treatments, although occasionally more or fewer than this number may be required. The number of ECT treatments necessary for remission does not appear to be a function of diagnosis, except possibly in chronic schizophrenia, for which ECT is rarely used. If onset of a therapeutic response is not present after six to eight ECT treatments, consideration should be given to alterations in the treatment plan, including the use of a different type of ECT technique when applicable.

The frequency of ECT treatments in the United States is now three per week. The severity of cognitive side effects with ECT is inversely proportional to the interval between ECT treatments; therefore, a frequency of three per week should not be exceeded with BL ECT, except for early in the treatment course in patients for whom a rapid onset of response is urgent. Because ULND ECT is associated with appreciably fewer cognitive side effects than BL ECT, it has been proposed that it may be administered at up to four to five treatments per week, although as yet there is little clinical experience with this practice.

A variation in ECT technique that has been suggested as a means to shorten time to clinical remission is multiple-monitored ECT (MMECT). This technique consists of induction of multiple adequate seizures within a single session of anesthesia. A typical treatment course with MMECT consists of two to four sessions (53). Although users of this technique have reported a more rapid therapeutic response, there has also been concern about an increased risk of prolonged seizures and an augmentation of the cardiovascular response. Particularly because no prospective controlled studies have yet been carried out comparing MMECT with standard ECT, the routine use of this technique has been limited.

SPECIAL CASES OF ELECTROCONVULSIVE THERAPY USE

Electroconvulsive Therapy in the Medically Ill

Given present referral patterns, it is not uncommon for patients with concurrent medical illnesses to be considered for ECT, particularly with the elderly.

As already stated, an assessment of potential risk is the major function of the pre-ECT evaluation, which should be tailored as needed to each patient's medical history and presenting symptomatology. Despite the presence of concurrent medical illness, ECT still often remains the safest and most effective form of treatment available, particularly because the ECT procedure can frequently be modified to diminish morbidity (20).

Electroconvulsive Therapy in the Elderly

In many facilities, the mean age for ECT patients is in the 50s or even 60s. This age distribution is not only due to the increased prevalence of severe, incapacitating depressive illness in the elderly, but also to the increased risks associated with psychotropic agents in this population (54). Although cognitive dysfunction with ECT may be increased in the elderly, particularly in those with baseline cerebral impairment, the presence of a dementia should not be considered a contraindication for ECT, particularly given the difficulties sometimes experienced in the evaluation of cases with coexisting dementia and depressive pseudodementia (55).

Pregnancy

Electroconvulsive therapy may be used in all three trimesters of pregnancy (56). The teratogenic risks during the first trimester for anticholinergic, anesthetic, and relaxant agents used with ECT are believed to be lower than those associated with psychotropic drugs. Obstetrical consultation is obtained before ECT, and noninvasive fetal monitoring of heart rate is carried out after 10 weeks of gestational age. Additional monitoring or the presence of an obstetrician may be indicated in high-risk situations.

Children and Adolescents

Electroconvulsive therapy may be helpful in the treatment of major depression, mania, or schizophrenia in adolescents, although utilization of ECT in this group is uncommon. Before beginning ECT, documented concurrence with the treatment plan should be obtained from a psychiatrist, not otherwise involved in the case, who is experienced with the treatment of adolescents. Use of ECT in children is exceedingly rare and should be reserved for extreme cases of affective disorder that are clearly unresponsive to all other available treatment modalities. In this situation, documented concurrence should be obtained from two psychiatrists, not otherwise involved in the case, who are experienced in the treatment of children.

POSTELECTROCONVULSIVE THERAPY MANAGEMENT

When effective, a course of ECT induces a remission, but does not, in itself, prevent the occurrence of relapse. Because risk of relapse with major depression, mania, or schizophrenia is high, particularly within the first 6 months following an index episode, it is important to provide continuation therapy during this time (57). Continuation therapy is usually prescribed in the form of psychotropic medication or, less commonly, with ECT (58). The precise timing of continuation ECT, which appears to be underutilized at present in the United States, varies considerably, but is often about one treatment per month. When risk of relapse remains high after 6 months, prophylactic "maintenance" therapy is indicated. In addition, brief series of ECT, if initiated rapidly, may be used to abort an incipient relapse.

The management of patients who have not responded therapeutically to ECT is problematic. Some practitioners prefer to utilize combination chemotherapy in such cases, whereas others consider a repeat ECT course with high-intensity stimuli and bilateral electrode placement. As noted earlier, the possible use of the combination of psychotropics plus ECT in such situations remains to be evaluated.

In addition to therapeutic outcome, cognitive effects should also receive attention after completion of the ECT course. If a confusional state is present after ECT, patients should not be discharged from the hospital until disorientation has diminished in severity. Patients who develop adverse cognitive effects after ECT should be counseled, as should their families, about any behavioral adjustments that may temporarily be indicated. When substantial amnesia is present, follow-up neuropsychological testing should also be considered.

MECHANISMS OF ACTION

The mechanism of action for therapeutic response with ECT is intimately related to the presence of generalized seizure activity. However, recent evidence has suggested that certain aspects of the induced seizure may be of more therapeutic importance than others. It may even be the brain's inhibitory response to the seizure, rather than the seizure itself, that is responsible for mediating beneficial effects (59).

Biochemically, electrically induced seizures produce a number of largely transient changes within the brain (60). Of particular importance, given the continued prominence of the monoaminergic hypothesis of depression, are observations from animal studies that a series of electrically induced seizures is associated with a cumulative downregulation of brain β_2-adrenoreceptors and an upregulation of brain α_2-adrenoreceptors. Still, findings suggesting an activation of central noradrenergic neurons with electrically induced seizures have not been corroborated in clinical populations.

The potent hypothalamic and pituitary activating effects of ECT (61) have been of great interest, given the high prevalence of hypothalamic-pituitary-adrenal axis dysregulation in depression. It is common for improvement in vegetative functioning to precede clinical elevation of mood in patients responding to ECT.

In addition to the foregoing work, considerable research activity is also being directed toward the possibility that endogenous peptide compounds with antidepressant, antimanic, or antipsychotic properties may be produced in response to induced seizure activity. Discovery of such products would go a long way toward the development of new, more potent psychotropic agents which might eventually replace ECT.

EDUCATION AND TRAINING

To assure that ECT is carried out in a safe and effective fashion, individuals involved in its administration, including anesthesia providers and nursing personnel, as well as psychiatrists, should receive adequate training. In addition, facilities providing ECT should exercise control over the competence of practitioners by means of local privileging.

Educational experiences related to ECT should be incorporated into medical and nursing school curricula. Exposure to ECT during psychiatric residency training should include both didactic presentations and practical experience. Such training should be provided by faculty who themselves are clinically privileged in ECT. Opportunity should also be provided for postgraduate continuing medical education in ECT. Such programs include practically oriented courses and symposia at regional and national professional meetings, and clinical ECT updates, courses, and fellowships at the local level. Examples of the latter type of programs are provided by the departments of psychiatry at Duke University Medical Center and State University of New York at Stony Brook.

REFERENCES

1. Abrams, R. (1988). *Electroconvulsive Therapy.* New York, Oxford Press.
2. Malitz, S. and Sackeim, H. A., eds. (1986). *Electroconvulsive Therapy: Clinical and Basic Research Issues.* New York, New York Academy of Sciences.
3. Glenn, M. D. and Weiner, R. D. (1985). *Practical Aspects of Electroconvulsive Therapy: A Programmed Text.* Washington, D.C., American Psychiatric Press, p. 147.

3a. American Psychiatric Assoc. (1990). *The Practice of ECT: Recommendations for Treatment, Training and Privileging.* Washington, D.C., American Psychiatric Press, Inc.

4. Nyro, J. and Jablonszky, A. (1929). Einige daten zur prognose der epilepsie: Mit

besonderer ruecksicht auf die konstitution. *Psychiatr. Neurol. Wochenschr. 31*: 547-549.

5. Wagner von Jauregg, J. (1922). The treatment of general paresis by inoculation of malaria. *J. Nerv. Ment. Dis. 55*:369-375.
6. Fink, M. (1984). Meduna and the origins of convulsive therapy. *Am. J. Psychiatry 141*:1034-1041.
7. Cerletti, U. and Bini, L. (1938). Un nuevo metodo di shockterapie "L'elettroshock." *Boll. Acad. Med. Roma 64*:136-138.
8. American Psychiatric Association Task Force on ECT (1978). *Electroconvulsive Therapy*. Task Force Report No. 14. Washington, D.C., American Psychiatric Association.
9. Thompson, J. W. and Blaine, J. D. (1987). Use of ECT in the United States in 1975 and 1980. *Am. J. Psychiatry 144*:557-562.
10. Consensus Conference, Electroconvulsive Therapy (1985). *JAMA 254*:2103-2108.
11. Weiner, R. D. and Coffey, C. E. (1988). Indications for use of electroconvulsive therapy. In *Review of Psychiatry*, Vol. 7. Edited by A. J. Francis and R. E. Hales. Washington, D.C., American Psychiatric Press, pp. 458-481.
12. Gregory, S., Shawcross, C. R., and Gill, D. (1985). The Nottingham ECT study: A double-blind comparison of bilateral, unilateral and stimulated ECT in depressive illness. *Br. J. Psychiatry 146*:520-524.
13. Zimmerman, M., Coryell, W., Stangl, D., and Pfohl, B. (1986). An American validation study of the Newcastle Scale. III. Course during index hospitalization and six-month prospective follow-up. *Acta Psychiatr. Scand. 73*:412-415.
14. Carney, M. W. P., Rolf, M., and Garside, R. F. (1965). The diagnosis of depressive reactions and the prediction of ECT response. *Br. J. Psychiatry 111*: 659-674.
15. Small, J. G. (1985). Efficacy of electroconvulsive therapy in schizophrenia, mania, and other disorders. II. Mania and other disorders. *Conv. Ther. 1*:271-276.
16. Small, J. G., Klapper, M. H., Kellams, J. J., Miller, M. J., Milstein, V., Sharpley, P. H., and Small, I. F. (1988). Electroconvulsive treatment compared with lithium in the management of manic states. *Arch. Gen. Psychiatry 45*:727-732.
17. Mukerjee, S., Sackeim, H. A., and Lee, C. (1988). Unilateral ECT in the treatment of manic episodes. *Conv. Ther. 4*:74-80.
18. Small, J. G. (1985). Efficacy of electroconvulsive therapy in schizophrenia, mania, and other disorders. I. Schizophrenia. *Conv. Ther. 1*:263-270.
19. Small, J. G., Milstein, V., Klapper, M. H., Kellams, J. J., and Small, I. F. (1982). ECT combined with neuroleptics in the treatment of schizophrenia. *Psychopharmacol. Bull. 18*:34-35.
20. Weiner, R. D. and Coffey, C. E. (1987). Electroconvulsive therapy in the medically ill. In *Principles of Medical Psychiatry*. Edited by A. Stoudemire and B. Fogel. New York, pp. 113-133.
21. Prudic, J., Sackeim, H. A., Decina, P., Hopkins, N., Ross, F., and Malitz, S. (1987). Acute effects of ECT on cardiovascular functioning: Relations to patient and treatment variables. *Acta Psychiatr. Scand. 75*:344-351.
22. Dec, G. W., Jr., Stern, T. A., and Welch, C. (1985). The effects of electroconvulsive therapy on serial electrocardiograms and serum cardiac enzyme values: A prospective study of depressed hospitalized inpatients. *JAMA 253*:2525-2529.

23. Ottosson, J.-O. (1962). Seizure characteristics and therapeutic efficiency in electroconvulsive therapy: An analysis of the antidepressive efficiency of grand mal and lidocaine-modified seizures. *J. Nerv. Ment. Dis. 135*:239-251.
24. Weiner, R. D. (1984). Does ECT cause brain damage? *Behav. Brain Sci. 7*:1-53.
25. Bolwig, T. (1988). Blood-brain barrier studies with special reference to epileptic seizures. *Acta Psychiatr. Scand. Suppl. 345*:15-20.
26. Meldrum, B. S., Vigouroux, R. A., and Bierley, J. B. (1973). Systemic factors in epileptic damage: Prolonged procedures in paralyzed artifically ventilated baboons. *Arch. Neurol. 29*:82-87.
27. Coffey, C. E., Figiel, G. S., Djang, W. T., Sullivan, D. C., Herfkens, R. J., and Weiner, R. D. (1988). Effects of ECT on brain structure: A pilot prospective magnetic resonance imaging study. *Am. J. Psychiatry 145*:701-706.
28. Hoyle, N. R., Pratt, R. T. C., and Thomas, D. G. T. (1984). Effect of electroconvulsive therapy on serum myelin basic protein immunoreactivity. *Br. Med. J. 288*:1110-1111.
29. Weiner, R. D. (1983). EEG related to electroconvulsive therapy. In *EEG and Evoked Potentials in Psychiatry and Behavioral Neurology*. Edited by J. R. Hughes, W. P. Wilson. Boston, Butterworth Publishers, pp. 101-126.
30. Weiner, R. D., Rogers, J. H., Davidson, J. R. T., and Kahn, E. M. (1986). Effects of ECT upon brain electrical activity. In *Electroconvulsive Therapy: Clinical and Basic Research Issues*. Edited by S. Malitz and H. A. Sackeim. New York, New York Academy of Sciences, pp. 270-281.
31. Abrams, R., Taylor, M. A., and Volovka, J. (1987). ECT-induced EEG assymmetry and therapeutic response in melancholia: Relation to treatment electrode placement. *Am. J. Psychiatry 144*:327-329.
32. Daniel, W. F. and Crovitz, H. F. (1982). The recovery of orientation after electroconvulsive therapy. A review. *Acta Psychiatr. Scand. 66*:421-428.
33. Daniel, W. F. and Crovitz, H. F. (1983). Acute memory impairment following electroconvulsive therapy. *Acta Psychiatr. Scand. 67*:1-7, 57-68.
34. Squire, L. R. (1986). Memory functions as affected by electroconvulsive therapy. In *Electroconvulsive Therapy: Clinical and Basic Research Issues*. Edited by S. Malitz and H. A. Sackeim. New York, New York Academy of Sciences, pp. 307-314.
35. Weiner, R. D., Rogers, H. J., Davidson, J. R. T., and Squire, L. R. (1986). Effects of stimulus parameters on cognitive side effects. In *Electroconvulsive Therapy: Clinical and Basic Research Issues*. Edited by S. Malitz and H. A. Sackeim. New York, New York Academy of Sciences, pp. 315-325.
36. Freeman, C. P. L. and Cheshire, K. E. (1986). Attitude studies on electroconvulsive therapy. *Conv. Ther. 2*:31-42.
37. Standish-Barry, H. M. A. S., Deacon, V., and Snaith, R. P. (1985). The relationship of concurrent benzodiazepine administration to seizure duration in ECT. *Acta Psychiatr. Scand. 71*:269-271.
38. Small, J. G., Kellams, J. J., Milstein, V. (1980). Complications with electroconvulsive treatment combined with lithium. *Biol. Psychiatry 15*:103-112.
39. Peters, S. G., Wochos, D. N., and Peterson, G. C. (1984). Status epilepticus complicating electroconvulsive therapy in the presence of theophylline. *Mayo Clin. Proc. 59*:568-570.

40. Culver, C. M., Ferrell, R. B., and Green, R. M. (1980). ECT and special problems of informed consent. *Am. J. Psychiatry 137*:586-591.
41. Bergsholm, P., Gran, L., and Bleie, H. (1984). Seizure duration in unilateral electroconvulsive therapy. The effect of hypocapnia induced by hyperventilation and the effect of ventilation with oxygen. *Acta Psychiatr. Scand. 69*:121-128.
42. Friedman, E. and Wilcox, P. H. (1942). Electrostimulated convulsive doses in intact humans by means of unidirectional currents. *J. Nerv. Ment. Dis. 96*:56-63.
43. Lancaster, N. P., Steinert, R. R., and Frost, I. (1958). Unilateral electroconvulsive therapy. *J. Ment. Sci. 104*:221-227.
44. Squire, L. R. and Slater, P. C. (1978). Bilateral and unilateral ECT: Effects on verbal and nonverbal memory. *Am. J. Psychiatry 135*:1316-1320.
45. Abrams, R. (1986). Is unilateral electroconvulsive therapy really the treatment of choice in endogenous depression? In *Electroconvulsive Therapy: Clinical and Basic Research Issues.* Edited by S. Malitz and H. A. Sackeim. New York, New York Academy of Sciences, pp. 50-55.
46. d'Elia, G. and Raotma, H. (1975). Is unilateral ECT less effective than bilateral ECT? *Br. J. Psychiatry 126*:83-89.
47. Weiner, R. D. and Coffey, C. E. (1986). Minimizing therapeutic differences between bilateral and unilateral nondominant ECT. *Conv. Ther. 2*:261-265.
48. d'Elia, G. (1970). Unilateral ECT. *Acta Psychiatr. Scand. 215*:1-98.
49. Liberson, W. T. (1948). Brief stimulus therapy. Physiological and chemical observations. *Am. J. Psychiatry 105*:28-39.
50. Robin, A. and de Tissera, S. (1982). A double-blind controlled comparison of the therapeutic effects of low and high energy electroconvulsive therapies. *Br. J. Psychiatry 141*:357-366.
51. Sackeim, H. A., Decina, P., Prohovnik, I., and Malitz, S. (1987). Seizure threshold in ECT: Effects of sex, age, electrode placement and number of treatments. *Arch. Gen. Psychiatry 44*:355-360.
52. Sackeim, H. A., Decina, P., Kanzler, M., Kerr, B., and Malitz, S. (1987). Effects of electrode placement on the efficacy of titrated, low-dose ECT. *Am. J. Psychiatry 144*:1449-1455.
53. Maletzky, B. M. (1981). *Multiple-Monitored Electroconvulsive Therapy.* Boca Raton, Fla., CRC Press.
54. Weiner, R. D. (1982). The role of ECT in the treatment of depression in the elderly. *J. Am. Geriatr. Soc. 30*:710-712.
55. Frances, A., Weiner, R. D., and Coffey, C. E. (1989). ECT for an elderly man with psychotic depression and concurrent dementia. *Hosp. Comm. Psychiatry 40*:237-242.
56. Wisner, K. L. and Perel, J. M. (1988). Pharmacologic agents and electroconvulsive therapy during pregnancy and the puerperium. In *Psychiatric Consultation in Childbirth Settings: Parent and Child-Oriented Approaches.* Edited by R. L. Cohen. New York, Plenum, pp. 165-206.
57. Imlah, N. W., Ryan, E., and Harrington, J. A. (1964). The influence of antidepressant drugs on the response to electroconvulsive therapy and on subsequent relapse rates. *Neuropsychopharmacology 4*:438-442.

58. Kramer, B. A. (1987). Maintenance ECT: A survey of practice (1986). *Conv. Ther. 3*:260-268.
59. Sackeim, H. A., Decina, P., Prohovnik, I., Malitz, S., and Resor, S. R. (1983). Anticonvulsant and antidepressant properties of electroconvulsive therapy: A proposed mechanism of action. *Biol. Psychiatry 18*:1301-1310.
60. Lerer, B. and Shapira, B. (1986). Neurochemical mechanisms of mood stabilization: Focus on electroconvulsive therapy. In *Electroconvulsive Therapy: Clinical and Basic Research Issues.* Edited by S. Malitz and H. A. Sackeim. New York. New York Academy of Sciences, pp. 366-375.
61. Fink, M. (1980). A neuroendocrine theory of convulsive therapy. *Trends Neurosci. 3*:25-27.

12

Lithium Potentiation of Antidepressants

JANUSZ K. RYBAKOWSKI

Medical Academy of Bydgoczcz
Bydgoszcz, Poland

DEPRESSION UNRESPONSIVE TO TREATMENT WITH ANTIDEPRESSANT DRUGS

Clinical Factors

The clinical efficacy of most antidepressant drugs in an average population of patients with unipolar or bipolar depressive disorder approaches only 65-70% (1), leaving a remaining 30% who require additional treatment. In addition, there is a relative lack of evidence for the superiority of any antidepressant drug in treating specific subtypes of depression, with the following exceptions: clomipramine in depression with obsessive-compulsive features (2) and monoamine oxidase inhibitors (MAOIs) in "atypical" depression with anxiety traits (3). Finally, many patients with delusional depression usually respond poorly to antidepressant drugs alone and have a better antidepressant response when a neuroleptic agent is used in combination or they are given electroconvulsive therapy (ECT) (4,5).

Pharmacokinetic Factors

With some antidepressant drugs, there is a relationship between the clinical efficacy and the plasma drug level (6-8). In addition, a dose-dependent effect has been demonstrated for MAOIs (9). It has been suggested that achieving a therapeutic plasma level with adequate doses of antidepressants may increase the response rate in depressed patients to 80-85% (10).

Pharmacodynamic Factors

Despite that they have received an adequate dose of an antidepressant, achieved optimal plasma levels, and maintained treatment for a sufficient period, 15-20% of depressed patients remain unresponsive to treatment. The reasons for this are not fully understood, but it may be due to insufficient interaction of the antidepressant drug at the receptor sites in the central nervous system (CNS). For example, in delusional depression, a disturbance of the dopaminergic receptor is postulated, which might not be appreciably affected by most antidepressant drugs (11). In addition, the development of tolerance to the therapeutic effects of antidepressants has also been described (12). Such patients may have a remission of symptoms with initial antidepressant treatment, but may relapse within weeks or months. Lieb and Balter (13) called this phenomenon "antidepressant tachyphylaxis" and postulated that it might result in an alteration of receptor function, depletion of neurotransmitter precursors, or calcium ion changes. Finally, Vinar (14) put forward a hypothesis, that certain immunodeficiencies, reflected by the disordered process of drug binding to the receptors, could be connected with the pharmacoresistance of some depressed patients.

Antidepressant Potentiation Measures

Various procedures have been proposed for depressions unresponsive to treatment with antidepressants. As early as 1963, Poldinger (15) described a potentiating effect of intramuscular reserpine in treatment-resistant depression. This effect is presumably caused by the rapid depletion of biogenic amines from intracellular compartments into synaptic clefts. The addition of the thyroid hormone, triiodothyronine, was found to potentiate the effect of antidepressant medication in female patients (16). In one study, three out of four tricyclic antidepressant-resistant patients improved significantly after the addition of triiodothyronine (17), and it was speculated that this antidepressant potentiation may result from the sensitization of central noradrenergic receptors by triiodothyronine. Finally, there is some recent experimental data suggesting the possibility of a synergistic effect of calcium channel blockers with antidepressants in animal models of depression (18).

LITHIUM AS AN ANTIDEPRESSANT DRUG

The role of lithium carbonate as an antidepressant and its ability to potentiate the antidepressant effect of other drugs will be briefly reviewed. The lithium ion has achieved a recognized place in the prevention of mania; however, the pharmacologic spectrum of lithium now also covers its antidepressant action. This refers to an acute antidepressant action as well as the prophylaxis of depressive episodes in both bipolar and recurrent unipolar affective illness.

Efficacy in an Acute Depressive Episode

Most controlled studies have shown an antidepressant action by lithium in certain subgroups of depressed patients (19); however, this is still somewhat controversial. The overall quality of acute antidepressant efficacy of lithium is lower than that of conventional antidepressants, with substantial effect in only 50-60% of patients (20). Thus, lithium is not a first-choice drug for the treatment of acute endogenous depression. Nevertheless, it does appear to be increasingly used as an initial antidepressant treatment in many bipolar depressed patients who would ultimately benefit from lithium prophylaxis.

A number of studies have attempted to identify specific clinical or biochemical features of lithium responders in acute depression. They showed some evidence that patients with a diagnosis or family history of bipolar illness might respond more favorably than those with a diagnosis of unipolar depression or without a family history of affective illness (21,22). Furthermore, it appears that a good therapeutic response to lithium may be more likely in patients with a classic endogenous symptom patterns and depressive episodes not linked to environmental events (23,24). Altered biochemical parameters, such as an increased erythrocyte/lithium ratio (25), lower urinary 3-methoxy-4-hydroxyphenylglycol (MHPG) excretion and cerebrospinal fluid 5-hydroxyindoleacetic acid (5-HIAA) level (26,27), have also been suggested as indicating a better response to lithium in depression.

In the search to delineate a lithium-responsive depression, some authors have advocated a lithium trial in patients previously unresponsive to tricyclic antidepressants, MAOIs, or ECT. Neubauer and Bermingham (28) described 20 depressive patients with a positive family history and clinical features of low energy, obsessional and hypochondriacal traits, who failed to respond to conventional antidepressant treatments, but rapidly responding to lithium. Kupfer et al. (29) identified the symptoms of hypersomnia and hyperphagia in depressed patients responsive to lithium and less so to tricyclic antidepressants.

The usual time course for therapeutic action of lithium in depression resembles that of tricyclic antidepressants, with a gradual improvement beginning in 2-4 weeks. However, a dramatic improvement of depression within several days has also been observed (19,28).

The plasma lithium level necessary for achieving optimal antidepressant response is not fully established; however, in most studies, a standard serum lithium concentration of 0.6-1.4 mmol/L was used (19). Some investigators recommend keeping the lithium level within the upper limit of this range while treating depression (24,30).

Prophylactic Efficacy Against Depression

Lithium remains the unsurpassed modality for the prophylaxis of depressive episodes in bipolar as well as unipolar affective illness (31). It has been suggested that lithium prevents the occurrence of depressive episodes in bipolar illness by preventing mania, and that its prophylactic effect is better in patients with a mania-depression sequence of episodes compared with those having a depression-mania sequence (32). The quality of this prophylactic effect may depend on gender (33). To date, no other drug has been found to have a better prophylactic efficacy against both depression and mania. The prophylactic action of the lithium-carbamazepine combination, which may be superior to lithium alone (34), has not been fully estimated. (A more complete discussion of carbamazepine in preventing affective episodes can be found in Chap. 8.)

Recent investigations clearly show that the quality of lithium's prophylactic effect in unipolar depression is similar to that in bipolar illness, and it has also been shown to be equal or better than that of other antidepressant drugs (35,36). Thus, for long-term prophylaxis of recurrent depressive episodes, lithium is still the drug of choice. Furthermore, it has been suggested that a good therapeutic effect of lithium in an acute depressive episode might also be an indicator of subsequent favorable prophylactic efficacy (37). Finally, there has been a tendency to keep the prophylactic lithium level within the lower range (i.e., 0.5-0.8 mmol/L) (38), to reduce the potential for renal damage and other side effects.

COMBINING LITHIUM AND ANTIDEPRESSANTS

Concomitant Administration

The first controlled study of the concomitant administration of lithium and antidepressants was published in 1974 (39). This comprised 45 patients randomly assigned to either a tricyclic antidepressant alone or to a combination with lithium. Lithium did not appear to interfere adversely with the therapeutic effect of the tricyclic antidepressant and, in some cases, appeared to synergize with its action. Two years later Nick et al. (40) compared the effect of clomipramine and lithium versus clomipramine alone in a double-blind trial in bipolar and unipolar patients and concluded that the combination was no better than treatment with clomipramine alone. This was in contrast with O'Flanagan (41), who observed a synergistic action of clomipramine and lithium. Similarly, Worall et al. (42) compared the antidepressant effect of tryptophan alone or in combination with lithium and found a superior antidepressant action with the combination. Thus, it may be concluded that lithium given jointly with antidepressants in an acute depressive episode may demonstrate a synergistic effect.

There have also been studies comparing the prophylactic efficacy of a combination of antidepressants and lithium with lithium alone in depression. These have shown no superiority for the lithium-antidepressant combination over that of lithium alone in unipolar and bipolar illness (43,44).

Adding Antidepressants to Lithium

Addition of an antidepressant to the lithium regimen has been a frequent practice when a patient relapses on prophylactic lithium. There is controversy over which antidepressant should be added, and for how long. Himmelhoch et al. (45) suggested using the MAOI, tranylcypromine, with lithium, if there was insufficient effect from adding a tricyclic. The successful use of lithium in combination with isocarboxazid was also described by Zall (46).

In contrast, reports have suggested that, in bipolar patients, the addition of antidepressants to lithium for a prolonged period may adversely affect the course of illness (e.g., by inducing rapid cycling) (47). At least one group of investigators (48) discourages adding antidepressants for patients who become depressed on a lithium regimen, because the combination could reduce the prophylactic effect of lithium.

Adding Lithium to Antidepressants

The addition of lithium to an antidepressant regimen may "potentiate" or "augment" the antidepressant effect (49,50). Subsequently, it was suggested that sequential administration of an antidepressant and then lithium may be necessary for this potentiation (49,50).

LITHIUM POTENTIATION OF ANTIDEPRESSANTS

Lingjaerde et al. (39) initially suggested that candidates for prophylactic lithium treatment should be started on lithium therapy during the depressive episode, while the patient is taking an antidepressant, but not yet in remission. Neubauer and Birmingham (28) demonstrated that of 20 refractory depressed patients experiencing a rapid effect from lithium, nine had lithium introduced while they were receiving a tricyclic antidepressant.

Subsequent studies of lithium potentiation have reported on more than 200 patients (49-75). Most have been small, uncontrolled studies, but several large well-designed trials have been presented by De Montigny et al. (53) in 39 patients and by Price et al. (69) in 84 patients.

The Type of Preceding Antidepressant

There have been a wide range of antidepressants used with lithium as shown in Table 1.

The most frequent have been tricyclic antidepressants. Trials of MAOIs, as well as a variety of atypical antidepressants have also been used in combination with lithium (73,74).

Although most reports have evaluated the addition of lithium to an antidepressant, there is also evidence that the reverse sequence can be beneficial. A lithium-tranylcypromine succession was described by Price et al. (62), in which tranylcypromine was added to lithium in patients showing unsuccessful

Table 1 Antidepressants Used with Lithium

Antidepressant	Ref. (No.)
Tricyclic antidepressants	
Imipramine	De Montigny et al. (53); Roy and Pickar (63)
Amitriptyline	De Montigny et al. (53); Rybakowski and Matkowski (71)
Desipramine	De Montigny et al. (53); Price et al. (69)
Clomipramine	Schreder and Levien (64); Rybakowski and Matkowski (71)
Trimipramine	De Montigny et al. (53)
Nortriptyline	Price et al. (69)
Noxiptyline	Rybakowski and Matkowski (71)
Doxepin	De Montigny et al. (53)
Dothiepin	Joyce et al. (55); Pai et al. (68)
MAOI	
Phenelzine	Nelson and Byck (52)
Tranylcypromine	Price et al. (62)
Atypical antidepressants	
Adinazolam	Price et al. (69)
Bupropion	Price et al. (69)
Carbamazepine	Post and Kramlinger (73); Rybakowski and Matkowski (74)
Fluvoxamine	Price et al. (69)
Iprindole	De Montigny et al. (61)
Maprotiline	Weaver (57); Kushmir (70)
Mianserin	Pai et al. (68); Price et al. (69)
Nomifensine	Rybakowski and Matkowski (71)
Trazodone	Birkhimer et al. (54); Price et al. (69)
Zimelidine	Joyce (65)

potentiation by other antidepressants, whereas Joyce et al. (55) added dothiepin to lithium after patients failed to respond to a phenelzine-lithium combination.

Finally, the few patients in these reports do not allow a definite conclusion about the superiority of one prelithium drug over another. However, the study of Price et al. (69) suggests that the use of trazodone before lithium may be less effective than other antidepressants. This, however, is in contrast with other reports describing good effects with the trazodone-lithium sequence (54,70).

The Type of Depression

Although most reports on lithium potentiation have examined unipolar depressives, this effect is also found in patients with bipolar illness. Price et al. (69) suggest a trend for better efficacy in unipolar depression. However, Nelson and Mazure (67) and Rybakowski and Matkowski (74) demonstrated better results in bipolar patients.

Patients with delusional depression have also been described in reports on lithium augmentation. Nelson and Mazure (67) studied 21 patients and found that the addition of lithium was successful when added to an antidepressant-neuroleptic combination. Furthermore, the addition of lithium to an antidepressant alone has also resulted in a substantial improvement or remission of symptoms in delusional depressives (57,68).

Regarding age limitations for lithium potentiation, several recent studies have demonstrated that the addition of lithium to another antidepressant in geriatric patients has been well tolerated (75,76), and Kushmir (70) achieved good results by the addition of small doses of lithium to antidepressants in five medically ill geriatric depressed patients aged 65-93 years.

Time Course of Lithium Potentiation

De Montigny et al. (49,53) observed a rapid onset of lithium potentiation within 48 hr, but this was not confirmed in subsequent studies. Although many patients showed marked improvement within the first week, most gradually improved over 4 weeks. In the study by Price et al. (69), only three patients out of 26 had marked improvement within the first few days. In our study 8 out of 24 patients showed significant improvement within the first week (74).

Lithium Dose and Serum Lithium Level

In most lithium potentiation studies the serum lithium level was kept within the recommended therapeutic range. However, beneficial effects have also been observed at lower concentrations. For example, De Montigny et al. (53) observed rapid potentiation with lithium levels of 0.4 mmol/L, and Kushmir (70) and others (76) showed that geriatric depressives had good response at lithium levels in the range of 0.2-0.3 mmol/L. Recently, Stein and Bernadt (72), compared the efficacy of the addition of 250 mg of lithium carbonate versus 750 mg, in 26 patients with tricyclic-resistant depression, and one-third of their patients responded at serum lithium levels in the range of 0.1-0.3 mmol/L.

Overall Efficacy

The cumulative data on efficacy of lithium potentiation may be misleading because the causistic and small sample studies bias the estimation toward more favorable results. De Montigny et al. (53) found more than 50% improvement within 48 hr in 72% of the unipolar patients. Price et al. (69) observed that 56% of their patients had significant response within 4 weeks, whereas Nelson and Mazure (67) reported their response rate was 53%. The small sample studies demonstrated efficacy in an even greater percentage of patients (58,71). Therefore, a beneficial effect of lithium might be anticipated in at least half of antidepressant-resistant depressives within 4 weeks and in a substantial proportion within the first week.

Side Effects

The addition of lithium to antidepressants is generally well tolerated and the prevalence of side effects does not appear to be high. De Montigny et al. (53) reported immediate side effects after lithium was added in 3 of 39 patients receiving tricyclics (including tremor, abdominal pain, pruritus), whereas Nelson and Mazure (67) observed tremor in only 4 of 21 patients in whom lithium was added. In our study of ten patients, tremor was observed in three patients and fatigue and muscle weakness in two (71). Hand tremor appears to be the most frequent side effect when lithium is introduced to tricyclic antidepressants. This symptom may be more intense with higher serum lithium levels or when lithium is added to an antidepressant-neuroleptic combination. Lithium-induced immediate side effects are usually transient and subside after the reduction of dose or a discontinuation of lithium.

A worsening of depression after lithium addition has been described in 4 of 84 patients (69), and several cases of lithium-induced hypomania in the course of lithium-antidepressant potentiation have also been reported (59, 60).

MECHANISMS OF LITHIUM POTENTIATION

Pharmacokinetic Factors

There is no evidence that lithium may exert an augmenting therapeutic effect by means of the increasing plasma levels of the antidepressant drug (53).

Serotoninergic Mechanisms

The most convincing hypothesis concerning the mechanism of lithium potentiation of antidepressants postulates a lithium-antidepressant interaction at central serotoninergic synapses (53). Some experimental studies have shown that pretreatment with different antidepressant drugs can cause an increased sensitivity of brain neurons to serotonin occurring by several mechanisms (77-79). Short-term lithium administration exerts a presynaptic serotoninergic effect by augmenting tryptophan transport into nerve cells and augmenting serotonin receptor sensitivity (80,81). Thus, interaction of lithium and antidepressant drugs will markedly potentiate the serotoninergic mechanisms. Such mechanisms may also operate in the potentiation of certain antidepressants by tryptophan (82,83), and in the antidepressant synergism of tryptophan and lithium (42). Therefore, it appears that the activity of serotonergic mechanisms are potentiated by lithium and play an important role both in the treatment of acute depression and in the prophylaxis of depression (but not in mania) (84,85).

Others

Central noradrenergic mechanisms may be of less significance in lithium-antidepressant protentiation (86).

Lithium has also been shown to have an attenuating effect on dopamine receptors (87), and this interaction may contribute to its therapeutic effect in delusional depression. Finally, the modifying effect of lithium on central synapses by means of other mechanisms, such as inhibition of phosphatidylinositol metabolism or calcium transport, cannot be excluded (88). A synergistic action of calcium antagonists and antidepressants on animals models of depression appears to be mediated, in part, through their effect on the serotonergic system (89).

PRACTICAL RECOMMENDATIONS

Patients

On the basis of this review, the introduction of lithium appears to be a therapeutic modality worth considering for a broad range of antidepressant-resistant patients. It may be expected that a substantial symptomatic improvement can be achieved in at least half of the patients. Such a trial would be especially recommended in patients whose course of the disease makes them candidates for subsequent lithium prophylaxis. This option could also be particularly helpful to the patient who is reluctant to undergo ECT treatment, or if such treatment has proved ineffective.

Old age is not a critical factor and lithium augmentation may achieve good results in older patients with concomitant medical illness.

Specific clinical or biochemical factors predicting a favorable effect of lithium potentiation have not yet been elucidated. Finally, it may be speculated that depressions with disordered function of central serotonergic synapses are the best target for lithium potentiation. This should be a subject of further studies.

Procedure

Lithium therapy may be started in doses appropriate for obtaining a serum concentration of 0.5-0.8 mmol/L. Initially, serum lithium levels should be monitored weekly, and the dose adjusted accordingly, then levels should be obtained at least every 6 weeks.

In geriatric patients or patients with medical conditions that could interfere with lithium therapy, it is advisable to begin with smaller doses (e.g., 150-300 mg of lithium carbonate daily), reaching serum lithium levels of 0.2-0.3 mmol/L. Then, the dose of lithium may be gradually increased, if therapeutic effect is not optimal within 2-3 weeks. Also, in patients with a "therapeutic" serum lithium level, the dose can be reduced in the event of troublesome side effects.

The assessment period for the efficacy of lithium addition should not exceed 4-6 weeks. If the response is poor, lithium should be discontinued, and another treatment approach should be implemented. With good results, lithium should be continued for at least 2-3 months. How long should the antidepressants be continued? This depends on whether the patient has unipolar or bipolar illness. Clinical experience suggests that in patients with bipolar illness, after achieving a normothymic state, the antidepressants (especially tricyclics) should be withdrawn and the patient left on lithium. In unipolar depression there is less concern about concomitant administration of lithium and antidepressant for a longer time, and withdrawal of the antidepressant may even precipitate a depressive relapse. Thus, in unipolar illness, the decision concerning the composition of drugs for prophylaxis should be judiciously considered.

REFERENCES

1. Ban, T. A. (1981). Chemotherapy of depression. In *Prevention and Treatment of Depression.* Edited by T. A. Ban, R. Gonzalez, A. S. Jablensky, N. A. Sartorius, and F. E. Vartanian. Baltimore, University Park Press, pp. 161-172.

2. Volavka, J., Neziroglu, F., and Yaryura-Tobias, J. A. (1985). Clomipramine and imipramine in obsessive-compulsive disorder. *Psychiatr. Res. 14*:83-91.
3. Liebowitz, M. R., Quitkin, F. M., Stewart, J. W., McGrath, P. J., Harrison, W., Rabkin, J., Tricamo, E., Markowitz, J. S., and Klein, D. F. (1984). Phenelzine v. imipramine in atypical depression. *Arch. Gen. Psychiatry 41*:669-676.
4. Glassman, A. H., Kantor, S. J., and Shostak, M. (1975). Depression, delusion and drug response. *Am. J. Psychiatry 132*:716-719.
5. Spiker, D. G., Perel, J. M., Hanin, I., Dealy, R. S., Griffin, S. J., Soloff, P. H., and Cofsky-Weiss, J. (1986). The pharmacological treatment of delusional depression: Part II. *J. Clin. Psychopharmacol. 6*:339-342.
6. Simpson, G. M., White, K. L., Boyd, J. L., Cooper, T. B., Halaris, A., Wilson, I. C., Raman, E. J., and Ruther, E. (1982). Relationship between plasma antidepressant levels and clinical outcome for inpatients receiving imipramine. *Am. J. Psychiatry 139*:358-360.
7. Ziegler, V., Co, B. T., Taylor, J., Clayton, P., and Biggs, J. (1976). Amitriptyline plasma levels and therapeutic response. *Clin. Pharmacol. Ther. 19*:795-801.
8. Burrows, G., Scoggins, G., Tuereck, L., and Davies, B. (1974). Plasma nortriptyline and clinical response. *Clin. Pharmacol. Ther. 16*:639-644.
9. Tyrer, P., Gardner, M., Lambourn, J., and Whitford, M. (1980). Clinical and pharmacokinetic factors affecting response to phenelzine. *Br. J. Psychiatry 136*:359-365.
10. Glassman, A., Perel, J., Shostak, M., Kantor, S., and Fleiss, J. (1977). Clinical implications of imipramine plasma levels for depressive illness. *Arch. Gen. Psychiatry 34*:197-204.
11. Exstein, I. and Bowers, M. B. (1975). The pharmacological meaning of successful antipsychotic-antidepressant combination. *Compr. Psychiatry 16*:427-431.
12. Cohen, B. M. and Baldessarini, R. J. (1985). Tolerance to therapeutic effects of antidepressants. *Am. J. Psychiatry 142*:489-490.
13. Lieb, J. and Balter, A. (1984). Antidepressant tachyphylaxis. *Med. Hypotheses 15*:279-291.
14. Vinar, O. (1987). Binding of drugs to receptors: A quasiimmune process. Presented at European College of Neuro-Psychopharmacology Conference, Brussels, May 7-8.
15. Poldinger, W. (1963). Combined administration of desipramine and reserpine or tetrabenazine in depressive patients. *Psychopharmacology 4*:308-310.
16. Prange, A. J., Wilson, I. C., Rabon, A. M., and Lipton, M. A. (1969). Enhancement of imipramine antidepressant activity by thyroid hormone. *Am. J. Psychiatry 126*:457-469.
17. Goodwin, F. K., Prange, A. J., Post, R. M., Muscattola, G., and Lipton, M. A. (1982). Potentiation of antidepressant effects by L-triiodothyronine in tricyclic non-responders. *Am. J. Psychiatry 139*:34-38.
18. Mogilnicka, E., Czyrak, A., and Maj, J. (1987). Dihydropyridine calcium channel antagonists reduce immobility in the mouse behavioral despair test: Antidepressants facilitate nifedipine action. *Eur. J. Pharmacol. 138*:413-416.
19. Ramsey, T. A. and Mendels, J. (1980). Lithium in the acute treatment of depression. In *Handbook of Lithium Therapy*. Edited by F. N. Johnson. Lancaster, MTP Press, pp. 17-25.

20. Nahunek, K., Svestka, J., and Rodova, A. (1970). Zur Stellung der Lithium in der Gruppe der Antidepressiva in der Behandlung von akuten endogenen und Involutionsdepressionen. *Int. Pharmacopsychiatry 5*:249-257.
21. Baron, M., Gershon, E. S., Rudy, W., Jonas, W. Z., and Buchsbaum, M. (1975). Lithium carbonate response in depression: Prediction by unipolar/bipolar illness, average evoked response, catechol-*O*-methyltransferase and family history. *Arch. Gen. Psychiatry 32*:1107-1111.
22. Goodwin, F. K., Murphy, D. L., Dunner, D. L., and Bunney, W. E., Jr. (1972). Lithium response in unipolar versus bipolar depression. *Am. J. Psychiatry 129*: 44-47.
23. Dyson, W. L. and Mendels, J. (1968). Lithium and depression. *Curr. Ther. Res. 10*:601-608.
24. Noyes, R., Jr., Dempsey, G. M., Blum, A., and Cavanaugh, G. L. (1974). Lithium treatment of depression. *Compr. Psychiatry 15*:187-193.
25. Mendels, J. and Frazer, A. (1973). Intracellular lithium concentration and clinical response: Toward a membrane theory of depression. *J. Psychiat. Res. 10*:9-18.
26. Beckmann, H., St-Laurent, J., and Goodwin, F. K. (1975). The effect of lithium on urinary MHPG in unipolar and bipolar depressed patients. *Psychopharmacology 42*:277-282.
27. Goodwin, F. K., Post, R. M., and Dunner, D. L. (1973). Cerebrospinal fluid amines metabolites in affective illness. The probenecid technique. *Am. J. Psychiatry 130*:73-79.
28. Neubauer, H. and Bermingham, P. (1976). A depressive syndrome responsive to lithium. *J. Nerv. Ment. Dis. 163*:276-281.
29. Kupfer, D. J., Pickar, D., Himmelhoch, J. M., and Detre, T. P. (1975). Are there two types of unipolar depression? *Arch. Gen. Psychiatry 32*:866-871.
30. Friedel, R. O. (1976). Lithium and depression. *Am. J. Psychiatry 133*:976.
31. Rybakowski, J. (1981). Lithium prophylaxis of depression. In *Prevention and Treatment of Depression*. Edited by T. A. Ban, R. Gonzalez, A. S. Jablensky, N. A. Sartorius, and F. E. Vartanian. Baltimore, University Park Press, pp. 173-182.
32. Grof, E., Haag, M., Grof, P., and Haag, H. (1987). Lithium response and the sequence of episode polarities: Preliminary report on a Hamilton sample. *Prog. Neuropsychopharmacol. Biol. Psychiatry 77*:199-204.
33. Rybakowski, J., Chlopocka-Wozniak, M., Kapelski, Z., and Strzyzewski, W. (1980). The relative prophylactic efficacy of lithium against manic and depressive recurrences in bipolar patients. *Int. Pharmacopsychiatry 15*:86-90.
34. Svestka, J., Nahunek, K., and Ceskova, E. (1987). Combined lithium and carbamazepine is more effective in the prophylaxis of affective psychoses than lithium alone. *Act. Nerv. Super.* (*Praha*) *29*:184-185.
35. Quitkin, F., Rifkin, A., and Klein, D. F. (1976). Prophylaxis of affective disorders: Current status of knowledge. *Arch. Gen. Psychiatry 33*:337-341.
36. Coppen, A., Ghose, K., Rao, R., Bailey, J., and Peet, M. (1978). Mianserin and lithium in the prophylaxis of depression. *Br. J. Psychiatry 133*:206-210.
37. Svestka, J. and Nahunek, K. (1975). The result of lithium therapy in acute phases of affective psychoses and some other prognostical factors of lithium prophylaxis. *Act. Nerv. Super.* (*Praha*) *17*:270-271.

38. Schou, M. (1984). Causes of and remedies for incomplete response to lithium. In *Frontiers in Biochemical and Pharmacological Research in Depression*. Edited by E. Usdin. New York, Raven Press, pp. 413-420.
39. Lingjaerde, O., Edlund, A. H., Gormsen, C. A., Gottfries, C. G., Haugstad, A., Hermann, I. L., Hollnagel, P., Makimattila, A., Rasmusen, K. E., Remvig, J., and Robak, O. H. (1974). The effects of lithium carbonate in combination with tricyclic antidepressants in endogenous depression. *Acta Psychiatr. Scand. 50*:233-242.
40. Nick, J., Luante, J. P., Des Lauriers, A., Moinet, A., and Monfort, J. (1976). L' association clomipramine-lithium, essai controle. *Encephale 2*:5-16.
41. O'Flanagan, P. M. (1973). Clomipramine infusion and lithium carbonate: A synergistic effect. *Lancet 2*:974.
42. Worall, E. P., Moody, J. P., Peet, M., Dick, P., Smith, A., Chambers, C., Adams, M., and Naylor, G. J. (1979). Controlled studies of the acute antidepressant effects of lithium. *Br. J. Psychiatry 135*:255-262.
43. Peselow, E. D., Gulbenkian, G., Dunner, D. L., Fieve, R. R., and Burdock, E. I. (1980). Lithium, tricyclics and lithium + tricyclics in the prophylaxis of unipolar illness. *IRCS Med. Sci. 8*:524-525.
44. Kane, J. M., Quitkin, F. M., Rifkin, A., Ramos-Lorenzi, J. R., Nayak, D. D., and Howard, A. (1982). Lithium carbonate and imipramine in the prophylaxis of unipolar and bipolar II illness. *Arch. Gen. Psychiatry 39*:1065-1069.
45. Himmelhoch, J. M., Detre, T., Kupfer, D. J., Schwartzburg, M., and Byck, R. (1972). Treatment of previously intractable depression with tranylcypromine. *J. Nerv. Ment. Dis. 155*:216-220.
46. Zall, H. (1971). Lithium carbonate and isocarbazid—an effective drug approach in severe depression. *Am. J. Psychiatry 127*:1400-1403.
47. Wehr, T. A. and Goodwin, F. K. (1979). Rapid cycling in manic-depressives induced by tricyclic antidepressants. *Arch. Gen. Psychiatry 36*:555-559.
48. Reginaldi, D., Tondo, L., Floris, G., Pignatelli, A., and Kukopulos, A. (1981). Poor prophylactic lithium response due to antidepressants. *Int. Pharmacopsychiatry 16*:124-128.
49. De Montigny, C., Grunberg, F., Mayer, A., and Dechenes, J. P. (1981). Lithium induced rapid relief of depression in tricyclic antidepressant drug non-responders. *Br. J. Psychiatry 138*:252-256.
50. Heninger, G. R., Charney, D. S., and Sternberg, D. E. (1983). Lithium carbonate augmentation of antidepressant treatment: An effective prescription for treatment-resistant depression. *Arch. Gen. Psychiatry 40*:1335-1342.
51. Ayd, F. J. (1981). New hope for tricyclic refractory unipolar depression. *Drug Ther. Newslett. 16*:25-27.
52. Nelson, J. C. and Byck, R. (1982). Rapid response to lithium in phenelzine nonresponders. *Br. J. Psychiatry 141*:85-86.
53. De Montigny, C., Cournoyer, G., Morissette, R., Langlois, R., and Caille, G. (1983). Lithium carbonate addition in tricyclic antidepressant-resistant unipolar depression. *Arch. Gen. Psychiatry 40*:1327-1334.
54. Birkhimer, L. J., Alderman, A. A., Schmitt, C. E., and Ednie, K. J. (1983). Combined trazodone-lithium therapy for refractory depression. *Am. J. Psychiatry 140*: 1382-1383.

55. Joyce, P. R., Hewland, H. R., and Jones, A. V. (1983). Rapid response to lithium in treatment-resistant depression. *Br. J. Psychiatry 142*:204-205.
56. Price, L. H., Conwell, Y., and Nelson, J. C. (1983). Lithium augmentation of combined neuroleptic-tricyclic treatment in delusional depression. *Am. J. Psychiatry 140*:318-322.
57. Weaver, K. E. C. (1983). Lithium for delusional depression. *Am. J. Psychiatry 140*:962-963.
58. Alvarez, E., Udina, C., Queralto, J. M., Ordonez, J., Rodriguez, J., and Casas, M. (1984). Factors indicating the favourable response of lithium added to the treatment of resistant depression. In *Abstracts of the 14th Collegium Internationale Neuro-Psychopharmacologicum Congress*, Florence, p. 75.
59. Louie, A. K. and Meltzer, H. Y. (1984). Lithium potentiation of antidepressant treatment. *J. Clin. Psychopharmacol. 4*:316-321.
60. Price, L. H., Charney, D. S., and Heninger, G. R. (1984). Manic symptoms following addition of lithium to antidepressant treatment. *J. Clin. Psychopharmacol. 4*:361-362.
61. De Montigny, C., Elie, R., and Caille, G. (1985). Rapid response to the addition of lithium in iprindole-resistant unipolar depression: A pilot study. *Am. J. Psychiatry 142*:220-223.
62. Price, L. H., Charney, G. S., and Heninger, G. R. (1985). Efficacy of lithium-tranylcypromine treatment in refractory depression. *Am. J. Psychiatry 142*: 619-623.
63. Roy, A. and Pickar, D. (1985). Lithium potentiation of imipramine in treatment-resistant depression. *Br. J. Psychiatry 147*:573-575.
64. Schrader, G. D. and Levien, H. E. M. (1985). Response to sequential administration of clomipramine and lithium carbonate in treatment-resistant depression. *Br. J. Psychiatry 147*:573-575.
65. Joyce, P. R. (1985). Mood response to methylphenidate and the dexamethasone suppression test as predictors of treatment of zimelidine and lithium in major depression. *Biol. Psychiatry 20*:598-604.
66. Garbutt, J. C., Mayo, J. P., Gilette, G. M., Little, K. Y., and Mason, G. A. (1986). Lithium potentiation following lack of T_3 potentiation. *Am. J. Psychiatry 143*:1038-1039.
67. Nelson, J. C. and Mazure, C. M. (1986). Lithium augmentation in psychotic depression refractory to combined drug treatment. *Am. J. Psychiatry 143*:363-366.
68. Pai, M., White, A. C., and Deane, A. G. (1986). Lithium augmentation in the treatment of delusional depression. *Br. J. Psychiatry 148*:736-738.
69. Price, L. H., Charney, D., and Heninger, G. R. (1986). Variability of response to lithium augmentation in refractory depression. *Am. J. Psychiatry 143*:1387-1392.
70. Kushmir, S. L. (1986). Lithium-antidepressant combination in the treatment of depressed, physically ill geriatric patients. *Am. J. Psychiatry 143*:378-379.
71. Rybakowski, J., and Matkowski, K. (1987). Synergistyczne dziattanie litu i tymoleptyków w depresji endogennej. *Psychiatr. Pol. 21*:115-120.
72. Stein, G. S. and Bernadt, M. (1987). A double-blind trial of very low doses of lithium in tricyclic-resistant depression. In *Abstracts of the Second British Lithium Congress.* (Wolverhampton Polytechnic, Sept. 6-9), p. 41.

73. Post, R. M. and Kramlinger, K. (1988). Carbamazepine-lithium combination: Clinical and laboratory effects. *Psychopharmacology 96* (suppl.):S101.
74. Rybakowski, J. K. and Matkowski, K. (1988). Lithium potentiation of various antidepressants. Presented at the First International Conference on Refractory Depression, Philadelphia, Oct. 6-7.
75. Katona, C. L. E. and Finch, E. J. L. (1988). Lithium augmentation for refractory depression in old age. Presented at the First International Conference on Refractory Depression, Philadelphia, Oct. 6-7.
76. Dumlao, M. S., Perl, E., Bagne, C. A., and Gurevich, D. (1988). Antidepressants and lithium in refractory depression in geriatric patients. Presented at the First International Conference on Refractory Depression, Philadelphia, Oct. 6-7.
77. De Montigny, C. and Aghajanian, G. K. (1978). Tricyclic antidepressants: Long-term treatment increases resposivity of rat forebrain neurons to serotonin. *Science 202*:1303-1306.
78. Blier, P., De Montigny, C., and Azzaro, A. J. (1984). Modification of serotonergic and noradrenergic neurotransmission by long-term administration of monoamine oxidase inhibitors. *Soc. Neurosci. Abstr. 10*(1):16.
79. Blier, P., De Montigny, C., and Tardif, D. (1984). Effect of the two antidepressant drugs mianserin and indalpine on the serotoninergic system: Single cell studies in the rat. *Psychopharmacology 84*:242-249.
80. Knapp, S. and Mandell, A. J. (1973). Short- and long-term lithium administration: Effects on the brain's serotonergic biosynthetic systems. *Science 180*:645-647.
81. Sangdee, C. and Franz, D. N. (1980). Lithium enhancement of central 5-HT transmission induced by 5-HT precursors. *Biol. Psychiatry 15*:59-75.
82. Wallinder, J., Skott, A., and Carlsson, A. (1976). Potentiation of the antidepressant action of clomipramine by tryptophan. *Arch. Gen. Psychiatry 33*:1384-1389.
83. Glassman, A. H. and Platman, S. R. (1969). Potentiation of a monoamine oxidase inhibitor by tryptophan. *J. Psychiatr. Res. 7*:83-88.
84. Muller-Oerlinghausen, B. (1985). Lithium long-term treatment—does it act via serotonin? *Pharmacopsychiatry 18*:214-217.
85. Van Praag, H. M. and De Haan, S. (1981). Chemoprophylaxis of depression. An attempt to compare lithium with 5-hydroxytryptophan. *Acta Psychiatr. Scand. Suppl. 290*:191-201.
86. Charney, D. S., Price, L. H., and Heninger, G. R. (1986). Desipramine-yohimbine combination treatment of refractory depression. *Arch. Gen. Psychiatry 43*: 1155-1161.
87. Bunney, W. E. and Garland, B. L. (1983). Possible receptor effects of chronic lithium administration. *Neuropharmacology 22*:367-372.
88. Berridge, M. J., Downes, C. P., and Hanley, M. R. (1982). Lithium amplifies agonist-dependent phosphatidylinositol responses in brain and salivary glands. *Biochem. J. 206*:587-595.
89. Czyrak, A., Mogilnicka, E., and Maj, J. (1988). The dihydropyridine calcium channel antagonist nimodipine as an antidepressant drug. *Psychopharmacology 96* (suppl.):S329.

13

Thyroid Hormones and Antidepressant Drugs

PETER T. LOOSEN and RICHARD S. SHELTON

Vanderbilt University Medical Center and Veterans Administration Medical Center
Nashville, Tennessee

INTRODUCTION

The associations between hormones and behavior have interested medical practitioners for centuries; for example, the effects of castration on personality and sexual function were known in antiquity. It was only in 1849, however, that an experimental basis for psychoendocrinology was established by Berthold, who observed behavioral and physical changes after castrating roosters and implanting testicles in hens (1).

In psychoneuroendocrinology, relationships between thyroid hormones (TH) and affective states have revealed clinically useful information. In 1825, Parry (2) delineated the importance of stress in the etiology of thyrotoxicosis, and in 1888 the Clinical Society of London provided evidence of the behavioral sequelae of myxedema (3).

More recent data have emphasized the association between TH and affective state (see Ref. 4 for a review). For example, depression is the most frequently observed psychiatric symptom in patients with hypothyroidism, and this symptom can often herald the onset of the condition (5). In addition, approximately 30% of euthyroid patients with major depression show a blunted thyrotropin (TSH) response after thyrotropin-releasing hormone (TRH) administration, suggesting evidence of abnormal regulation of thyroid responsiveness in this disorder (4,6). Furthermore, administration of TRH may induce an increased sense of well-being and relaxation in some depressed patients and healthy volunteers (7,8). Finally, the addition of TH to tricyclic antidepresssants (TCAs) may increase the speed of antidepressant response, as well as the therapeutic efficacy of the TCA.

THYROID HORMONE AS ADJUNCT TO ANTIDEPRESSANT THERAPY

Acceleration of the Antidepressant Actions of Tricyclic Antidepressants by Thyroid Hormone

Four studies (9-12) involving 127 patients have shown that when imipramine (IMI) or amitriptyline (AMI) were given in usual doses and accompanied by as little as 20 μg triiodothyronine (T_3) per day, the antidepressant effect occurred faster than with the TCA alone. The addition of TH to IMI or AMI thus appeared to ameliorate one of the major drawbacks of these TCAs (i.e., delayed onset of therapeutic action) (Table 1). The acceleration of response

Table 1 Thyroid Hormones in Combination with Tricyclic Antidepressants in Untreated Depressed Patients

Study	Dose	Patients	Results and comment
10	150 mg IMI, plus 25 μg T_3 or Pbo	20 F with MAD	Remission with T_3 twice as fast
9	150 mg IMI, plus 25 μg T_3 or Pbo	10 M with MAD	No T_3 advantage
13	200 mg IMI, plus 25 μg T_3 or Pbo	49 patients with MAD	Nonsignificant T_3 advantage
11	100 mg AMI, plus 20 or 40 μg T_3 or Pbo	57 M or F depressed outpatients	T_3 advantage with both doses, more toxicity with higher dose
12	150 mg IMI, plus 25 μg T_3 or Pbo	30 M or F with MAD	T_3 advantage, limited to F
14	150 mg IMI, plus 25 μg T_3 or Pbo; ECT alone	12 F with MAD	No difference between treatments

Studies are listed as they are referenced. All doses per diem. IMI, imipramine; AMI, amitriptyline; Pbo, placebo; MAD, major affective disorder; M, male; F, female. All studies are double-blind.

by TH appears more marked in women than in men, and it has been observed in patients with unipolar or bipolar depression, agitated or retarded depression, and in women who are pre- or postmenopausal. Whether or not the addition of TH to other antidepressants is equally effective has not been systematically studied.

Two investigations have, however, shown less promising results. Feighner et al. (13) found a statistical trend only for T_3 to hasten the IMI response, whereas Steiner et al. (14) also found no difference in response rates between three groups of four depressed women each, one receiving IMI alone, another IMI plus T_3,and the third electroconvulsive therapy (ECT) alone. In all of these studies, the patients were euthyroid at the outset of treatment and remained so throughout the course of therapy. Finally, T_3 has not been associated with an increased rate of TCA side effects, and in one study (12), T_3 actually appeared to reduce side effects of the antidepressant.

Practical Aspects

These aforementioned studies utilized T_3 rather than thyroxine (T_4) for three practical reasons: (1) it is a more potent form of thyroid hormone; (2) it acts more rapidly; and (3) it is eliminated faster than T_4 (15). Thus, if toxicity from TH were to occur, the T_3 could be discontinued and safety regained promptly. Nonetheless, many clinicians have also used T_4 with excellent results, although this has not been systematically studied. Indeed, the effect of T_4 may be "smoother" because of its longer elimination half-life. However, two to four times as much T_4 as T_3 is necessary to achieve the same effects; therefore, the recommended daily dosages of T_4 are up to 50-100 μg.

The Use of Thyroid Hormone in Tricyclic Antidepressant Failures

In addition to delayed therapeutic action, TCAs are ineffective in as many as 35% of depressed patients. During the past decade, seven studies involving 273 patients have examined the effect of TH as an adjunct in treating patients who have failed to respond to treatment with a TCA (16-22). All of these studies have yielded positive results (8) (Table 2). Furthermore, the conversion rate from nonresponse to response was as high in men as in women. Goodwin et al. (22) showed that T_3 could convert treatment "failures" to "successes," even when TCA blood levels were in the "therapeutic range."

In view of these findings, the question arises of whether or not the addition of TH to a TCA regimen does something that is not obtained by simply increasing the TCA dose. To address this issue, Banki (19,20) randomly assigned a large series of TCA nonresponders to one of two treatment groups: either the addition of T_3 or an increase in TCA dose. In these studies, the addition of T_3 was more effective.

Table 2 Thyroid Hormones in Combination with Tricyclics in Depressed Patients Who Are Treatment Nonresponsive

Study	Dose	Patients	Results and comment
16	IMI, AMI or NT, 25 μg T_3	25 M and F with depression	70% improved when given T_3
17	Various TCA, 20-30 μg T_3	44 M and F with MAD	66% improved when given T_3
18	Various, AMI, or CIMI; various T_4 and T_3 regimens	16 M and F	Both T_4 and T_3 effective
19	75-200 mg AMI, 100-300 mg TRIM, 20-40 μg T_3	96 M and F	75% improved when given T_3
20	75-200 mg AMI, 20-40 μg T_3	49 F with MAD	70% improved when given T_3
21	Six TCAs, 10-25 μg T_3	11 M with MAD, all showing TSH blunting	10 improved when given T_3

Studies are listed as they are referenced. All doses per diem. IMI, imipramine; AMI, amitriptyline; NT, nortriptyline; CIMI, chlorimipramine; MAD, major affective disorder; M, male; F, female. TSH blunting defined as delta max TSH less then 5.0 μU/mL after TRH stimulation.

Practical Aspects

It is advisable to add TH to the TCA treatment regimen only after a reasonable trial has been completed, that is, after the TCA has been maintained at therapeutic doses (and, when appropriate, therapeutic plasma concentrations) for at least 6 weeks. If, after this time, no beneficial effect has been observed, then T_3 (recommended dose: 25 μg) or T_4 (recommended dose: 50-100 μg) should be added. The antidepressant effect should be rapid, with notable improvement within a few days. If, after about 10 days, no change in mood is noted, we suggest discontinuing TH and adding lithium carbonate.

Pathophysiologic Considerations

How does T_3 accelerate the TCA response in women and convert TCA nonresponders in both sexes? It is unlikely that T_3 exerts an effect on TCA metabolism because (1) TCA toxicity is unchanged or reduced with TH; (2) T_3 can exert its effect even when TCA plasma levels are therapeutic; and (3) T_3 shows no effects on IMI blood levels (23). However, it is possible that T_3 in the presence of TCA enhances the activity of central noradrenergic receptors (24). Furthermore, T_3-responsive patients may have a dysregulation in their hypothalamic-pituitary thyroid (HPT) axis. Tsutsui et al. (21) identified 11 patients with persistent depression who had poor response to TCAs as well as a blunted TSH response after TRH stimulation. Ten of these patients improved when given adjunct T_3, indicating the possibility that an inadequate response of the HPT axis may contribute to TCA failure and that, when this abnormality is corrected by the addition of T_3, TCA nonresponders begin to improve.

BEHAVIORAL EFFECTS OF THYROTROPIN-RELEASING HORMONE

Behavioral effects of TRH administration in animals include reversal of hibernation and sedation with barbiturates; stimulation of locomotor activity; complex effects on thermoregulation as well as the cardiovascular and respiratory system (including increases in blood pressure and respiratory rate); antinociceptive actions; and gastrointestinal effects including suppression of food and water intake and increase in gastric motility. In addition, there appears to be a complex interaction of TRH with several central nervous system neurotransmitters (including dopamine, acetylcholine, and serotonin) and neuropeptides (including opioid peptides and neurotensin) (7,8,25,26). However, there is less convincing evidence that exogenous TRH administration substantially influences human behavior (25). The behavioral effects of TRH in humans may not be observed for several reasons (25,26), including the fact that peripherally injected TRH does not appreciably cross the blood-brain barrier, and the determination of the direct behavioral effects of TRH may be altered by the endocrine effects in the periphery. In addition, TRH is rapidly degraded in plasma (the elimination half-life being 5 min), and interactions with other neuropeptides and neurotransmitters may mitigate the behavioral effects.

Depression

Prange et al. (27) were the first to report mood changes after an injection of TRH in ten women with unipolar depression. These investigators observed a brief, though partial, improvement in affect. Patients improved within a few hours and tended to relapse to baseline severity within 1 week of TRH administration. In this study, the maximum improvement (as measured by the Hamilton Rating Scale for Depression) was about 50% over pretreatment ratings. Subsequently, others examined the antidepressant effects of TRH in depression with inconsistent results (Table 3) (7,8,28). These studies indicated that the behavioral effects of TRH were not limited to depression and were often nonspecific. However, Furlong et al. (29) suggested that the differences in results might be attributed to endocrinologically distinct subtypes of depression. For example, Kieley et al. (30) gave large doses of oral

Table 3 Behavioral Studies of TRH in Depression

Studies	Positive	Negative
Oral TRH		
Single-blind	1 (1 patient)	0
Double-blind	1 (4 patients)	5 (75 patients)
Intravenous TRH		
Single-blind	4 (188 patients)	5 (61 patients)
Double-blind	7 (133 patients)	9 (129 patients)

TRH, which resulted in hyperthyroidism in some patients, and noted that the behavioral effects of TRH were related to the level of circulating thyroid hormones. Karlberg et al. (31) showed that the behavioral improvement after TRH in depression was negatively correlated with the pretreatment serum free T_4 index, and Loosen et al. (32) demonstrated that pretreatment with a single dose of TH could abolish the behavioral response to TRH in depression. Because repeated oral doses of TRH [but not a single intravenous (IV) dose] often led to a sustained thyroid stimulation (33), it seemed plausible that this might have contributed to the negative findings of TRH in depression. A review of the literature (4,8) indicates a positive behavioral response after oral TRH in one of five studies; whereas after a single IV injection of TRH the number of positive studies increased to seven of nine. The significance of this observation remains unclear, although the possibility of TRH-induced behavioral effects in a subgroup of depressives with subtle thyroid axis dysregulation is intriguing.

Mania

There is a paucity of TRH trials in patients with mania. However, in one double-blind, placebo-controlled study in five euthyroid manic men, Huey et al. (34) observed an augmentation of manic symptoms after TRH administration.

INTERACTIONS BETWEEN THYROID HORMONES AND DRUGS USED IN AFFECTIVE ILLNESS

Lithium

Among psychotropic drugs, lithium clearly has the most profound effects on thyroid function. The concentration of lithium in the thyroid gland is 1.5

to 5 times higher than it is in serum. In healthy subjects, administration of lithium results in a 60% increase of TSH response to TRH (35). This inhibitory effect of lithium on the thyroid gland (with a compensatory increase of TSH secretion) is probably the result of intrathyroidal inhibition of thyroid hormone release (36-38).

Observations from depressed patients on lithium maintenance are consistent with this view. During the course of lithium treatment, reduced levels of T_3 and T_4, increased resting levels of TSH, and exaggerated TSH responses to TRH stimulation may be observed (39-44). Clinical hypothyroidism may also occur in 5-30% of patients taking lithium (45,46), and this phenomenon may be more evident in female patients (39,42,43). Moreover, 14-23% of lithium patients may show persistent elevation of serum TSH levels in the presence of normal T_4 levels (47). Wolff (48) reported that the incidence of euthyroid goiter and goiter with hypothyroidism was 6% and 4%, respectively in 876 patients taking lithium, whereas Mannisto (49) found the incidence of goiter to be 5% in 800 lithium patients. Two prospective studies have assessed the time course of lithium-induced thyroid changes. Smigan et al. (50) studied 51 patients before lithium administration, and at 4 and 12 months during therapy. By 4 months, the levels of serum T_3 and T_4 had diminished, whereas TSH had increased. By 12 months into treatment, T_3 and T_4 had returned to baseline levels; however, TSH remained increased. Fyroe et al. (39) studied 43 lithium-treated patients and found that protein-bound iodine (PBI) levels were reduced after 2, 3, and 6 weeks of lithium treatment, but returned to pretreatment levels by 3 months of treatment. These studies suggest that lithium maintenance can temporarily suppress thyroid function in some patients (in particular women); however, these effects seem to reverse, even when lithium is continued, and they virtually always reverse after it is discontinued. Nevertheless, it appears useful to monitor thyroid function during lithium therapy. Although the best indications for frequency and type of testing remain controversial, at the very least, assessment of thyroid function before beginning lithium appears necessary to identify preexisting thyroid abnormalities that could change during treatment. Lithium-induced hypothyroidism may be supplemented with TH if discontinuation of lithium is not feasible.

Assessment of the TSH response to TRH stimulation will allow clinicians to identify subclinical hypothyroidism. This diagnosis may be important in certain affective disorder patients because it is sometimes associated with rapid cycling in bipolar illness (47).

Monoamine Oxidase Inhibitors

There is remarkably little clinical information concerning the effects of monoamine oxidase inhibitors (MAOI) on thyroid hormones. In general, MAOIs do not appear to have any profound effect on thyroid function; however, one may caution against the use of MAOIs in the presence of hyperthyroidism. Increased TH concentration results in increased myocardial sensitivity to a number of central and peripheral mediators of cardiac activity, including catecholamines and indoleamines. Thus, cardiac toxicity could potentially result from the use of MAOIs in patients with hyperthyroidism.

Tricyclic Antidepressants

Although the toxicity of TCAs is increased in the presence of hyperthyroidism (8,28), there appear to be no morphological or functional changes in thyroid axis function after TCA administration. In healthy controls, the TRH-induced TSH response remains normal after brief administration of IMI (50 mg IV) or chlorimipramine and nortriptyline (orally) daily for 1 week (51,52). Similarly, Coppen et al. (53) and Karlberg et al. (31) found that treatment with AMI for 3 weeks does not appear to have an effect on TSH response in depressed patients (31,53) and indicate that routine monitoring of thyroid function in patients taking TCAs is not necessary.

Finally, TCAs should be used with caution, in patients with hyperthyroidism, as the TCA may exacerbate tachycardia and cardiac arrhythmias in this condition. The physiological basis for these effects is speculated to be similar to that described for MAOIs.

Carbamazepine

Carbamazepine, an anticonvulsant drug that is used increasingly in the management of bipolar disorder, decreases thyroid function in both epileptic and affectively ill patients. Roy-Bourne et al. (54) observed a decrease in serum TH levels in depressed patients after 4 weeks of carbamazepine treatment, and this decrease was even greater in carbamazepine responders compared with nonresponders. Joffe et al. (55) demonstrated a reduced TRH-induced TSH response during carbamazepine treatment and speculated that carbamazepine may decrease thyroid function primarily by reducing TSH secretion at the pituitary level. Thus, although lithium appears to act directly on the thyroid gland, carbamazepine exerts its effect at the pituitary gland. These findings are of clinical importance because side effects of carbamazepine, such as sedation, lethargy, and fatigue, could be interpreted as signs of early hypothyroidism. Therefore, it appears useful to carefully monitor thyroid function before and during carbamazepine treatment. Whether or not the thyroid suppressing effects of carbamazepine or lithium are related to their therapeutic effects remains to be demonstrated.

ADDITION OF LITHIUM TO THE TRICYCLIC ANTIDEPRESSANT REGIMEN

In addition to TH augmentation of TCA, several investigators have shown a similar effect by the addition of lithium to the TCA regimen (56,57). Because TH and lithium have been found to convert many TCA treatment failures, there now appears to be a substantial number of patients for whom either treatment may be effective. Unfortunately, no direct prospective comparison of TH and lithium augmentation in TCA failures has been reported. A more detailed description of lithium potentiation of antidepressants is provided in Chapter 12.

Pathophysiologically, the clinical usefulness of both "prothyroid" (TH) and "antithyroid" (lithium, carbamazepine) treatment regimens poses puzzling questions. For example, how can both achieve the same results? Joffe and his colleagues (58) have tried to answer this intriguing question by suggesting that an antidepressant effect can be produced by *reducing* the "thyroid state" of brain. They speculate that the antidepressant effects of lithium and carbamazepine may, in part, be due to their antithyroid effect. They suggest that the antidepressant effects of adjunctive TH do not contradict this hypothesis because T_3 administration produces a reduction in T_4 levels, making less T_4 available to the brain (for conversion to in situ T_3). This hypothesis is based upon the observation that the brain depends largely on the availability of T_4, rather than of T_3 (59). To clarify these issues, controlled studies with small doses of T_4 to amplify the antidepressant effects of TCAs must be performed.

CONCLUSIONS

Studies of the relationship between brain and thyroid function have produced a variety of findings. Thyroid abnormalities may be associated with affective and cognitive disorders, and manipulation of the thyroid axis may be effective in treating these conditions. Furthermore, drugs, such as lithium and carbamazepine, that have therapeutic effects in affective disorders, also affect peripheral and central thyroid axis functioning. These actions may be relevant to the mechanism of action of antidepressant drugs and may provide a clue to the ultimate relationships between thyroid activity and behavior.

REFERENCES

1. Berthold, A. A. (1849). Transplantation der Hoden. *Arch. Anat. Physiol. Wiss. Med. 16*:42-51.

2. Parry, C. H., ed. (1825). *Collections from the Unpublished Writings of the Late Caleb Hillier Parry,* Vol. 1. London, Underwoods.
3. Clinical Society of London (1888). Report on myxedema. *Trans. Clin. Soc. Lon. 21*(suppl.). London, Longmans.
4. Loosen, P. T. (1986). Hormones of the hypothalamic-pituitary-thyroid axis: A psychoneuroendocrine perspective. *Pharmacopsychiatry 19*:401-415.
5. Sachar, E. J. (1975). Psychiatric disturbances associated with endocrine disorders. In *American Handbook of Psychiatry,* Vol. 4. Edited by D. X. Freedman and J. E. Dyrud. New York, Basic Books, pp. 299-313.
6. Kirkegaard, C. (1981). The thyrotropic response to thyrotropin-releasing hormone in endogenous depression. *Psychiatry Res. 3*:253-364.
7. Prange, A. J., Loosen, P. T., and Nemeroff, C. B. (1979). Peptides: Application to research in nervous and mental disorders. In *New Frontiers of Psychotropic Drug Research.* Edited by S. Fielding. New York, Futura Publishing, pp. 117-189.
8. Loosen, P. T., and Prange, A. J. (1984). Hormones of the thyroid axis and behavior. In *Peptides, Hormones and Behavior.* Edited by C. B. Nemeroff and A. J. Dunn. New York, Spectrum Publishers, pp. 533-577.
9. Prange, A. J., Jr., Wilson, I. C., Rabon, A. M., and Lipton, M. A. (1969). Enhancement of imipramine antidepressant activity by thyroid hormone. *Am. J. Psychiatry 126*:457-469.
10. Wilson, I. C., Prange, A. J., Jr., McClane, T. K., Rabon, A. M., and Lipton, M. A. (1970). Thyroid hormone enhancement of imipramine in non-retarded depression. *N. Engl. J. Med. 282*:1063-1067.
11. Wheathley, D. (1972). Potentiation of amitriptyline by thyroid hormone. *Arch. Gen. Psychiatry 26*:229-233.
12. Coppen, A., Whybrow, P. C., Noguera, R., Maggs, R., and Prange, A. J., Jr. (1972). The comparative antidepressant value of L-tryptophan and imipramine with and without attempted potentiation by liothyronine. *Arch. Gen. Psychiatry 26*:234-241.
13. Feighner, J. P., King, L. J., Schuckit, M. A., Croughan, J., and Briscoe, W. (1972). Hormonal potentiation of imipramine and ECT in primary depression. *Am. J. Psychiatry 128*:1230-1238.
14. Steiner, M., Radwan, M., Elizur, A., Blum, I., Atsmon, A., and Davidson, S. (1978). Failure of L-triiodothyronine (T_3) to potentiate tricyclic antidepressant response. *Curr. Ther. Res. 23*:655-659.
15. Ingbar, S. H. and Woeber, K. A. (1981). The thyroid gland. In *Textbook of Endocrinology.* Edited by R. H. Williams. Philadelphia, W. B. Sanders, pp. 117-248.
16. Earle, B. V. (1970). Thyroid hormone and tricyclic antidepressants in resistant depressions. *Am. J. Psychiatry 126*:1667-1669.
17. Ogura, C., Okuma, T., Uchida, Y., Imai, S., Yogi, H., and Sunami, Y. (1974). Combined thyroid (triiodothyronine)-tricyclic antidepressant treatment in depressive states. *Folia Psychiat. Neurol. Jpn. 28*:179-186.
18. Cavalca, G. G., Covezzi, E., and Boncinelli, A. (1974). Clinical experiences with the combination of thyroid extract and tricyclics in the treatment of depressed patients. *Riv. Sper. Freniatr. 98*:271-300.

19. Banki, C. M. (1975). Triiodythyronine in the treatment of depression. *Orv. Hetil. 116*:2543-2546.
20. Banki, C. M. (1977). Cerebrospinal fluid amine metabolites after combined amitriptyline-triiodothyronine treatment of depressed women. *Eur. J. Pharmacol. 41*:311-315.
21. Tsutsui, S., Yamazaki, Y., Namba, Y., and Tsushima, M. (1979). Combined therapy of T_3 and antidepressants in depression. *J. Int. Med. Res. 7*:138-146.
22. Goodwin, F. K., Prange, A. J., Jr., Post, R. M., Muscettola, G., and Lipton, M. A. (1982). Potentiation of antidepressant effect by L-triiodothyronine in tricyclic nonresponders. *Am. J. Psychiatry 139*:34-38.
23. Garbutt, J., Malekpour, B., Brunswick, D., Jonnalagadda, M. R., Jolliff, L., Podolak, R., Wilson, I., and Prange, A. J., Jr. (1979). Effects of triiodothyronine on drug levels and cardiac function in depressed patients treated with imipramine. *Am. J. Psychiatry 136*:980-982.
24. Frazer, A., Pandey, G., Mendels, J., Neeley, S., Kane, M., and Hess, M. E. (1974). The effect of triiodothyronine in combination with imipramine on (^{3}H)-cyclic AMP production in slices of rat cerebral cortex. *Neuropharmacology 13*: 1131-1140.
25. Nemeroff, C. B., Kalivas, P. W., Golden, R. N., and Prange, A. J. (1984). Behavioral effects of hypothalamic hypophysiotropic hormones, neurotensin, substance P and other neuropeptides. *Pharmacol. Ther. 24*:1-56.
26. Griffiths, E. C. (1985). TRH: Endocrine and central effects. *Psychoneuroendocrinology 10*:225-235.
27. Prange, A. J., Jr., Wilson, I. C., Lara, P. O., Alltop, L. B., and Breese, G. R. (1972). Effect of thyrotropin-releasing hormone in depression. *Lancet 2*:999-1002.
28. Prange, A. J., Jr., and Loosen, P. T. (1984). Peptides in depression. In *Frontiers of Psychotropic Drug Research.* Edited by E. Usdin, M. Asberg, L. Bertilsson, and F. Sjoeqvist. New York, Raven Press, pp. 127-145.
29. Furlong, F. W., Brown, G. M., and Beeching, F. M. (1976). TRH: Differential antidepressant and endocrinological effects. *Am. J. Psychiatry 133*:1187-1190.
30. Kieley, W. F., Adrian, A. D., Lee, J. H., and Nicoloff, J. T. (1976). Therapeutic failure of oral TRH in depression. *Psychosom. Med. 38*:233-241.
31. Karlberg, B. E., Kjellman, B. F., and Kagedol, B. (1978). Treatment of endogenous depression with oral thyrotropin. *Acta Psychiatr. Scand. 58*:389-400.
32. Loosen, P. T., Wilson, I. C., and Prange, A. J., Jr. (1980). Endocrine and behavioral changes in depression after TRH: Alteration by pretreatment with thyroid hormones. *J. Affect. Disord. 2*:267-278.
33. Burger, A. G., and Patel, Y. C. (1977). TSH and TRH: Their physiological regulation and the clinical application of TRH. In *Clinical Neuroendocrinology.* Edited by L. Martini and G. M. Besser. New York, Academic Press, pp. 69-131.
34. Huey, L. Y., Janowsky, D. S., Mandell, A. J., Judd, L. L., and Pendery, M. (1975). Preliminary studies on the use of TRH in manic states, depression, and the dysphoria of alcohol withdrawal. *Psychopharmacol. Bull. 11*:24-27.
35. Lauridsen, U. B., Kirkegaard, C., and Nerup, J. (1974). Lithium and pituitary-thyroid axis in normal subjects. *J. Clin. Endocrinol. Metab. 39*:383-385.

36. Burrow, G. N., Burke, W. R., Himmelhoch, J. M., Spencer, R. P., and Hershman, R. P. J. M. (1971). Effect of lithium on thyroid function. *J. Clin. Endocrinol. Metab. 32*:647-652.
37. Spaulding, S. W., Burrow, G. N., Bermudez, F., and Himmelhoch, J. M. (1972). The inhibitory effect of lithium on thyroid hormone release in both euthyroid and thyrotoxic patients. *J. Clin. Endocrinol. Metab. 35*:905-911.
38. Carlson, H. E., Temple, R., and Robbins, J. (1973). Effect of lithium on thyroxine disappearance in man. *J. Clin. Endocrinol. Metab. 36*:12-1254.
39. Fyroe, B., Petterson, U., and Sedvall, G. (1973). Time course for the effect of lithium on thyroid function in men and women. *Acta Psychiatr. Scand. 49*:230-236.
40. McLarty, D. G., O'Boyle, J. H., Spencer, C. A., and Ratcliffe, J. G. (1975). Effects of lithium on hypothalamic-pituitary thyroid function in patients with affective disorders. *Br. Med. J. 3*:623-626.
41. McLarty, D. G., Ratcliffe, W. A., Ratcliffe, J. G., Shiminins, J. G., and Goldberg, A. (1978). Effects of lithium on hypothalamic-pituitary-thyroid function in patients with affective disorders. *Br. J. Psychiatry 133*:211-218.
42. Lindstedt, G., Nilsson, L., Walinder, J., Skott, A., and Ohman, R. (1977). On the prevalence, diagnosis and management of lithium-induced hypothyroidism in psychiatric patients. *Br. J. Psychiatry 130*:452-458.
43. Cho, J. T., Bone, S., Dunner, D. L., Colt, E., and Fieve, R. R. (1979). The effect of lithium treatment on thyroid function in patients with primary affective disorder. *Am. J. Psychiatry 136*:115-116.
44. Yamaguchi, N., Tanimoto, K., and Kuromaru, S. (1980). Growth hormone (GH) release following thyrotropin-releasing hormone (TRH) injection in manic patients receiving lithium carbonate. *Psychoneuroendocrinology 5*:253-259.
45. Jefferson, J. W., Greist, J. H., and Ackerman, D. C. (1983). *Lithium Encyclopedia for Clinical Practice.* Washington, D.C., American Psychiatric Press.
46. Hullin, R. P. (1978). The place of lithium in biological psychiatry. In *Lithium in Medical Practice.* Edited by F. N. Johnson and S. M. Johnson. Lancaster, Eng., TP Press, pp. 433-454.
47. Cowdry, R. W., Wehr, T. A., Zis, A. P., and Goodwin, F. K. (1983). Thyroid abnormalities associated with rapid-cycling bipolar illness. *Arch. Gen. Psychiatry 40*:414-420.
48. Wolff, J. (1979). Lithium interactions with the thyroid gland. In *Lithium: Controversies and Unresolved Issues.* Edited by T. B. Cooper, S. Gershon, and N. S. Kline. Princeton, Excerpta Medica, pp. 552-564.
49. Mannisto, P. T. (1980). Endocrine side effects of lithium. In *Handbook of Lithium Therapy.* Edited by F. N. Johnson and S. M. Johnson. Lancaster, Eng., TP Press, pp. 310-322.
50. Smigan, L., Wahlin, A., Jacobson, L., and von Knorring, L. (1984). Lithium therapy and thyroid function tests: A prospective study. *Neuropsychobiology 2*:39-43.
51. Kirkegaard, C., Bjorum, N., Cohn, D., Faber, J., Lauridsen, U. B., and Nerup, J. (1977). Studies on the influence of biogenic amines and psychoactive drugs on the pronostic value of the TRH stimulation test in endogenous depression. *Psychoneuroendocrinology 2*:131-136.

52. Widerlow, E., Wide, L., and Sjostrom, R. (1978). Effects of tricyclic antidepressants on human plasma levels of TSH, GH and prolactin. *Acta Psychiatr. Scand. 58*:449-456.
53. Coppen, A., Montgomery, S., Peet, M., and Bailey, J. (1974). Thyrotropin-releasing hormone in the treatment of depression. *Lancet 2*:433-434.
54. Roy-Byrne, P. P., Joffee, R. T., Uhde, T. W., and Post, R. M. (1984). Carbamazepine and thyroid function in affectively ill patients. *Arch. Gen. Psychiatry 41*:1150-1153.
55. Joffe, R. T., Gold, P. W., Uhde, T. W., and Post, R. M. (1984). The effects of carbamazepine on the thyrotropin response to thyrotropin-releasing hormone. *Psychiatry Res. 12*:161-166.
56. De Montigny, C., Cournoyer, G., Morisette, R., Langlois, R., and Caille, G. (1983). Lithium carbonate addition in tricyclic antidepressant-resistant unipolar depression. *Arch. Gen. Psychiatry 40*:1327-1334.
57. Heninger, G. R., Charney, D. S., and Sternberg, D. E. (1983). Lithium carbonate augmentation of antidepressant therapy. *Arch. Gen. Psychiatry 40*:1335-1342.
58. Joffe, R. T., Blank, D. W., Post, R. M., and Uhde, T. W. (1985). Decreased triiodothyronines in depression. *Biol. Psychiatry 20*:922-925.
59. Reed Larsen, P. (1982). Thyroid-pituitary interaction: Feedback regulation of thyrotropin secretion by thyroid hormones. *N. Engl. J. Med. 306*:23-32.

14

Use of Antidepressants in the Medically Ill Patient

THOMAS A. BAN and MARK KUTCHER

Vanderbilt University, Nashville, Tennessee

INTRODUCTION

Depression is one of the most common psychiatric disorders, with a worldwide prevalence of 3%. In a study, carried out in the United States, it was found that 10% of patients consulting a primary care physician were depressed (1). European surveys from Bavaria (2) and Switzerland (3) have yielded even higher figures for depression in patients seeking some form of medical treatment—17% and 18%, respectively. However, the diagnosis of depression can be a challenge in this population because of difficulty in distinguishing depressive from somatic symptoms and signs. Some physical illness can produce symptoms suggestive of depression (4); and depression may be manifested in symptoms suggestive of physical illness (5).

MEDICAL ILLNESS MIMICKING DEPRESSION

Many neurological, endocrine, nutritional, and metabolic disorders produce symptoms that can be mistaken for refractory depression (6). Among the neurological disorders, some of the episodic symptoms of multiple sclerosis, such as fatigue, weakness and somatosensory complaints, may be confused with depression (7). Normal-pressure hydrocephalus may resemble a form of agitated depression, and the headaches, vague paresthesias, and lapses of memory following unrecognized seizures may suggest a diagnosis of depression in temporal lobe tumor (8).

Endocrine disorders mimic depression more frequently than neurological diseases. Patients with hypothyroidism may look depressed because of their slow movements and speech; and patients with adrenal insufficiency are often misdiagnosed as depressed because of their persistent complaints of fatigue, weight loss, and diminished activity (9). The same applies to patients with hyperparathyroidism who exhibit symptoms of lethargy, fatigue, and aspontaneity (10).

Metabolic disorders characterized by decreased serum concentrations of sodium or potassium, as well as conditions with increased serum calcium levels, may simulate depression. Among the nutritional disorders, anemia caused by iron, folate, or vitamin B_{12} deficiency can frequently present with symptoms suggestive of depression in the early stages of evaluation. Furthermore, depressive manifestations often precede other signs of malignancies in patients with cancer of the pancreas or the gastrointestinal tract (6).

DEPRESSION MIMICKING MEDICAL ILLNESS

Although medical illness may mimic depression, the reverse situation is far more common. It is estimated that one-half to two-thirds of patients over 40 years of age seen by primary care physicians may suffer from *masked depression* (11), a term indicating that the clinical picture strongly suggests depressive illness. Originally, this "diagnosis" was applied to only endogenous depression; later it was extended to include psychogenic depression (3). Characteristic features of masked depression include the phasic appearance of autonomic or other somatic signs and symptoms (diurnal fluctuations), diminished cognitive abilities and memory impairment, mood changes, fatigue, sleep disturbance, and anxious, obsessive, or phobic symptoms.

Depressive "pseudodementia" mimics organic dementia just as masked depression mimics medical illness and, thus, should be regarded as a variety of masked depression. In differentiating depression from dementia, probably the most important factor is that the severity of cognitive impairment fluctuates in depressed patients, whereas it remains constant in dementia. Somatic symptoms such as anorexia, weight loss, insomnia, and headache, are typical of depression, but not of dementia. Furthermore, only depressed patients communicate a sense of distress, and only in depression will memory, comprehension, and retention respond to electroconvulsive or cyclic antidepressant therapy.

DEPRESSION COEXISTENT WITH MEDICAL ILLNESS

In a study of 2000 psychiatric outpatients, Koranyi (12) found that 43% had one or more physical illnesses. When antidepressants are used in the medically ill, consideration must be given to the interactional effects of the drugs, including their interactions with the pathophysiology of the disease, the interactive mechanisms of the drug used for disease treatment, and the pharmacodynamic properties of the antidepressant drug itself. Importantly, the relative potency of their effects on adrenergic (α_1 and α_2), acetylcholine (muscarinic), and histamine (H_1 and H_2) receptors should be a particular consideration (Table 1).

Central Nervous System Disorders

Alzheimer's Disease

Caution is necessary when using antidepressants in patients with Alzheimer's disease and other primary degenerative dementias, because the drugs may aggravate the cholinergic deficit in these disorders and result in an exacerbation of symptoms, as well as a spectrum of adverse anticholinergic effects including delirium, blurred vision, dry mouth, urinary retention, and constipation. There is no definitive study on which tricyclic antidepressant (TCA) preparation is best in this circumstance, but there is a consensus that whatever compound is chosen should be prescribed at the lowest effective dose. Some clinicians prefer the use of monoamine oxidase inhibitors

Table 1 Rank Order of the Relative Potency of Antidepressants for Neurotransmitter Receptors

	Adrenergic			Histamine	
	α_1	α_2	Muscarinic	H_1	H_2
High	Doxepin/ trimipramine	Trazodone	Amitriptyline	Doxepin	Doxepin
	Amitriptyline	Trimipramine	Protriptyline	Trimipramine	Amitriptyline
	Trazodone	Amitriptyline	Trimipramine	Amitriptyline	Trimiperamine
	Amoxapine	Doxepin	Doxepin	Maprotiline	Imipramine
	Notriptyline	Nortriptyline	Imipramine	Nortriptyline	Protriptyline
	Imipramine/ maprotiline	Amoxapine	Nortriptyline	Imipramine	Maprotiline
	Protriptyline/ desipramine	Imipramine	Desipramine	Protriptyline/ amoxapine	Amoxapine
	Fluoxetine	Protriptyline	Maprotiline	Desipramine	Desipramine
		Desipramine	Amoxapine	Trazodone	Trazodone
↓		Maprotiline	Fluoxetine	Fluoxetine	Nortriptyline
Low			Trazodone		

Source: Based on Refs. 13, 14 and Richelson, E. (1982). Pharmacology of antidepressants in use in the United States. *J. Clin. Psychiatry 43*:4-11; Snyder, S. and Yamamura, H. I. (1977). Antidepressants and the muscarinic acetylcholine receptor. *Arch. Gen. Psychiatry 34*:236-239.

(MAOI) because of their lower anticholinergic potential, whereas others continue to advocate TCAs for these patients. Desipramine and maprotiline offer some advantages because of their low anticholinergic properties, and newer antidepressants, such as trazodone and fluoxetine, have few anticholinergic side effects (13,14).

Stroke

Depressive disorders occur in approximately 20-25% of poststroke patients, and Robinson et al. (15) have revealed a significant relationship between depression and the site of the lesion. In a study of right-handed patients with single ischemic lesions and no previous history of depressive disorder, six of ten patients with left frontal lesion had symptoms of depression, whereas only 2 of 20 patients with other lesion locations manifested depressive symptoms. Among the patients with left frontal lesions, there was a strong correlation between the proximity of the lesion, on computed tomography (CT) scan, to the frontal pole and severity of depression. The depression seen in these patients has been attributed to the depletion of norepinephrine (NE) because left anterior, but not right anterior lesions (induced experimentally in rats) appear to be associated with a depletion of NE in the locus ceruleus.

In favor of the NE deficiency hypothesis of depression in poststroke patients are the results of a double-blind clinical study in which nortriptyline, a specific NE-reuptake inhibitor was found to be superior in its therapeutic effect to placebo in the treatment of poststroke depressions (16).

Parkinson's Disease

Patients suffering from Parkinson's disease frequently have concomitant depressive symptoms. It is uncertain whether levodopa, the agent most commonly used to treat Parkinson's disease, reduces depressive symptoms by stimulating catecholamine release or aggravates the depressive symptomatology by decreasing serotonin levels. One must be cautious, however, in prescribing an MAOI antidepressant for a patient taking levodopa because the concurrent use of these drugs can produce a substantial rise in blood pressure.

In patients being treated with antiparkinsonian agents that have anticholinergic properties, prolonged TCA administration may produce excessive anticholinergic effects, which can often be avoided by decreasing the antiparkinsonian drug dosage or by employing an antiparkinsonian or antidepressant drug with little or no anticholinergic activity (17).

Epilepsy

Seizure disorders are not a contraindication to the use of TCAs or MAOIs. However, because TCAs tend to lower the seizure threshold, cautious titration of both antidepressant and anticonvulsant medications is necessary (18). In addition, this problem is compounded by metabolic interactions between

TCAs and phenytoin, resulting in elevated serum phenytoin levels (19). On the other hand, phenytoin can interact with antidepressants by displacing them from plasma protein-binding sites, resulting in an increased free fraction of the antidepressant. Furthermore, barbiturates, carbamazapine, and phenytoin may also decrease TCA plasma levels by increasing their metabolic elimination rate (20).

There are no apparent differences in seizure potential among TCAs. Thus, there is no evidence that there is a lower incidence of seizures with older TCAs, such as amitriptyline and imipramine, than with the newer antidepressant compounds (21). In fact, there may be a greater risk of seizures with the use of some of the newer antidepressants, such as maprotiline and amoxapine (22,23).

Endocrine Disorders

Although hypothyroidism frequently mimics depressive illness, *diabetes mellitus* is frequently encountered in depressive disease to the extent that in a sample of 203 manic-depressive patients the prevalence of diabetes was approximately five times higher (10%) than in the general population (2%) (24).

When diabetes mellitus is associated with depression, the primary choice of antidepressant treatment is with a conventional TCA or one of the second-generation antidepressant drugs. The MAOI antidepressants should be used with caution because they significantly modify the response to insulin: the hydrazine MAOIs potentiate and prolong insulin-induced hypoglycemia, whereas the nonhydrazines MAOI compounds delay the time of recovery. As a result, the likelihood of hypoglycemic stupor or hypotensive collapse can be diminished by adjusting the dosage of insulin when a MAOI is added to the treatment regimen (25).

Respiratory Disorders

The use of TCA or MAOI antidepressants appears to have little deleterious effect on respiratory mechanisms or on pulmonary gas exchange at usual therapeutic doses (26). Consequently, treatment with antidepressants should not be withheld in chronic obstructive pulmonary disease.

For bronchial asthma, treatment with some of the tertiary amine TCAs, such as amitriptyline, imipramine, and doxepin, may potentiate the therapeutic action of concomitant bronchodilators, because of their atropinelike effects. In spite of this, treatment with MAOIs should be avoided and TCAs should be given with caution because of the frequent need for direct- or indirect-acting sympathomimetic agents (e.g., epinephrine, α-adrenergic agonists) in asthmatic patients (27). Because decongestants frequently contain

α-adrenergic agonist drugs, the use of topical, rather than oral, decongestants is recommended in patients requiring a decongestant, to minimize the potential for adverse interactions including hypertension, tachycardia, and hyperpyrexia (28).

Cardiovascular Disorders

In spite of their cardiovascular effects, TCAs or MAOI antidepressants should not be withheld from cardiac patients. However, cardiac decompensation, even if not fully controlled, should always be treated before the initiation of treatment with an antidepressant.

Myocardial Infarction

Antidepressants have no effect on "cardiac ejection fraction," even in ventricular dysfunction (29). However, if possible, the use of antidepressant drugs in patients with acute myocardial infarction should be avoided until the cardiovascular status has stabilized. If treatment for depression is essential during this period, electroconvulsive therapy should be considered as the initial treatment modality.

Angina Pectoris

Antidepressants increase heart rate by their anticholnergic effect and may, thereby, precipitate or aggravate attacks of angina pectoris. Because of this, with ischemic chest pain, concurrent administration of a β-adrenergic receptor blocker may be necessary (30). An alternative possibility is treatment with trazodone, which, rather than acceleration, may cause a deceleration of heart rate (31).

Conduction Disorders

Tricyclic antidepressants can delay cardiac conduction and produce an increase in the PR, QRS, and QTc intervals (27,32). Consequently, patients with cardiac conduction disorders characterized by a prolonged QT interval are at an increased risk to develop atrioventricular (AV) block and malignant arrhythmia (33). Doxepin is frequently preferred for treatment of patients with cardiac conductance changes, because it interferes considerably less, with distal intracardiac conduction, as evidenced by HIS bundle electrocardiography, than amitriptyline, nortriptyline, or imipramine (34). An alternative possibility is treatment with MAOIs, which affect cardiac conduction to a considerably lesser degree than TCAs (35,36).

Cardiac Arrhythmia

Tricyclic antidepressants share common properties with type I antiarrhythmic medications, such as quinidine and procainamide. Hence, when TCAs are administered in combination with procainamide, significant interaction ensues.

Although TCAs have been reported to decrease premature ventricular contractions (29), they also have been reported to produce atrial arrhythmias, including atrial fibrillation. Patients, especially the elderly, with cardiac disease, particularly those with mitral valve prolapse, are particularly prone to atrial fibrillation or flutter (37-39).

For a more detailed discussion of the use of antidepressants in patients with cardiovascular disease, see Chapter 15.

Hypertensive Disease

Tricyclic antidepressants inhibit the uptake of guanethidine and similar compounds into the neuronal terminal and prevent their accumulation at the synaptic junction. Consequently, TCAs can antagonize the antihypertensive effect of guanethidinelike drugs. However, as doxepin, at low doses (100 mg/day), does not block the uptake of guanethidine, some clinicians have considered it to be the drug of choice for concurrent therapy of depression in a patient treated for preexisting hypertension with guanethidinelike drugs (40).

Among the other available antihypertensive agents, clonidine may cause a paradoxical rise in blood pressure in patients treated with TCAs (5); and reserpine or α-methyldopa may induce or aggravate depression to the extent that treatment with these substances may prevent or interfere with the therapeutic effect of antidepressant drugs.

Liver Disease

Tricyclic antidepressants are primarily metabolized by the liver, and any medical illness that interferes with normal liver function can lead to increased concentrations of circulating antidepressants. Consequently, in hepatic insufficiency, there is a marked CNS sensitivity and intolerance to antidepressant drugs (41). Furthermore, MAOIs should be given with caution to patients with a history of liver disease or abnormal liver function tests because hydrazine MAOI compounds have been reported to produce hepatocellular injury, which may, in turn, lead to acute or chronic liver disease with fatal consequences (42).

Gastrointestinal Disorders

Some TCAs (e.g., doxepin and amitriptyline) are also potent histamine (H_1 and H_2) receptor antagonists and, therefore, they have been employed in the treatment of several gastrointestinal disorders (43,44).

Peptic Ulcer

Tricyclic antidepressants can produce a reduction of gastric secretion and acid production and, thereby, have a favorable effect in peptic ulcer disease. Conversely, H_2 receptor antagonists, such as cimetidine and ranitidine, commonly used in peptic ulcer disease may induce depression in predisposed patients (45). Furthermore, cimetidine interferes with the hepatic metabolism of antidepressants to the extent that, for example with doxepin, the dosage may need to be decreased by 20-30% to prevent toxic effects (46,47).

Irritable Bowel Syndrome

By slowing gastric emptying time and small bowel transit time, TCAs may have a beneficial effect on irritable bowel syndrome (43,48). However, they must be administered with caution, because the decrease of intestinal motility may induce or exacerbate constipation, which, if ignored can lead to adynamic ileus or colonic pseudo-obstruction (i.e., Ogilvie's syndrome; 49,50).

Renal Disorders

Tricyclic antidepressants are well tolerated in renal disease because they are primarily metabolized by the liver. However, a dosage adjustment (usually down) may be necessary in depressed patients with renal failure, because of the somewhat higher antidepressant blood level that result from "inhibited" protein binding (51).

Other Disorders

In narrow-angle glaucoma, even small doses of TCAs can precipitate an acute attack with disasterous effects on vision. Because of the possibility of precipitating an acute-angle closure, TCAs should be administered with extreme caution to patients with this condition. The same does not apply to other forms of glaucoma which can be managed by cholinergic eye drops.

In prostatic hypertrophy, TCAs, particularly those with substantial anticholinergic activity, should be administered with caution because they may precipitate or aggravate urinary retention. New compounds or MAOIs with less anticholinergic activity may be more appropriate in patients with prostatic hypertrophy.

By relaxing the esophageal sphincter, TCAs may aggravate hiatal hernia (52). Again, newer antidepressant compounds, or a switch to MAOIs, may be helpful in depressed patients with esophageal pathology.

Tricyclic antidepressants can potentiate the effect of narcotic analgesics (53), as well as that of phenylbutazone, which is frequently employed in the treatment of rheumatoid arthritis. With phenylbutazone there may be an increase in blood concentration, despite the compromised absorption, because of interference with the metabolism of the drug (54).

Procarbazine, one of the chemotherapy agents employed in the treatment of Hodgkin's disease, is also an MAOI (55).

CONCLUSIONS

The use of antidepressants in patients with various medical illness has been reviewed. Obviously, this represents only a partial list of the medical problems the general physician will encounter in his depressed patients. Nevertheless, a working knowledge of the interactions between depression, medical illness, and the concomitant treatment of both disorders is essential in the outpatient setting. Therefore, we have emphasized some of the possible interactions between antidepressants and other medications, interactions between antidepressants and underlying medical illnesses, and how some antidepressant compounds can be used to treat both depression and a coexisting medical illness. Other chapters in this volume will expand upon many of the subjects touched on in this chapter.

REFERENCES

1. Barrett, J., Barrett, J. A., Oxman, T. E., and Gerber, P. D. (1988). The prevalence of psychiatric disorders in a primary care practice. *Arch. Gen. Psychiatry* *45*:1100-1106.
2. Dilling, H., Weyerer, S., and Enders, J. (1978). Patienten mit psychischen Storungen in der Allgemeinpraxis und ihre psychiatrische Uberweisungsbedurfigkeit. In *Psychiatrische Epidemiologie*. Edited by H. Hafner. Berlin, Springer-Verlag.
3. Kielholz, P., Poldinger, W., and Adams, C. (1982). *Masked Depression*. Koln-Lovenich, Deutscher Arzte-Verlag.
4. Ban, T. A. (1984). Chronic disease and depression in the geriatric population. *J. Clin. Psychiatry* *45*:18-23.
5. Ban, T. A., Guy, W., and Wilson, W. H. (1984). The psychopharmacological treatment of depression in the medically ill patient. *Can. J. Psychiatry* *29*:461-465.
6. Hollister, L. (1980). Depressed medical patients: Diagnostic and treatment challenges. In *Clinical Depressions*: *Diagnostic and Therapeutic Challenges*. Edited by F. J. Ayd. Baltimore, Ayd Medical Communications.
7. Goodstein, R. K. and Ferrell, R. B. (1977). Multiple sclerosis—presenting a depressive illness. *Dis. Nerv. Syst.* *38*:127-131.
8. Rosen, H. and Swigar, M. E. (1976). Depression and normal pressure hydrocephalus: A dilemma in neuropsychiatric diagnosis. *J. Nerv. Ment. Dis.* *163*: 35-40.
9. Taylor, J. W. (1975). Depression and thyrotoxicosis. *Am. J. Psychiatry* *132*: 552-553.
10. Nobel, P. (1974). Depressive illness and hyperparathyroidism. *Proc. R. Acad. Med.* *67*:1066-1067.
11. Lesse, S. (1980). Unmasking the masks of depression. In *Clinical Depression*: *Diagnostic and Therapeutic Challenges*. Edited by F. J. Ayd. Baltimore, Ayd Medical Communications.

12. Koranyi, E. K. (1979). Morbidity and the rate of undiagnosed physical illness in a psychiatric clinic population. *Arch. Gen. Psychiatry 36*:414-419.
13. Richardson, J. W. and Richelson, E. (1984). Antidepressants: A clinical update for medical practitioners. *Mayo Clin. Proc. 59*:330-337.
14. Stark, P., Fuller, R. W., and Wong, D. T. (1985). The pharmacologic profile of fluoxetine. *J. Clin. Psychiatry 46*:7-13.
15. Robinson, R. G., Lipsey, J. R., and Price, T. R. (1985). Diagnosis and clinical management of post-stroke depression. *Psychosomatics 26*:769-788.
16. Lipsey, J. R., Robinson, R. G., Pearlson, G. D., Rao, I., and Price, T. R. (1984). Nortriptyline treatment of post-stroke depression: A double-blind study. *Lancet 1*:297-300.
17. Ban, T. A. and Hollender, M. (1981). *Psychopharmacology for Everyday Practice.* Basel, Karger.
18. Edwards, J. G. (1979). Antidepressants and convulsions. *Lancet 2*:1368-1369.
19. Perucca, E. and Richens, A. (1977). Interaction between phenytoin and imipramine. *Br. J. Clin. Pharmacol. 4*:485-486.
20. Salzman, C. (1984). *Clinical Geriatric Psychopharmacology.* New York, McGraw-Hill, pp. 77-115.
21. Ban, T. A. (1981). *Psychopharmacology of Depression.* Basel, Karger.
22. Blackwell, B. (1987). Side effects of antidepressant drugs. In *APA Annual Review*, Sect. VI, Vol. 6. Edited by R. E. Hales and A. J. Frances. Washington, D.C., American Psychiatric Press.
23. Kulig, K. (1985). Cyclic antidepressant overdose. *J. Clin. Psychiatry 3*:19-23.
24. Lilliker, S. L. (1980). Prevalence of diabetes in a manic-depressive population. *Compr. Psychiatry 21*:270-275.
25. Cooper, A. J. and Aschcroft, G. (1966). Potentiation of insulin hypoglycemia by MAOI antidepressant drugs. *Lancet 1*:407-409.
26. Borson, S., Gayle, T., McDonald, G., Raskin, M. A., and Veith, R. C. (1987). Secondary depression in mentally ill elderly. Presented at the 140th Annual Meeting of the American Psychiatric Association, Chicago, Ill.
27. Risch, S. C., Groom, G. P., and Janowsky, D. S. (1981). Interfaces of psychopharmacology and cardiology—Part one. *J. Clin. Psychiatry 42*:23-34.
28. Saklad, S. R. (1984). Drug interaction with antidepressants. *Med. Psychiatry 1*:4-5.
29. Veith, R. C., Raskind, M. A., Caldwell, J. H., Barnes, R. F., Gumbrecht, G., and Ritchie, J. L. (1982). Cardiovascular effects of tricyclic antidepressants in depressed patients with chronic heart disease. *N. Engl. J. Med. 306*:954-959.
30. Jefferson, J. W. (1975). A review of the cardiovascular effects and toxicity of tricyclic antidepressants. *Psychosom. Med. 37*:160-179.
31. Jefferson, J. W. (1985). Biologic treatment of depression in cardiac patients. *Psychosomatics 26* (suppl.):31-37.
32. Bigger, J. T., Jr., Giardina, E. G. V., Perel, J. M., Kantor, S. J., and Glassman, A. (1977). Cardiac antiarrhythmic effect of imipramine hydrochloride. *N. Engl. J. Med. 296*:206-208.
33. Flugelman, M. Y., Tal, A., Pollack, S., Hefez, A., Weisstub, E. B., Gotsman, M. S., and Lewis, B. S. (1985). Psychotropic drugs and long QT syndromes: Case reports. *J. Clin. Psychiatry 46*:290-291.

34. Burrows, G. D., Vohra, J., and Hunt, D. (1976). Cardiac effects of different tricyclic antidepressant drugs. *Br. J. Psychiatry 129*:335-341.
35. Goldman, L. S., Alexander, R. C., and Luchins, D. J. (1986). Monoamine oxidase inhibitors and tricyclic antidepressants. Comparison of their cardiovascular effects. *J. Clin. Psychiatry 47*:225-227.
36. McGrath, P. J., Blood, D. K., Stewart, J. W., Harrisons, W., Quitkin, F. M., Tricamo, E., and Markowitz, J. (1987). A comparative study of the electrocardiographic effects of phenelzine, tricyclic antidepressants, mianserin, and placebo. *J. Clin. Psychopharmacol. 7*:335-339.
37. Murray, G. B. (1985). Atrial fibrillation/flutter associated with amoxapine: Two case reports. *J. Clin. Psychopharmacol. 5*:124-125.
38. Pariser, S. F., Reynolds, J. C., Falko, J. M., Jones, B. A., and Mercer, D. L. (1981). Arrhythmia induced by a tricyclic antidepressant in a patient with undiagnosed mitral valve prolapse. *Am. J. Psychiatry 138*:507-523.
39. White, W. B. and Wong, S. H. Y. (1985). Rapid atrial fibrillation associated with trazodone hydrochloride. *Arch. Gen. Psychiatry 42*:424.
40. Oates, J. A., Fann, W. E., and Cavanaugh, J. H. (1969). Effect of doxepin on the norepinephrine pump. A preliminary report. *Psychosomatics 10*:12-13.
41. Larry, D., Roeff, B., Pessayre, D., Danan, G., Algard, M., Geneve, J., and Benhamou, J. P. (1986). Cross hepatoxicity between tricyclic antidepressants. *Gut 27*:726-727.
42. Zimmerman, H. J. and Ishak, K. G. (1987). The hepatic injury of monoamine oxidase inhibitors. *J. Clin. Psychopharmacol. 7*:211-213.
43. Cunha, U. V. (1986). Antidepressants: Their uses in nonpsychiatric disorders of aging. *Geriatrics 41*:63-74.
44. Richelson, E. (1982). Tricyclic antidepressant: Drugs for other diseases. *Arch. Intern. Med. 142*:231-232.
45. Billings, R. F. and Stein, M. B. (1986). Depression associated with ranitidine. *Am. J. Psychiatry 143*:915-916.
46. Abernethy, D. R. and Todd, E. L. (1986). Doxepin-cimetidine interaction: Decreased doxepin bioavailability during cimetidine treatment. *J. Clin. Psychopharmacol. 6*:8-12.
47. Miller, M. E., Perry, C. J., and Siris, S. G. (1987). Psychosis in association with combined cimetidine and imipramine treatment. *Psychosomatics 28*:217-219.
48. Greenbaum, D. S. (1984). Preliminary report on antidepressant treatment of irritable bowel syndrome: Comments on comparison with anxiolytic therapy. *Psychopharmacol. Bull. 20*:622-628.
49. Clarke, I. M. C. (1971). Adynamic ileus and amitriptyline. *Br. Med. J. 2*:531.
50. Hayes, J. R., Bojrab, S. L., and McCarthy, M. C. (1987). Gastrointestinal effects of tricyclic antidepressants: Ogilvie's syndrome. *Psychosomatics 28*:442-443.
51. Levy, M. B. (1985). Use of psychotropics in patients with kidney failure. *Psychosomatics 26*:699-709.
52. Tyber, M. A. (1975). The relationship between hiatal hernia and tricyclic antidepressants: A report of five cases. *Am. J. Psychiatry 132*:653-654.

53. Ventafridda, V., Ripamonti, C., De Conno, F., Bianchi, M., Pazzuconi, F., and Panerni, A. E. (1987). Antidepressants increase bioavailability of morphine in cancer patients. *Lancet 1*:1204.
54. Bassuk, E. and Schoonover, S. (1978). Rampant dental caries in the treatment of depression. *J. Clin. Psychiatry 29*:163-165.
55. Goldberg, R. J. and Cullen, L. O. (1986). Use of psychotropics in cancer patients. *Psychosomatics 27*:687-700.

15

Cardiovascular Effects of Tricyclic Antidepressants in Depressed Patients with and without Heart Disease

STEVEN P. ROOSE and ALEXANDER H. GLASSMAN

College of Physicians and Surgeons of Columbia University
and New York State Psychiatric Institute
New York, New York

There has been long-standing concern about the cardiovascular effects of tricyclic antidepressants (TCAs), prompted by the observation that patients who took fatal overdoses of TCAs frequently died from heart block or arrhythmias (1). Although it was originally believed that similar cardiovascular effects would occur in an attenuated form when these drugs were administered at usual therapeutic doses to vulnerable patients, this has not proved to be the case. It has taken 20 years to acquire an accurate understanding of the cardiovascular effects of TCAs, and only now are we in a position to make more informed clinical judgments regarding the treatment of depressed patients with preexisting cardiovascular disease. In this chapter, we will review our current knowledge of the cardiovascular effects of TCAs, as well as the management of patients with and without heart disease who are taking these compounds.

NORMAL CARDIAC ELECTROPHYSIOLOGY

Under normal conditions, the sinus node (SN) acts as the pacemaker for the heart. The sinus impulse is rapidly distributed over the heart by a specialized conduction system to trigger a synchronized contraction. The impulse arising in the SN is transmitted to the atrioventricular node (AVN) through three specialized atrial internodal tracts. Conduction through the AVN is very slow, and this allows time to complete atrial contraction before the beginning of ventricular contraction. Below the AVN the impulse enters a short, cablelike structure called the bundle of His. At the top of the intraventricular septum, the bundle of His divides into the left and right bundle branches, which repeatedly branch to produce millions of peripheral Purkinje fibers. Together, the bundle of His, bundle branches, and peripheral Purkinje fibers are known as the ventricular specialized conducting system (VSCS).

The standard 12-lead electrocardiogram (ECG) reflects electrical activity of only the cardiac muscle. Depolarization of the SN is not seen. The P wave is the first event in a normal ECG and represents depolarization of the atria. The next event seen on the ECG is the QRS complex which represents the depolarization of the ventricular muscle. The time between these two events is measured as the PR interval and represents activation of the AVN and the VSCS. Activation of these structures causes no deflection in the ECG. The final event on the ECG is the T wave, which represents repolarization of the ventricular muscle. The QT interval measures total electrical systole in the ventricle (i.e., the time from depolarization to full repolarization of ventricular tissues).

Conduction disturbances can cause disassociation between the normal sinus pacemaker and ventricular contraction. Partial or complete block can result from anatomical lesions or drug effects at the AVN, the bundle of His, and the upper bundle branches. Delay at any site manifests itself as a lengthening of the PR interval as recorded on the ECG. A block at more distal sites (i.e., in the subendocardial Purkinje system) is very unlikely because of the extensive anastomoses in this portion of the VSCS.

In 1969, a technique was introduced that made it possible to record the electrical activity from the bundle of His by cardiac catheterization. Recordings from the bundle of His now permit the PR interval to be partitioned into the following two time intervals: the atria-His (AH) and the His-ventricle (HV) intervals, representing conduction time through the AVN and the VSCS, respectively. Recently, His bundle ECG has become an important tool in understanding the action of TCAs on the heart.

EFFECTS OF THERAPEUTIC DOSES OF TRICYCLIC ANTIDEPRESSANTS ON CARDIAC CONDUCTION

Therapeutic plasma concentrations of TCAs can produce an increase in the PR interval, QRS complex, and QT (rate corrected) interval (2-4). Additionally, the use of the His bundle ECG has established the site where TCAs affect the atrioventricular conducting system. Vohra et al. observed a "quinidine-like" action with nortriptyline; that is, the AH interval was unaffected, whereas the HV interval was prolonged (5).

Glassman et al. considered the possibility that the prolongation of the PR interval and QRS complex with imipramine might represent a clinical estimation of the plasma concentration of imipramine and its demethylated metabolite. Although there was a significant correlation between the plasma level of imipramine and the change in the QRS duration within some patients, changes in the ECG could not generally be interpreted to indicate the presence of a therapeutic level of TCA (4).

The data from several studies indicate that TCAs at, or just above, therapeutic plasma concentrations frequently prolong PR and QRS intervals and exert their major action on intraventricular (HV) conduction. In depressed patients with normal cardiac conduction (as reflected by a normal pretreatment ECG), the clinician can expect TCAs at therapeutic plasma levels to increase the PR or QRS intervals moderately to a clinically insignificant extent.

HEART RATE

The literature abounds with references to TCA-induced tachycardia, but there is a paucity of systematic data to support this contention. Freyschuss et al. (6) and Ziegler et al. (7) reported that a therapeutic plasma level of nortriptyline resulted in an average increase of 16 beats/min in 57 patients who were free of heart disease. Subsequently, Ziegler et al. (8) and Peet et al. (9) reported similar increases in heart rate in depressed patients treated with amitriptyline. However, the method used in all these studies was simply to determine the heart rate from a single pulse or ECG measurement. With use of the more definitive method of 24-hr ECG recording, Glassman et al. (4) reported that imipramine caused only trivial increases in heart rate after 4 weeks of treatment at therapeutic plasma levels. Additionally, the increase in heart rate over baseline, measured over a 24-hr period, averaged less than 3 beats/min. However, Glassman's data also agreed with previous reports indicating larger increases in patients who had lower initial heart rates.

In summary, although there may be differences among TCAs in their propensity to cause small increases in heart rate, more importantly, none of the TCAs has been shown to produce tachycardia on a regular basis. If clinically significant tachycardia does occur from a TCA, the data would suggest that it is an uncommon event.

ORTHOSTATIC HYPOTENSION

One of the most frequent and potentially serious side effects of TCA treatment is orthostatic hypotension. Fractures, lacerations, myocardial infarctions, and sudden death, all have been reported (10,11). Imipramine has been considered the TCA most likely to cause this side effect, but this probably is because imipramine is the most studied TCA in this context. Muller et al. (11) observed "moderate to severe" postural hypotension in 24% of 82 depressed patients treated with imipramine. Most of the untoward reactions attributed to orthostatic hypotension, including two myocardial infarctions in patients with preexisting angina, occurred in older patients with a mean age of 70 (11). Subsequently, Glassman et al. (10), measured the orthostatic effect of imipramine in 44 depressed patients with an average age of 59. In this study patients were in the hospital, and orthostatic blood pressures were measured three times daily in a 6-week study that included 2 weeks of drug-free baseline data. These investigators found that 1 min after standing, the average fall in systolic blood pressure was 25 mmHg, a significant ($p < 0.001$) increase compared with predrug orthostatic drop. There were several important clinical characteristics of this on-drug orthostatic drop including (1) an inability of patients to accommodate to this side effect, and (2) that the orthostatic blood pressure drop was maximally present below the therapeutic plasma level of imipramine.

Although the available data on the orthostatic effect of other TCAs are not as extensive, the work of Nelson et al. (12), Hayes et al. (13), Kopera et al. (14), and Glassman and Roose (15), all indicate that this orthostatic effect also exists for amitriptyline, desmethylimipramine, and doxepin.

For reasons that are still unclear, the story is different with nortriptyline. Early studies (6,16,17) reported that the postural systolic drops in patients treated with nortriptyline were negligible when compared with other TCAs. In the most extensive study of nortriptyline, Roose et al. (18), measured the change in blood pressure in 33 patients in a retrospective study and 15 patients in a prospective study. The retrospective group had a mean age of 67 years and a mean daily nortriptyline dosage of 85 mg and a mean plasma concentration of 98 ng/mL. None of the 33 patients developed orthostatic hypotension. The prospective study compared the orthostatic effect of nortriptyline in 15 patients, with an average age of 59, with a comparable group of patients taking imipramine. The average orthostatic blood pressure drop on nortriptyline (13 mmHg) was significantly less than that of imipramine (26 mmHg). Furthermore, some patients were treated with imipramine and nortriptyline at separate times, thereby allowing a comparison of the orthostatic effect within each individual. In this group, nortriptyline caused less orthostatic hypotension. Additionally, patients who were unable to tolerate the orthostatic effects of imipramine rarely showed similar orthostatic hypotension when switched to nortriptyline.

Thus, it appears that the most frequent cardiovascular effect of TCAs in a physically healthy depressed patient, is orthostatic hypotension. This problem is best documented for imipramine, which appears to cause severe orthostatic hypotension in approximately 10% of patients, but probably occurs with a similar frequency with desmethylimipramine, amitriptyline, and doxepin. Nortriptyline, however, appears to cause less orthostatic hypotension and, generally, can be used when the other TCAs are not tolerated.

In summary, (1) TCAs do not appear to have a robust effect on heart rate; (2) at therapeutic plasma levels they do appear to prolong the PR and QRS intervals, which is not usually clinically significant if the patient has a normal conduction system; and (3) the most frequent severe cardiovascular effect is orthostatic hypotension.

THE USE OF TRICYCLIC ANTIDEPRESSANTS IN PATIENTS WITH HEART DISEASE

Antiarrhythmic Effect of Tricyclic Antidepressants and Their Use in Patients with Cardiac Arrhythmias

Because TCAs can cause severe arrhythmias when taken in an overdose, it had been erroneously concluded that the TCAs intrinsically are arrhythmogenic and that their use in patients with preexisting arrhythmias is contraindicated. It has now been established that TCAs have powerful antiarrhythmic activity that is of potential clinical importance. The antiarrhythmic effect of imipramine was first reported by Bigger et al. (19) in two depressed patients with ventricular premature depolarizations (VPDs). These investigators subsequently confirmed this observation in 11 depressed patients with VPDs, 10 of whom had 90% VPD suppression at imipramine plasma concentrations of 100-300 ng/mL (20). However, the consideration remained whether the arrhythmic activity itself was intrinsically related to the presence of affective disorder, and therefore its subsequent suppression by imipramine was a byproduct of imipramine's antidepressant effect. This was disproved by cardiologists studying the antiarrhythmic effect of TCAs. Giardina et al. (21) reported that 17 of 22 cardiac patients with VPDs and without depression had more than 75% VPD suppression during imipramine treatment. The antiarrhythmic profile of imipramine also produced a reduction in the complex features of arrhythmias such as bigeminy, pairs, and unsustained ventricular tachycardia.

Subsequent studies have demonstrated that nortriptyline is similar to imipramine in its antiarrhythmic activity (22), and one might assume that the other TCAs also share this property (23).

The observation that imipramine affects the initial inward sodium current of the Purkinje fiber (24,25), and that His bundle studies demonstrate a depression of conduction velocity (5), give TCAs an electrophysiological profile that is characteristic of type 1A antiarrhythmic compounds, such as quinidine and procainamide. This electrophysiological profile also extends to desmethylimipramine and the TCA hydroxy metabolites (25,26). In fact,

2-hydroxyimipramine is equipotent with imipramine in slowing conduction blocks of the isolated Purkinje fibers and suppressing ouabain-induced arrhythmias (24,25). These data support the view that TCAs exert their antiarrhythmic effect by direct action on the heart. However, other studies suggest the possibility that some arrhythmic activity (particularly by TCAs) may be mediated, in part, by central nervous system mechanisms.

The clinical significance of the antiarrhythmic effect of the TCAs is that depressed patients with VPD activity are likely to derive a double benefit from their use. However, two cautionary notes should be taken: (1) Patients with preexisting arrhythmic activity are likely to be taking an antiarrhythmic agent when they initially consult the psychiatrist and, therefore, it must be remembered that adding a TCA is tantamount to giving an additional type 1A antiarrhythmic. If the patient is already taking a type 1A antiarrhythmic, such as quinidine or procainamide, then one is effectively increasing the dosage of the antiarrhythmic drug and, therefore, must be aware that these compounds can have a paradoxical effect at high concentrations (27). (2) A knowledge of the antiarrhythmic effect of the TCAs necessitates a reconsideration of how to conceptualize and treat a TCA overdose. Malignant ventricular arrhythmias are uncommon in more mild TCA overdoses, but are more commonly seen in severe and, subsequently, fatal overdoses (28). In a patient who has taken a TCA overdose and who is having significant ventricular arrhythmia, the emergency room physician may consider treatment with quinidine or a similar agent. Only if the physician realizes that TCA is a type 1A antiarrhythmic drug does the danger of this procedure become apparent. Although systematic data are not yet available, given the antiarrhythmic profile of TCAs, it would seem most reasonable to consider the TCA overdose equivalent to a "quinidine overdose" relative to the develop- of arrhythmias and if such arrhythmias develop, one would treat the overdose as one would a quinidine overdose (29).

THE USE OF TRICYCLIC ANTIDEPRESSANTS IN PATIENTS WITH CONGESTIVE HEART FAILURE

Early studies investigating the effects of TCAs on left ventricular function concluded that the TCA adversely affected cardiac output (30-32). However, all earlier studies used the systolic time interval (STI) as the method for evaluating left ventricular performance. Unfortunately, the interpretation of the STI as an indicator of myocardial function in patients taking TCAs that prolong intraventricular conduction time has been problematic (33). The advent of radionuclide angiography provides a relatively noninvasive procedure for the evaluation of left ventricular function not dependent on conduction time. Using this methodology, Veith et al. (34) evaluated the effect of imipramine and doxepin in 17 depressed patients and found no evidence of impaired left ventricular function. However, this study used relatively low doses of TCA and included few patients with ejection fractions below 40% (i.e., patients with significant impairment of left ventricular function). Subsequent studies (35,36) reported radionuclide data from a series of depressed patients with moderate to severe impairment of left ventricular function and a mean ejection fraction baseline 33% (which included patients with ejection fractions as low as 12%) taking therapeutic doses of imipramine or nortriptyline. The TCAs had no deleterious effect on any measure of left ventricular function, even in the patients with severe left ventricular impairment.

Although the TCAs do not decrease cardiac output, they are far from safe in patients with congestive heart failure because of unexpectedly high rates of orthostatic hypotension. The extent of orthostatic hypotension induced by imipramine, and the magnitude of the difference between imipramine and nortriptyline, increase dramatically between physically healthy depressed patients and those with congestive heart failure. Glassman and Roose (35,37) reported that a total of 25 depressed patients with significant preexisting left heart failure treated with imipramine, had a rate of drug-induced orthostatic hypotension approaching 50%. However, the same authors also reported that in 21 comparable patients with preexisting failure treated with nortriptyline, only 4.8% developed orthostatic hypotension (36). Furthermore, in 19 of the 21 nortriptyline-treated patients who had previously been treated with imipramine, eight demonstrated severe hypotensive symptoms while taking imipramine.

Although the mechanism by which TCAs induce orthostatic hypotension is still unclear, it seems apparent that the presence of affective illness may be a significant risk factor for the development of orthostatic hypotension with TCAs. In contrast to nearly 50% of depressed patients with congestive heart failure who developed orthostatic hypotension when treated with imipramine, Giardina et al. (21,38) reported that only 1 of 22 nondepressed cardiac patients (4%) with congestive heart failure treated with comparable doses of imipramine for arrhythmia control had serious symptoms of orthostatic hypotension. Thus, it is possible that those endogenously depressed patients with heart disease who are treated with imipramine are at greater risk of developing orthostatic hypotension than those patients with heart disease alone.

In summary, it appears that only nortriptyline is relatively safe in patients with congestive heart failure. However, three caveats should be mentioned: (1) Although it was concluded that TCAs generally do not have a robust effect on heart rate, special consideration should be given to TCA-induced tachycardia when treating patients with coronary artery disease. Increasing heart rate increases oxygen consumption, and the resulting oxygen demand can be met only by increased coronary blood flow. If coronary flow cannot keep pace with the increased demand, angina pectoris can result. Thus, what may be an insignificant heart rate increase in a patient with no preexisting cardiac disease, may be problematic if the patient has marginally compensated congestive heart failure. (2) One must be sure that the congestive heart failure does not exist concurrently with conduction disease (specifically bundle-branch block); this unfortunate sequence of myocardial infarction producing congestive heart failure and permanent damage to the conduction system is a frequent event. TCAs have the potential to cause increased degrees of atrioventricular bundle-branch block in patients with preexisting bundle-branch block (39). (3) There is reason for concern that specific drug-drug interactions might develop when using a TCA in a patient with congestive heart failure. Specifically, there is an interaction between digoxin and quinidine in which quinidine induces a significant rise in digoxin plasma levels, thereby causing digoxin toxicity. Although the effect of TCAs on digoxin plasma levels has not been specifically evaluated, it would seem prudent to monitor digoxin plasma levels in patients in whom a TCA is subsequently added.

TREATMENT OF THE PATIENT WITH PREEXISTING CONDUCTION DISEASE

Therapeutic plasma concentrations of TCAs can frequently prolong the PR and QRS intervals, but rarely, if ever, cause symptomatic conduction disturbance. However, the propensity of TCAs to reduce conduction velocity raises the question of whether or not patients with preexisting conduction disease would be at risk to develop atrioventricular (AV) block when treated with a TCA. This concern was strengthened by the frequency of AV block observed after TCA overdose and by case reports of patients with preexisting bundle-branch block who developed 2:1 AV block when treated with imipramine (40). Roose et al. (39) reported the only prospective study of TCA use in patients with preexisting conduction disease to determine if they were at greater risk to develop AV block than patients with normal pretreatment ECGs. In that study, 41 depressed patients with first-degree AV block or bundle-branch block were compared with 151 patients with normal ECGs during treatment with imipramine or nortriptyline. The risk of developing a 2:1 AV block was higher (9%) in patients with preexisting bundle-branch block, compared with the rate (0.7%) in patients with normal pretreatment ECGs. Thus, there is no TCA that can be used without substantial risk of inducing a potentially fatal conduction complication when treating patients with preexisting bundle-branch block. When use of a TCA is necessary for treating a depressed patient with bundle-branch block, measures of cardiac conduction (ECGs, 24-hr continuous ECG recordings), blood pressure recordings, and TCA plasma concentrations should be routinely monitored.

However, given the risks of TCA use in such patients, electroconvulsive therapy could be considered for severe depression in this group.

CARDIOVASCULAR EFFECTS OF NEWER ANTIDEPRESSANTS: ARE THEY SAFER?

Newer antidepressants have recently become available to the clinician and many of them claim to have fewer cardiovascular effects than the TCAs. After considering those compounds that have cardiovascular effect profiles similar to the TCAs (41,42) and compounds that have a prominent adverse effect profile, such as amoxapine (43,44), there emerge several compounds that are intriguing in terms of cardiovascular effects. Specifically, this group would include trazodone, bupropion, and fluoxetine.

Before considering these drugs individually, it is worth noting some methodological considerations which apply to all of them. First of all, there is limited cardiovascular data on these drugs even in healthy depressed patients, and an extraordinary paucity of data when it comes to their effects in patients with preexisting cardiac disease. That a drug may produce no significant complications when used in healthy depressed patients, should not be taken to mean that the same drug also will not produce any problems when used in patients with preexisting cardiac disease. Though pharmaceutical companies would like to promote the concept that "if it is safe in healthy depressed patients it will be safe as well in patients with heart disease," a more prudent position would be that safety in healthy depressed patients can only allow you to conclude that we do not know whether or not it will be dangerous in patients with preexisting heart disease. Furthermore, even if a new drug is established as having a safer cardiac profile, one has to make sure that the benefits gained in this area are not overshadowed by significant side effects involving other organ systems. And, of course, one has not even mentioned the issue of the relative efficacy of these new compounds compared with the TCAs, an important consideration when one is trying to establish a risk/benefit ratio for a drug. Given all these theoretical considerations, one can now proceed to consider the data available on these compounds.

Trazodone

Trazodone, a triazolopyridine derivative, appears to have a different cardiovascular profile than conventional TCAs. It does not appear to substantially affect cardiac conduction (45), although there have been several case reports of conduction abnormalities with trazodone. Furthermore, in the limited data available from overdose studies (46-48) trazodone does not appear to produce significant cardiac effects, despite extremely toxic doses of the drug involved. However, there have been several reports suggesting an arrhythmogenic effect of trazodone (49). Therefore, until this issue is resolved, it would seem prudent to avoid using trazodone in patients with ventricular arrhythmias. Similarly, this has a bearing on the use of trazodone in patients with bundle-branch block, many of whom may have concurrent ventricular irritability, thereby making the use of trazodone less attractive.

Fluoxetine

There is a lack of data on the cardiovascular effects of this compound. The little available data suggest that fluoxetine does not have a substantial effect on PR or QRS intervals and actually may induce a slight decrease in heart rate (50-52). However, the only prudent conclusion is that if the cardiovascular profile of fluoxetine is still unknown in healthy depressed patients, then caution should be exercised when using fluoxetine in patients with preexisting heart disease.

Bupropion

It is ironic that of the new drugs the one with the most extensive cardiovascular literature (including preexisting arrhythmia, congestive heart failure, and conduction disease) is not yet available to the clinician. In physically healthy depressed patients, bupropion appears to have no substantial effect on heart rate, orthostatic blood pressure, or cardiac conduction (53). In a study comparing bupropion with imipramine in patients with congestive heart failure, Roose et al. (37) found that neither drug impaired left ventricular function (as measured by radionuclide angiography) and that bupropion did not induce orthostatic hypotension, in contrast with the 50% rate induced by imipramine. Thus, the cardiovascular profile of bupropion is promising and deserves further investigation in depressed patients with cardiovascular disease.

CONCLUSION

In summary, depressed patients with severe cardiac disease can often be safely and effectively treated with a conventional TCA. The most critical issue is to be forewarned of possible adverse effects and to monitor the patient closely for early signs of problems.

REFERENCES

1. Williams, R. B., Jr. and Sherter, C. (1971). Cardiac complications of tricyclic antidepressant therapy. *Ann. Intern. Med. 74*:395-398.

2. Vohra, J., Burrows, G. D., Hunt, D., and Sloman, G. (1975). The effect of toxic and therapeutic doses of tricyclic antidepressant drugs on intracardiac conduction. *Eur. J. Cardiol. 3*:219-227.
3. Burrows, G. D., Vohra, J., Dumovic, P., Maguire, K., Scoggins, B. A., and Davies, B. (1977). Tricyclic antidepressant drugs and cardiac conduction. *Prog. Neuropsychopharmacol. 1*:329-334.
4. Kantor, S. J., Glassman, A. H., Bigger, J. T., Jr., Perel, J. M., and Giardina, E. V. (1978). The cardiac effects of therapeutic plasma concentrations of imipramine. *Am. J. Psychiatry 135*:534-538.
5. Vohra, J., Hunt, D., Burrows, G. D., and Sloman, G. (1975). Intracardiac conduction defects following overdose of tricyclic antidepressant drugs. *Eur. J. Cardiol. 2*:443-452.
6. Freyschuss, U., Sjoqvist, F., Tuck, D., and Asberg, M. (1970). Circulatory effects in man of nortriptyline, a tricyclic antidepressant drug. *Pharmacol. Clin. 2*:68-71.
7. Ziegler, V. E., Co, B. T., and Biggs, J. T. (1977). Plasma nortriptyline levels and ECG findings. *Am. J. Psychiatry 134*:441-443.
8. Ziegler, V. E., Co, B. T., and Biggs, J. T. (1977). Electrocardiographic findings in patients undergoing amitriptyline treatment. *Dis. Nerv. Syst. 38*:697-699.
9. Peet, M., Tienari, P., and Jaskari, M. O. (1977). A comparison of the cardiac effects of mianserin and amitriptyline in man. *Pharmakopsychiatr. Neuropsychopharmakol. 10*:309-312.
10. Glassman, A. H., Bigger, J. T., Jr., Giardina, E. V., Kantor, S. J., Perel, J. M., and Davies, M. (1979). Clinical characteristics of imipramine-induced orthostatic hypotension. *Lancet 1*:468-472.
11. Muller, O. F., Goodman, N., and Bellet, S. (1961). The hypotensive effect of imipramine hydrochloride in patients with cardiovascular disease. *Clin. Pharmacol. Ther. 2*:300-307.
12. Nelson, J. C., Jatlow, P., Quinlan, D. M., Bowers, M. B., Jr. (1982). Desipramine plasma concentration and antidepressant response. *Arch. Gen. Psychiatry 39*:1419-1422.
13. Hayes, J. R., Born, G. F., and Rosenbaum, A. H. (1977). Incidence of orthostatic hypotension in patients with primary affective disorders treated with tricyclic antidepressants. *Mayo Clin. Proc. 52*:509-512.
14. Kopera, H. (1978). Anticholinergic and blood pressure effects of mianserin, amitriptyline and placebo. *Br. J. Clin. Pharmacol. 5* (suppl. 1):29S-34S.
15. Roose, S. P., Glassman, A. H., Siris, S. G., and Bruno, R. L. (1980). Tricyclic-induced postural hypotension: Comparative studies. New Research presented at A.P.A., San Francisco.
16. Vohra, J., Burrows, G. D., and Sloman, G. (1975). Assessment of cardiovascular side effects of therapeutic doses of tricyclic anti-depressant drugs. *Aust. N. Z. J. Med. 5*:7-11.
17. Thayssen, P., Bjerre, M., Kragh-Sorensen, P., Moller, M., Petersen, O. L., Kristensen, C. B., and Gram, L. F. (1981). Cardiovascular effects of imipramine and nortriptyline in elderly patients. *Psychopharmacology 74*:360-364.

18. Roose, S. P., Glassman, A. H., Siris, S. G., Walsh, B. T., Bruno, R. L., and Wright, L. B. (1981). Comparison of imipramine- and nortriptyline-induced orthostatic hypotension: A meaningful difference. *J. Clin. Psychopharmacol. 1*:316-319.
19. Bigger, J. T., Jr., Giardina, E. G. V., Perel, J. M., Kantor, S. J., and Glassman, A. H. (1977). Cardiac antiarrhythmic effect of imipramine hydrochloride. *N. Engl. J. Med. 296*:206-208.
20. Giardina, E. G., Bigger, J. T., Jr., Glassman, A. H., Perel, J. M., and Kantor, S. J. (1979). The electrocardiographic and antiarrhythmic effects of imipramine hydrochloride at therapeutic plasma concentrations. *Circulation 60*:1045-1052.
21. Giardina, E. G. V. and Bigger, J. T., Jr. (1982). Antiarrhythmic effect of imipramine hydrochloride in patients with ventricular premature complexes without psychological depression. *Am. J. Cardiol. 50*:172-179.
22. Giardina, E. G. V., Barnard, T., Johnson, L. L., Saroff, A. L., Bigger, J. T., Jr., and Louie, M. (1986). The antiarrhythmic effect of nortriptyline in cardiac patients with ventricular premature depolarizations. *J. Am. Coll. Cardiol. 7*:1363-1369.
23. Raeder, E. A., Zinsli, M., and Burckhardt, D. (1979). Effect of maprotiline on cardiac arrhythmias. *Br. Med. J. 2*:102.
24. Weld, F. M. and Bigger, J. T., Jr. (1980). Electrophysiological effects of imipramine on ovine cardiac Purkinje and ventricular muscle fibers. *Circ. Res. 46*: 167-175.
25. Wilkerson, R. D. (1978). Antiarrhythmic effects of tricyclic antidepressant drugs in ouabain-induced arrhythmias in the dog. *J. Pharmacol. Exp. Ther. 205*:666-674.
26. Muir, W. W., Strauch, S. M., and Schaal, S. F. (1982). Effects of tricyclic antidepressant drugs on the electrophysiological properties of dog Purkinje fibers. *J. Cardiovasc. Pharmacol. 4*:82-90.
27. Hoffman, B. F. and Bigger, J. T., Jr. (1971). Antiarrhythmic drugs. In *Drill's Pharmacology in Medicine*, 4th ed. Edited by J. R. DiPalma. New York, McGraw-Hill, pp. 824-852.
28. Langou, R. A., Van Dyke, C., Tahan, S. R., and Cohen, L. S. (1980). Cardiovascular manifestations of tricyclic antidepressant overdose. *Am. Heart J. 100*: 458-464.
29. Glassman, A. H. and Bigger, J. T., Jr. (1981). Cardiovascular effects of therapeutic doses of tricyclic antidepressants. A review. *Arch. Gen. Psychiatry 38*: 815-820.
30. Burckhardt, D., Raeder, E., Muller, V., Imhof, P., and Neubauer, H. (1978). Cardiovascular effects of tricyclic and tetracyclic antidepressants. *JAMA 239*: 213-216.
31. Raeder, E. A., Burckhardt, D., Neubauer, H., Walter, R., and Gastpar, M. (1978). Long-term tri- and tetra-cyclic antidepressants, myocardial contractility, and cardiac rhythm. *Br. Med. J. 2*:666-667.
32. Taylor, D. J. and Braithwaite, R. A. (1978). Cardiac effects of tricyclic antidepressant medication: A preliminary study of nortriptyline. *Br. Heart J. 40*: 1005-1009.
33. Giardina, E. G. V., Bigger, J. T., Jr., and Glassman, A. H. (1982). Comparison between imipramine and desmethylimipramine on the electrocardiogram and left ventricular function. *Clin. Pharmacol. Ther. 31*:230.

34. Veith, R. C., Raskind, M. A., Caldwell, J. H., Barnes, R. F., Gumbrecht, G., and Ritchie, J. L. (1982). Cardiovascular effects of tricyclic antidepressants in depressed patients with chronic heart disease. *N. Engl. J. Med. 306*:954-959.
35. Glassman, A. H., Johnson, L. L., Giardina, E. G. V., Walsh, B. T., Roose, S. P., Cooper, T. B., and Bigger, J. T., Jr. (1983). The use of imipramine in depressed patients with congestive heart failure. *JAMA 250*:1997-2001.
36. Roose, S. P., Glassman, A. H., Giardina, E. G. V., Johnson, L. L., Walsh, B. T., Woodring, S., and Bigger, J. T., Jr. (1986). Nortriptyline in depressed patients with left ventricular impairment. *JAMA 256*:3253-3257.
37. Roose, S. P., Glassman, A. H., Giardina, E. G. V., Johnson, L. L., Walsh, B. T., and Bigger, J. T., Jr. (1987). Cardiovascular effects of imipramine and bupropion in depressed patients with congestive heart failure. *J. Clin. Psychopharmacol. 7*:247-251.
38. Giardina, E. G. V., Johnson, L. L., Vita, J., Bigger, J. T., Jr., and Brem, R. F. (1985). Effect of imipramine and nortriptyline on left ventricular function and blood pressure in patients treated for arrhythmias. *Am. Heart J. 109*:992-998.
39. Roose, S. P., Glassman, A. H., Giardina, E. G. V., Walsh, B. T., Woodring, S., and Bigger, J. T., Jr. (1987). Tricyclic antidepressants in depressed patients with cardiac conduction disease. *Arch. Gen. Psychiatry 44*:273-275.
40. Kantor, S. J., Bigger, J. T., Jr., Glassman, A. H., Macken, D. L., and Perel, J. M. (1975). Imipramine-induced heart block: A longitudinal case study. *JAMA 231*:1364-1366.
41. Crome, P. and Newman, B. (1979). Fatal tricyclic antidepressant poisoning. *J. R. Soc. Med. 72*:649-653.
42. Edwards, J. G. and Goldie, A. (1983). Mianserin, maprotiline, and intracardiac conduction. *Br. J. Clin. Pharmacol. 15*:249s-254s.
43. Kulig, K. (1986). Management of poisoning associated with "newer" antidepressant agents. *Ann. Emerg. Med. 15*:1039-1045.
44. Litovitz, J. L. and Troutman, W. G. (1983). Amoxapine overdose: Seizures and fatalities. *JAMA 250*:1069-1071.
45. Burgess, C. D., Hames, T. K., and George, C. F. (1982). The electrocardiographic and anticholinergic effects of trazodone and imipramine in man. *Eur. J. Clin. Pharmacol. 23*:417-421.
46. Henry, J. A. and Ali, C. J. (1983). Trazodone overdosage: Experience from a poisons information service. *Hum. Toxicol. 2*:353-356.
47. Lesar, T., Kingston, R., Dahms, R., and Saxena, K. (1983). Trazodone overdose. *Ann. Emerg. Med. 12*:221-223.
48. Lippmann, S., Bunch, S., Abuton, J., Embry, C., Manshadi, M., and Surender, E. (1982). A trazodone overdose [Letter]. *Am. J. Psychiatry 139*:1373.
49. Janowsky, D., Curtis, G., Zisook, S., Kuhn, K., Resovsky, K., and LeWinter, M. (1983). Ventricular arrhythmias possibly aggravated by trazodone. *Am. J. Psychiatry 140*:796-797.
50. Fisch, C. (1985). Effect of fluoxetine on the electrocardiogram. *J. Clin. Psychiatry 46*:42-44.
51. Wernicke, J. F. (1985). The side effect profile and safety of fluoxetine. *J. Clin. Psychiatry 46*:59-67.

52. Benfield, P., Heck, R. C., and Lewis, S. P. (1986). Fluoxetine: A review of its pharmacodynamic and pharmacokinetic properties, and therapeutic efficacy in depressive illness. *Drugs 32*:481-508.
53. Wenger, T. L. and Stern, W. C. (1983). The cardiovascular profile of bupropion. *J. Clin. Psychiatry 44*:176-182.

16

Use of Antidepressants in Geriatric Patients

MARCELLA PASCUALY

Seattle Veterans Administration Medical Center and
University of Washington School of Medicine
Seattle, Washington

RICHARD C. VEITH

American Lake Veterans Administration Medical Center and
University of Washington School of Medicine
Seattle, Washington

INTRODUCTION

Most elderly individuals traverse late life free of significant psychological disability. For those who encounter psychiatric difficulties severe enough to warrant diagnosis, the most common disturbance is depression (1-3). Traditional clinical lore has suggested that rates of depression are increased in the aged (1,4), compared with those in the young. However, this perception is not supported by recent studies of the prevalence of major depressive illness that indicate no age-related increase in depression in community populations (2,3,5). These findings do not, however, imply that depression is unimportant in the aged. On the contrary, compelling evidence indicates that suicide is overrepresented in the elderly (6,7) and that depression compromises the quality of life and contributes to the morbidity of chronic medical illness that often accompanies advanced age.

EPIDEMIOLOGY OF DEPRESSION IN LATE LIFE: MAGNITUDE OF THE PROBLEM

Affective disturbances span a spectrum of severity from transient depressive symptoms to unremitting melancholia and acute mania. Surveys on the prevalence of "depression" as a symptom and a diagnosis are highly variable

(1,4,5) because depression is a troublesome term that can be applied to many conditions, including normal fluctuations in mood state, feelings of despondency, episodes of bereavement, transient psychological reactions to injury or loss, or the neurovegetative syndrome that characterizes a major depressive episode. Differentiation of these states within the context of chronic illness, multiple losses, medication effects, and functional impairment, which often accompany aging, is a formidable challenge.

Recent studies, with DSM-III criteria (8) for major depressive epidoses, indicate that approximately 4% of the population over age 65 have major depression (5), a rate that is comparable with studies in younger individuals (2,3). An additional 15% of older individuals living independently in the community have significant depressive symptomatology (1,5). Rates for depression among older patients enrolled in outpatient medical clinics and on inpatient medical services range between 20 and 30% (9-11), and the rates for institutionalized elderly patients suggest that depression is especially prevalent (4,12).

Suicide rates, however, are disproportionately high in the aged (6,7,13). Individuals over age 65 composed 11% of the United States population in 1985, but accounted for 17% of the suicides (7). Moreover, suicide is a particularly serious problem in the "oldest-old" (6), those individuals aged 85 and over, who represent the fastest-growing segment of the population. In addition, studies in younger individuals suggest that depression is associated with increased mortality from cardiovascular causes (14), and this risk probably extends to older patients. Thus, depression represents an important, potentially preventable cause of mortality and morbidity in the elderly.

DIAGNOSIS AND DIFFERENTIAL DIAGNOSIS

Aging in our society often requires individuals to adjust psychologically to multiple losses, financial hardships, altered family roles, or chronic medical illness. In this context, the process of discerning the presence of a pathological depressive state can be problematic. The principal goal of the clinician considering pharmacotherapy for the older patient is to determine if the form of "depression" present is likely to require antidepressant treatment. The need for accurate diagnosis is particularly important when considering antidepressant treatment for the elderly because of the need to avoid unnecessarily exposing older patients to the potential adverse effects antidepressant treatment.

For the purpose of considering antidepressant therapy, we will use the term *depression* to connote the DSM-III-R criteria (15) for major depressive episode (Table 1). These criteria, however, are not necessarily *synonymous* with a clinical indication for antidepressant treatment. Because of the broad, in-

Table 1 DSM-III-R Diagnostic Criteria for Major Depressive Episode

A. At least five of the following symptoms have been present during the same 2-week period and represent a change from previous functioning; at least one of the symptoms is either (1) depressed mood, or (2) loss of interest or pleasure.
   1. Depressed mood most of the day, nearly every day, as indicated either by subjective account or observation by others.
   2. Markedly diminished interest or pleasure in all, or almost all, activities most of the day, nearly every day (as indicated either by subjective account or observation by others of apathy most of the time).
   3. Significant weight loss or weight gain when not dieting (e.g., more than 5% of body weight in a month), or decrease or increase in appetite nearly every day.
   4. Insomnia or hypersomnia nearly every day.
   5. Psychomotor agitation of retardation nearly every day (observable by others, not merely subjective feelings of restlessness or being slowed down).
   6. Fatigue or loss of energy nearly every day.
   7. Feelings of worthlessness or excessive or inappropriate guilt (which may be delusional) nearly every day (not merely self-reproach or guilt about being sick).
   8. Diminished ability to think or concentrate, or indecisiveness, nearly every day (either by subjective account or as observed by others).
   9. Recurrent thoughts of death (not just fear of dying), recurrent suicidal ideation without a specific plan, or a suicide attempt or a specific plan for committing suicide.

B. 1. It cannot be established that an organic factor initiated and maintained the disturbance.
   2. The disturbance is not a normal reaction to the death of a loved one (uncomplicated bereavement).

C. At no time during the disturbance have there been delusions or hallucinations for as long as 2 weeks in the absence of prominent mood symptoms (i.e., before the mood symptoms developed or after they have remitted).

D. Not superimposed on schizophrenia, schizophreniform disorder, delusional disorder.

clusive nature of these criteria, patients experiencing an array of affective disturbances might fulfill them, but might also respond satisfactorily to supportive psychotherapy, rather than pharmacotherapy.

Clinical studies indicate that the best predictors of response to antidepressant drug therapy are "endogenous symptoms," such as sleep disturbance, appetite change, psychomotor change, and insidious onset (16). This neurovegetative syndrome conforms more closely to the DSM-III-R criteria for melancholia (Table 2) than for major depressive episode.

This does not suggest that this differentiation can be easily made in the presence of the medical, medication, and psychosocial problems usually en-

Table 2 DSM-III-R Diagnostic Criteria for Major Depressive Episode, Melancholic Type

A. Meets criteria for major depressive episode.
B. The presence of at least five of the following:
   1. Loss of interest or pleasure in all, or almost all, activities
   2. Lack of reactivity to usually pleasurable stimuli (does not feel much better, even temporarily, when something good happens)
   3. Depression regularly worse in morning
   4. Early morning awakening (at least 2 hr before usual time of awakening)
   5. Psychomotor retardation or agitation (not merely subjective complaints)
   6. Significant anorexia or weight loss (e.g., more than 5% of body weight in a month)
   7. No significant personality disturbance before first major depressive episode
   8. One or more previous major depressive episodes followed by complete, or nearly complete, recovery
   9. Previously good response to specific and adequate somatic antidepressant therapy (e.g., tricyclics, ECT, MAOI, lithium)

countered in the older patient. However, such a conceptual approach to depression is an important first step in considering pharmacotherapy for these patients. We are not suggesting that individuals whose depression fulfills DSM-III-R criteria, without endogenous symptoms or melancholia, are not candidates for pharmacotherapy, because some of these patients will benefit from such therapy; rather, we would emphasize that meeting the DSM-III-R criteria for major depression need not be synonymous with a requirement for drug treatment.

Clinical studies that have examined the differential efficacy of pharmacotherapy and psychotherapy, mostly performed in young patients over the past 10 years, bear out this interpretation (17-19). The conclusions from these studies are further confirmed by those of Gallagher and Thompson (20) who found that depressed elderly patients with endogenous symptoms responded to psychotherapy less well than to pharmacotherapy and had higher relapse rates than did those with nonendogenous depression.

How, then, should we conceptualize the other, highly prevalent, forms of depression in our older patients? We have adopted a conceptual framework (Table 3) that describes several conditions, which often might be subsumed under the diagnosis of depression, that are commonly encountered in the elderly patient. This model combines our clinical experience with that of others (21-23). The psychological states outlined in Table 3 should not supplant the need for specific diagnostic criteria (e.g., DSM-III-R), but are a

Table 3 Conceptual Classification of Conditions Commonly Termed "Depression" in the Elderly

Bereavement
Despondency
Secondary depression
Medical illness
Medications
Nonmelancholic major depression
Melancholic major depression

proposed classification scheme for the initial *conceptual* appraisal of the various forms of depression often encountered in the elderly.

Bereavement

Loss of loved ones and acquaintances through death is a universal experience of advanced age, when multiple losses over brief periods are common. Death of a loved one is normally accompanied by a period of acute grieving that typically persists for several months. Such periods can be associated with intense sadness, emotional lability, and sleeplessness, but the identifiable onset of bereavement provides a benchmark useful to differentiate this "normal" psychological reaction from a pathological depression. However, protracted, unremitting grief may also be a precipitant for the development of major depression. The presence of prolonged grieving, if associated with anhedonia, guilt, impaired social functioning, or vegetative symptoms, should prompt a careful appraisal for presence of a major depression that might complicate normal bereavement.

Despondency

Despondency is a construct that can be used to characterize a mood disturbance in individuals who are struggling to cope with potentially overwhelming stress (e.g., multiple losses, chronic illness). The concept of despondency has been promoted by Hackett and Cassem (23) for its usefulness in the hospital setting where depressive reactions to medical illness may present an affective continuum, ranging from depressive adjustment disorders to major depression. The obvious implication is that some forms of depression are situationally determined psychological reactions and may be responsive to elimination of the stressful circumstances or to supportive psychotherapy. Patients whose symptoms persist or are unresponsive to supportive strategies may require antidepressant therapy.

Secondary Depression

Medical Illness

The increased presence of medical illness and medication use in the elderly complicates the differential diagnosis of depression. Numerous medical diseases (Table 4) are often associated with behavioral disturbances that include depressive symptoms or might present initially as depressive illness.

Medical disease in the elderly presents several problems for the clinician considering treatment with antidepressant medication. First, one must determine that the patient's apparent depression is not simply a manifestation of medical disorder or a consequence of associated metabolic disturbances. Therefore, all older patients with suspected depression should receive a thorough medical, neurological, and laboratory evaluation for identification and treatment of underlying medical conditions. Alternatively, the medical illness, itself, might produce symptoms (e.g., lethargy, sleep or appetite disturbance) that are indistinguishable from those of a primary depression. Thus, the clinician must decide to what degree the mood disturbance is a reasonable psychological response to the illness (e.g., DSM-III-R adjustment disorder with depressed mood, despondency) and which symptoms

Table 4 Medical Illnesses Commonly Associated with Depressive Symptoms

Endocrine or metabolic	
Hypothyroidism	Hypoglycemia
Hyperthyroidism	Hyponatremia
Cushing's disease	Hypocalcemia
Addison's disease	Hepatic failure
Hypo/hyperparathyroidism	Uremia
Diabetes	
Central Nervous System	
Tumor or mass lesion	Alzheimer's disease
Multiple sclerosis	Parkinson's disease
Vascular disease	
Miscellaneous	
Alcoholism	Infections
Congestive heart failure	Carcinoma
Pernicious anemia	Porphyria
Systemic lupus erythematosus	

should be attributed to the underlying clinical condition. Such differentiation usually requires stabilization of the patient's medical status.

If after careful treatment of the primary medical illness the patient develops a persistent depression, he or she may well be a candidate for antidepressant treatment, despite the fact that the depression is secondary to the medical illness. Here, it is the presence of the neurovegetative depressive syndrome and not the presence or absence of an obvious environmental precipitant that provides the indication for antidepressant intervention. This conclusion is borne out in studies of patients with heart disease (24) and with depressed patients after a stroke (25,26). Although depression in these studies was usually considered "secondary," both groups of patients benefited from tricyclic antidepressants.

Finally, it is possible that patients might develop depression coexistent with a primary medical disease. For example, Robinson et al. (25-27) observed a high frequency of depression following stroke, particularly strokes affecting the left frontal lobe region. Similarly, depression has been reported in 25% of patients with Alzheimer's disease (28). In such settings, patients who exhibit persistent mood disturbance associated with neurovegetative symptoms of depression deserve serious consideration for an antidepressant trial in conjunction with other supportive measures.

Medications

Medication use is common in older patients and is an additional source of diagnostic confusion. Table 5 lists medications most commonly alleged to produce depression. The true magnitude of drug-induced depression is unknown because of the anecdotal nature of many surveys (29). However, it is likely that many drugs may cause depression, particularly in patients with a prior history of mood disturbance. In this context, the clinician must first consider the possibility that the symptoms that appear as major depression

Table 5 Drugs Commonly Associated with Depressive Symptoms

Antihypertensives: reserpine, guanethidine, propranolol
Anxiolytics
Alcohol
Sedative-hypnotics
Steroids: glucocorticoids, oral contraceptives
Analgesics: opiates
Neuroleptics: (akinesia, masked faces)
Antiparkinsonian agents
Antineoplastics

might be drug-induced adverse effects. This requires that the clinical indication for each medication be carefully reviewed and all unnecessary drugs discontinued before a final diagnosis of depression is made. The other major complication of the increased medication use in the depressed elderly patient is the potential for drug-drug interactions that can complicate antidepressant treatment. This is discussed in greater detail later.

Nonmelancholic Major Depression

It is important that the clinician weigh the potential benefits and risks of antidepressant treatment in older patients with major depression who do not appear to have prominent endogenous or melancholic symptoms. We would reemphasize that some patients, particularly those with less severe major depression, might well benefit from antidepressant therapy. Nevertheless, it remains in the patient's best interest to avoid unnecessary medication use, particularly in older patients with concurrent medical illness. Thus, for such patients, a reasonable strategy might be to institute nonpharmacologic treatment before starting antidepressant medication. If symptoms persist, however, adjunctive pharmacologic treatment should be offered with the confidence that combined psychotherapy and pharmacotherapy generally appears to be preferable to pharmacologic treatment alone (17-19).

Melancholic Major Depression

The decision to initiate antidepressant treatment in elderly patients represents a distillation process that identifies patients who exhibit neurovegetative symptoms of DSM-III-R melancholia. This approach may exclude some depressed patients who might initially benefit from antidepressants, but in our opinion, the increased hazards of psychotropic use in the aged justify this conservative approach.

AGE EFFECTS ON THE PHARMACOKINETIC METABOLISM OF ANTIDEPRESSANTS

Normal aging is associated with alterations in several physiological systems that influence the pharmacokinetic and pharmacodynamic effects of antidepressants (31-33). In general, psychotropic agents are highly lipid-soluble and protein bound. They bind with high affinity to brain, heart, and adipose tissue and are metabolized by liver microsomal enzymes by demethylation, hydroxylation, or glucuronide formation, which increases their water solubility and renal excretion.

Age-related changes in body composition result in an increase in body adipose tissue relative to lean body mass, which can increase the distribution volume of lipid-soluble drugs (such as tricyclic antidepressants) and prolong their elimination half-life. In addition, the effectiveness of the hepatic microsomal enzymes diminish and this can also prolong drug action, foster drug accumulation, and delay its elimination. Age and nutritional or disease-related reductions in plasma proteins can increase the concentration of free, unbound drug at receptor sites, thereby altering its therapeutic and its toxic profiles (34). Aging is also associated with a generalized slowing (35) of renal clearance, which could prolong the elimination of drugs and their metabolites. Collectively, these changes probably contribute to the increased frequency of adverse effects and the variable drug responses among older patients. It is also possible that the age-related changes in neuronal systems within the central nervous system, and their response to drug administration might account for the increased sensitivity of older patients to these agents.

Several studies have directly explored the effects of these age-related physiological changes on the pharmacokinetic characteristics of antidepressants. Although not all studies are in agreement (36-39), a positive correlation between age and steady-state plasma levels has been found with several antidepressants (33), and the clearance and elimination half-life of imipramine has been shown to be prolonged in the elderly (40).

Most tricyclic antidepressants are biotransformed in the liver to form hydroxylated metabolites. These compounds are pharmacologically active (41) and can occur in high concentrations in some patients. Interestingly, these "hydroxy metabolites" may correlate more closely with the cardiovascular effects of these agents than the parent antidepressant (42). In addition, the plasma levels of the hydroxylated metabolites increase with age reflecting a reduction in glomerular filtration rate (43). Although these observations require additional study, they support the use of lower doses of tricyclic antidepressants in the elderly.

TRICYCLIC, TETRACYCLIC, AND SECOND-GENERATION ANTIDEPRESSANTS

Drug Selection

The drugs of first choice for the treatment of major depression in the elderly are tricyclic antidepressants or related agents (Table 6). Although relatively few controlled studies have specifically investigated the therapeutic or adverse effects of these drugs in elderly patients (30,44), their efficacy in appropriately selected older patients is well established.

Intense research activity has focused on the possibility that subgroups of depressed patients might respond differentially to specific antidepressants, based on differences in pharmacologic structure or profile (45-50). To date,

Table 6 Tricyclic and Second-Generation Antidepressants

Structure	Trade name	Usual dose (mg/day) Adult	Usual dose (mg/day) Elderly
Tricyclic			
Tertiary			
amitriptyline	Elavil	100-300	25-150
imipramine	Tofranil	100-300	25-150
doxepin	Sinequan	100-300	25-150
trimipramine	Surmontil	100-300	25-150
Secondary			
nortriptyline	Pamelor	50-100	10-60
desipramine	Norpramine	100-300	25-150
protriptyline	Vivactil	20-60	5-30
Second-generation antidepressants			
Tricyclic			
Dibenzoxazepine			
amoxapine	Ascendin	150-300	25-150
Triazolopyridine			
trazodone	Desyrel	150-400	50-300
Tetracyclic			
maprotiline	Ludiomil	100-300	25-150
Methylphenylpropylamine			
fluoxetine	Prozac	20	20 (qod)
Phenylaminoketone			
bupropion	Wellbutrin	225-450	225-450

however, these intriguing research questions remain unresolved and should not be applied on a routine clinical basis. Therefore, the selection among the available agents for older patients is customarily determined by differences in their potential side effect profiles.

Dosages

Regardless of the drug selected, starting doses should be lower for older patients. It is particularly important to individualize treatment, recognizing that the presence of concurrent medical disease, concomitant medication, and age-related pharmacokinetic alterations impart a greater variability of drug metabolism and response in the elderly. A typical starting dose for tertiary amine tricyclics, such as amitriptyline, imipramine, and doxepin, would be 25-50 mg at bedtime; for frail patients, 10 mg might be more appropriate. The elimination half-life of the new antidepressant fluoxetine, is 2-3 days and its active metabolite (norfluoxetine) is 7-9 days. Thus, this agent should be used with caution in older patients. In fact, these individuals might require only every-other-day administration to achieve a good therapeutic effect.

Dosage increments for all antidepressants should be instituted more slowly than in younger patients (i.e., 10-25 mg increments every 4-5 days until a therapeutic effect is achieved). Moreover, it is important to employ an adequate trial before concluding that treatment is unsuccessful. Because steady-state doses will be achieved more gradually in these patients, several more weeks of treatment may be required to observe a therapeutic effect.

The optimal duration of maintenance therapy for patients who achieve a good response has not been established for older patients, but treatment is customarily maintained for 6-9 months before tapering the antidepressant. If symptoms recur, treatment can be resumed for several additional months.

Inadequate Therapeutic Response

Several possible explanations might be considered for patients who fail to achieve a satisfactory clinical response. The most common cause is the adverse effects of the antidepressant, usually the result of anticholinergic or hypotensive properties of these agents.

The possibility that some subtypes of depressed patients might demonstrate variability of response to certain antidepressants has been studied. Additionally, for example, differences in neuronal uptake inhibition of serotonin or norepinephrine might be related to differences in antidepressant response (46-50), although these theories have not been of practical clinical value. Nevertheless, the possibility of administering a different pharmacologic agent (i.e., tertiary versus secondary amine, tricyclic versus nontricyclic, or norepinephrine versus serotonin reuptake inhibitor) remains a reasonable strategy if a patient fails to respond to the initial drug therapy.

An inadequate therapeutic response that is not directly attributable to adverse effects should always prompt a diagnostic reappraisal. If an antidepressant continues to be indicated, the usual strategy is to select an alternative agent (as suggested earlier). Furthermore, a substantial number of severely depressed elderly patients will have delusional depression, a condition which responds poorly to conventional doses of tricyclic antidepressants (51-54). Careful titration to high doses of these agents might be required for such patients or concomitant treatment with a neuroleptic might be beneficial (51). However, it is also important to recognize the increased risk of tardive dyskinesia in older patients (55), and this factor requires judicious and time-limited use of the neuroleptics in this population.

There has been little systematic investigation of treatment-resistant depression in the elderly. Studies in younger patients have indicated the value of adjunctive lithium carbonate with tricyclic antidepressants (56,57). However, this work has not been extended to the elderly, and the casual use of lithium in older individuals is not recommended because of age-related reductions in renal clearance.

In contrast, electroconvulsive therapy (ECT) is often well tolerated in older patients, when applied during careful anesthesiological management. This treatment option deserves serious consideration for the treatment-resistant patient, for those unable to tolerate antidepressant medication, and for those too suicidal to await the response of medication treatment.

Adverse Effects

Sedation

Depressed elderly patients are particularly sensitive to the adverse effects of the tricyclic and tetracyclic antidepressants. The sedative, anticholinergic, and cardiovascular side effects are of most concern. These agents vary in their sedative properties (Table 7). Sedation can be an advantage in the agitated

Table 7 Tricyclic and Second-Generation Antidepressants: Side Effect Profiles

		Adverse effects		
Structure	Trade name	Sedation	Anticholinergic	Hypotension
Tricyclic				
Tertiary				
amitriptyline	Elavil	+ + +	+ + + +	+ + +
imipramine	Tofranil	+ +	+ + +	+ + +
doxepin	Sinequan	+ + +	+ + + +	+ + +
trimipramine	Surmontil	+ + +	+ + +	+ + +
Secondary				
nortriptyline	Pamelor	+	+ +	+ +
desipramine	Norpramine	0	+ +	+ + +
protriptyline	Vivactil	0	+ + +	+ + +
Second-generation antidepressants				
Tricyclic				
dibenzoxazepine				
amoxapine	Ascendin	+ +	+ + +	+ + +
triazolopyridine				
trazodone	Desyrel	+ + +	+	+ + +
Tetracyclic				
maprotiline	Ludiomil	+	+ + +	+ + +
Methylphenylpropylamine				
fluoxetine	Prozac	0	0	0
Phenylaminoketone				
bupropion	Wellbutrin	0	0	0

[a]FDA approval pending.

patient who is not sleeping, but it is an unwanted nuisance in the withdrawn patient with psychomotor retardation. In contrast, the less-sedating agents potentially subject older patients to restlessness, tremulousness, or sleep disturbance, which also is not well received. Although great interindividual variability is present, sedation is largely dose-related, which often restricts the maximal dose that older patients are able to tolerate.

Anticholinergic Effects

The anticholinergic effects include dry mouth, constipation, urinary obstructive symptoms, and exacerbation of narrow-angle glaucoma. The potential for CNS anticholinergic toxicity leading to the development of confusion or delirium is particularly worrisome. Hence, it is often preferable to avoid the more anticholinergic of these agents (e.g., amitriptyline, doxepin) in favor of agents that are less potent (e.g., nortriptyline, desipramine); however, in high doses these latter agents also impart a substantial anticholinergic effect, albeit less than would occur with amitriptyline or doxepin. Trazodone has less anticholinergic activity, but can produce priapism (58) and ventricular arrhythmias at conventional doses (59), which offset its potential value in treating older patients. Fluoxetine also has fewer anticholinergic properties, but, because of its long duration of action and its tendency to cause weight loss (60,61), it must be used cautiously in older patients. Bupropion is essentially devoid of cholinergic or α_1-adrenergic receptor antagonism (62); however, it has not yet received widespread clinical use in the elderly. If proven both safe and effective, its pharmacologic profile offers several potential advantages in the treatment of older patients.

Cardiovascular Effects

The cardiovascular risks from antidepressant drugs have traditionally posed an additional obstacle to their use in older patients. More recent research, however, has clarified the specific concerns related to these agents (24,63-71). The three major cardiovascular effects of tricyclic antidepressants are (1) an anticholinergic effect that increases heart rate, (2) intraventricular conduction delay, and (3) orthostatic hypotension. Concern that these agents might exert a negative inotropic effect on the heart has not been substantiated by several studies of patients with cardiac disease that found no significant effect of imipramine, doxepin, or nortriptyline on the left ventricular ejection fraction, a measure of ventricular pumping efficiency (24,66,68).

The tendency to increase heart rate by antagonism of vagal slowing of the heart is variable among the drugs and is a function of their anticholinergic properties. Although increases of 5-10 beats/min are common (65), this rarely causes problems in patients who have no heart failure or coronary artery disease.

The tricyclic antidepressants also possess antiarrhythmic properties at therapeutic doses (24,66,68). In contrast, trazodone has been reported to exacerbate ventricular arrhythmias (59), interestingly, this compound lacks the tendency to delay intraventricular conduction common to the other antidepressants that share an antiarrhythmic property. This is also true for fluoxetine, which has little, if any, effect on cardiac rhythm in dogs (70).

The tricyclic antidepressants delay conduction through the distal His-Purkinje specialized conduction system of the heart (64,71), which is reflected on the electrocardiogram (ECG) as a dose-related prolongation of the QRS and QTc intervals (65). This property, shared by quinidine which also stabilizes heart rhythm at therapeutic doses, has led to clinical trials of several tricyclics as antiarrhythmic agents in cardiac patients with refractory ventricular arrhythmias. However, such "quinidinelike" action can also be potentially hazardous for patients with preexisting conduction delay (72). Of greatest concern are those patients with bundle-branch or fascicular blocks who are prone to develop complete heart block when treated with antidepressants. Electroconvulsive therapy or the use of the monoamine oxidase inhibitors, which do not delay cardiac conduction (73), might be preferable for patients with pretreatment conduction defects. Fluoxetine also offers the potential benefit of no apparent effects on cardiac conduction, but this agent should be used cautiously in the elderly until its general safety profile is better established by widespread use in patients without cardiac disease.

Orthostatic hypotension poses a substantial risk for older patients for whom antidepressants have been prescribed (67), an effect thought to be mediated by the α_1-adrenergic receptor-blocking effects of these drugs. This side effect often limits the maximal tolerated doses and is an important cause of falls in the elderly (74). Clinical predictors for those patients most likely to develop orthostatic hypotension include the presence of pretreatment hypotension (67), congestive heart failure (68), deconditioning from bed rest, or the use of other drugs that lower blood pressure (e.g., antihypertensives, nitrates) (24). In our experience, the development of hypotension is dose-related, but not all investigators share this view (67). Importantly, it has been demonstrated (63) that within its usually recommended optimal plasma levels of 50-150 ng/mL, nortriptyline may produce less orthostatic hypotension than other antidepressants. This characteristic of nortriptyline offers a useful therapeutic advantage for older patients. Fluoxetine is less potent than the tricyclic antidepressants in antagonizing α_1-adrenoreceptors and has less effect on blood pressure (70,75), although this has not been systematically investigated in older patients. Bupropion causes less hypotension than imipramine in therapeutically effective doses (76), and it might represent a useful treatment alternative for older patients.

The cardiovascular hazards of these agents can be minimized by careful monitoring of orthostatic blood pressure before and during treatment and by cautious dosing (i.e., starting with low doses, progressing slowly, using divided doses, and avoiding high doses if possible). A pretreatment ECG is useful to identify patients with preexisting conduction disturbances or poorly controlled arrhythmias. Subsequent ECGs, obtained during incremental dosing, should be examined for evidence of clinically significant conduction disturbances that might warrant a reduction in dose or termination of treatment.

MONOAMINE OXIDASE INHIBITORS

The monoamine oxidase inhibitors (MAOI) have received renewed interest over the past several years (77). However, this has not led to widespread use of these agents in the elderly (78). The MAOI pose two distinct risks for older patients: dietary restrictions, which add complexity to the use of these agents for older patients, and orthostatic hypotension (73,79), which is a particular risk for the older patient. However, these agents do not delay intraventricular conduction (73) and might offer a useful advantage for patients unable to tolerate the tricyclic antidepressants because of preexisting conduction defects.

STIMULANT DRUGS

The stimulants have received a limited degree of clinical popularity as a treatment of depression (80). Methylphenidate and dextroamphetamine are generally thought to be less effective than the tricyclic antidepressants and the MAOIs in treating depression, and they also have the potential of producing adverse cardiovascular effects, insomnia, and paranoid reactions with prolonged use. However, in low doses and on a time-limited basis these agents may be a useful alternative for the treatment of some elderly patients who are unable to tolerate traditional antidepressants. Several uncontrolled clinical trials have reported clinical benefits from the use of the stimulants in treating either medically ill depressed patients or the withdrawn, apathetic dementia patients, and our own clinical experience supports these impressions (80-84). We tend to consider a stimulant trial in frail, bedridden, withdrawn, and apathetic depressed patients who have failed an antidepressant trial or who cannot tolerate the hypotensive properties of even low doses of these agents. Typically, we initiate treatment with 5-10 mg/day of methylphenidate and assess the response over several days, possibly increasing the dosage to 15-20 mg/day if tolerated. By giving medication in the morning and early afternoon, the potential disruption of sleep can be minimized. Not uncommonly, such patients improve, with an increase in ability to participate in their care, increased energy, brightening of mood and, surprisingly, an improvement in appetite. As has been reported by others (81), patients who benefit from such trials usually respond within 2-4 days after starting treatment. It is important to emphasize that these drugs have a potential for abuse and should not be used indiscriminately. Thus, treatment should be implemented on a time-limited basis, with the expectation that a lack of convincing evidence of therapeutic benefit will result in stopping treatment within several days or 1-2 weeks. We have treated such patients for several months, with apparent benefit and minimal side effects.

DRUG INTERACTIONS

The antidepressants pose a special risk for older patients, for whom multiple medications are often prescribed. The tricyclic antidepressants interfere with the antihypertensive effects of guanethidine by blocking its uptake into CNS neurons. These agents also attenuate the hypotensive effects of clonidine, possibly by the production of α_2-adrenergic receptor subsensitivity following prolonged treatment. However, our studies indicate (unpublished findings) that desipramine can antagonize the blood pressure-lowering effect of clonidine after only 2 days of desipramine treatment. The antihypertensive effects of methyldopa, hydralazine, or the diuretics do not appear to be affected by the tricyclic antidepressants.

The sedative and anticholinergic effects of the tricyclic antidepressants may also accentuate similar properties of other centrally acting medications and produce an additive effect with other drugs that reduce blood pressure. It seems reasonable that these agents would also produce an additive effect with other class 1-A antiarrhythmic agents, but we are unaware of any data supporting this theoretical possibility.

In summary, the careful diagnosis of depressive illness in elderly patients, together with the judicious application of the proper antidepressant treatment modality, can lead to a dramatic clinical improvement in a population of patients at substantial risk for increased morbidity and mortality.

ACKNOWLEDGMENT

This work was supported in part by the Research Service of the Department of Veterans Affairs.

REFERENCES

1. Gurland, B., Dean, L., Cross, P., and Golden, R. (1980). The epidemiology of depression and dementia in the elderly: The use of multiple indicators of these

conditions. In *Psychopathology in the Aged.* Edited by J. O. Cole and J. E. Barrett. New York, Raven Press, pp. 37-60.

2. Myers, J. K., Weissman, M. W., Tischler, G. L., Holzer, C. E., Leaf, P. J., Kramer, M., and Stolzman, R. (1984). Six-month prevalence of psychiatric disorders in three communities. *Arch. Gen. Psychiatry 41*:959-967.
3. Robins, L. N., Helzer, J. E., Weissman, M. M., Orvaschel, H., Gruenberg, E., Burke, J. D., and Regier, D. A. (1984). Lifetime prevalence of specific psychiatric disorders in three sites. *Arch. Gen. Psychiatry 41*:949-958.
4. Blazer, D. B. (1982). *Depression in Late Life.* St. Louis, C. V. Mosby, pp. 105-117.
5. Blazer, D. and Williams, C. D. (1980). Epidemiology of dysphoria and depression in an elderly population. *Am. J. Psychiatry 137*:439-444.
6. Manton, K. G., Blazer, D. G., and Woodbury, M. A. (1987). Suicide in middle age and later life: Sex and race specific life table and cohort analyses. *J. Gerontol. 42*:219-227.
7. McIntosh, J. L. (1985). Suicide among the elderly: Levels and trends. *Am. J. Orthopsychiatry 55*:188-193.
8. American Psychiatric Association (1980). *Diagnostic and Statistical Manual of Mental Disorders*, 3rd ed. Washington, D.C., American Psychiatric Association.
9. Borson, S., Barnes, R. A., Kukull, W. A., Okimoto, J. T., Veith, R. C., Inui, T. S., Carter, W. C., and Raskind, M. A. (1986). Symptomatic depression in elderly medical outpatients. *J. Am. Geriatr. Soc. 34*:341-347.
10. Kitchell, M. A., Barnes, R. F., Veith, R. C., Okimoto, J. T., and Raskind, M. A. (1982). Screening for depression in hospitalized geriatric medical patients. *J. Am. Geriatr. Soc. 30*:174-177.
11. Rodin, G. and Voshart, K. (1986). Depression in the medically ill: An overview. *Am. J. Psychiatry 143*:696-705.
12. Dovenmuehle, R. H., Reckless, J. B., and Newpan, G. (1970). Depressive reactions in the elderly. In *Depressive Reactions in the Elderly, Normal Aging.* Edited by E. Palmore. Durham, N. C., University Press.
13. Asgood, N. J. (1985). *Suicide in the Elderly: A Practitioners Guide to Diagnosis and Mental Health Intervention.* Rockville, Md., Aspen Press. pp. 3-13.
14. Avery, D. and Winokur, G. (1976). Mortality in depressed patients treated with electroconvulsive therapy and antidepressants. *Arch. Gen. Psychiatry 33*:1029-1037.
15. American Psychiatric Association (1987). *Diagnostic and Statistical Manual of Mental Disorders*, 3rd ed., revised. Washington, D.C., American Psychiatric Association.
16. Bielski, R. J. and Friedel, R. O. (1976). Prediction of tricyclic antidepressant response: A critical review. *Arch. Gen. Psychiatry 33*:1479-1489.
17. Weissman, M. M. (1979). The psychological treatment of depression. Evidence for the efficacy of psychotherapy alone, in comparison with, and in combination with pharmacotherapy. *Arch. Gen. Psychiatry 36*:1261-1269.
18. DiMascio, A., Weissman, M. M., Prusoff, B. A., Neu, C., Swilling, M., and Klerman, G. L. (1979). Differential symptom reduction by drugs and psychotherapy in acute depression. *Arch. Gen. Psychiatry 36*:1450-1456.

19. Prusoff, B. A., Weissman, M. M., Klerman, G. L., and Rounsaville, B. J. (1980). Research diagnostic criteria subtypes of depression. Their role as predictors of differential response to psychotherapy and drug treatment. *Arch. Gen. Psychiatry 37*:796-801.
20. Gallagher, D. E. and Thompson, L. W. (1983). Effectiveness of psychotherapy for both endogenous and non-endogenous depression in older adult outpatients. *J. Gerontol. 38*:707-712.
21. Maletta, G. (1988). Commentary on review by Veith and Raskind: The many faces of depression. *Neurobiol. Aging 9*:122-124.
22. Koenig, H. (1986). Depression and dysphoria among the elderly: Dispensing a myth. *J. Fam. Pract. 23*:383-385.
23. Cassem, N. H. (1978). Depression. In *Handbook of General Hospital Psychiatry*. Edited by T. P. Hackett and N. H. Cassem. St. Louis, C. V. Mosby, pp. 209-225.
24. Veith, R. C., Raskind, M. R., Caldwell, J. H., Barnes, R. F., Gumbrecht, G., and Ritchie, J. L. (1982). Cardiovascular effects of the tricyclic antidepressants in depressed patients with chronic heart disease. *N. Engl. J. Med. 306*:954-959.
25. Lipsey, W. R., Robinson, R. E., Pearlson, G. D., Rao, K., and Price, T. R. (1984). Nortriptyline treatment of post-stroke depression: A double-blind study. *Lancet 1*:297-300.
26. Robinson, R. G., Lipsey, J. R., and Price, T. R. (1985). Mood disorders in post-stroke patients. In *Treatment of Affective Disorders in the Elderly*. Washington, D. C., American Psychiatric Press, pp. 65-74.
27. Robinson, R. G., Kubos, K. L., Starr, L. B., Rao, K., and Price, T. R. (1984). Mood disorders in stroke patients: Importance of location of lesion. *Brain 107*: 81-93.
28. Reifler, B. V., Larsen, E., and Hanley, R. (1982). Coexistence of cognitive impairment and depression in geriatric outpatients. *Am. J. Psychiatry 139*:623-626.
29. Pascualy, M. and Veith, R. C. (1989). Drug-induced depression. In *Depression in Aging and Chronic Illness*. Edited by R. G. Robinson and P. V. Rabins. New York, Igaku-Shoin Medical Publishers, pp. 132-151.
30. Veith, R. C. (1982). Depression in the elderly: Pharmacologic considerations in treatment. *J. Am. Geriatr. Soc. 30*:581-586.
31. Vestal, R. E. (1982). Pharmacology and aging. *J. Am. Geriatr. Soc. 30*:191-200.
32. Plein, J. B. and Plein, E. M. (1981). Aging and drug therapy. *Annu. Rev. Gerontol. Geriatr. 2*:211-254.
33. Nies, A., Robinson, D. S., Friedman, M. J., Green, R., Cooper, T., Ravaris, C. L., and Ives, J. O. (1977). Relationship between age and tricyclic antidepressant plasma levels. *Am. J. Psychiatry 134*:790-793.
34. Sjöqvist, F. and Bertilsson, L. (1981). Clinical pharmacology of tricyclic antidepressants: Facts, controversies, and future challenges. In *Clinical Pharmacology in Psychiatry*. Edited by E. Usdin. New York, Elsevier, pp. 141-153.
35. Lindeman, R. D., Tobin, J., and Shock, N. W. (1985). Longitudinal studies on the rate of decline in renal function with age. *J. Am. Geriatr. Soc. 33*:278-285.

36. Cutler, N. R., Zavadil, A. P., Eisdorfer, C., Ross, R. J., and Potter, W. Z. (1981). Concentrations of desipramine in elderly women. *Am. J. Psychiatry 138*: 1235-1237.
37. Dawling, S., Crome, P., Braithwaite, R. A., and Lewis, R. R. (1980). Nortriptyline therapy in elderly patients: Dosage prediction after single dose pharmacokinetic study. *Eur. J. Clin. Pharmacol. 18*:147-150.
38. Montgomery, B., Braithwaite, R., Dawling, S., and McAuley, R. (1978). High plasma nortriptyline levels in the treatment of depression. I. *Clin. Pharmacol. Ther. 23*:309-314.
39. Turbott, J., Normal, T. R., Burrows, G. D., Maguire, K. P., and Davies, B. M. (1980). Pharmacokinetics of nortriptyline in elderly volunteers. *Commun. Psychopharmacol. 4*:225-231.
40. Hrdina, P. D., Rovei, V., Henry, J. F., Gomeni, R., Forette, F., and Morselli, P. I. (1980). Comparison of single-dose pharmacokinetics of imipramine and maprotiline in the elderly. *Psychopharmacology 70*:29-34.
41. Potter, W. Z., Calil, H. M., Sutfin, B. S., Zavadil, A. P., Jusko, W. J., Rapoport, J., and Goodwin, F. X. (1982). Active metabolites of imipramine and desipramine in man. *Clin. Pharmacol. Ther. 31*:393-401.
42. Jandhyala, B. S., Steenberg, M. L., and Perel, J. M. (1977). Effects of several tricyclic antidepressants on the hemodynamics and myocardial contractility of the anesthetized dog. *Eur. J. Pharmacol. 42*:403-410.
43. Kitanaka, J., Ross, R. J., Cutler, N. R., Zavadil, A. P., and Potter, W. Z. (1982). Altered hydroxydesipramine concentrations in elderly depressed patients. *Clin. Pharmacol. Ther. 31*:51-55.
44. Jarvik, L. F. and Gerson, S. (1985). Outcome of drug treatment in depressed patients over the age of fifty. In *Treatment of Affective Disorders in the Elderly*. Edited by C. A. Shamoian. Washington, D.C., American Psychiatric Press, pp. 29-36.
45. Veith, R. C. and Raskind, M. A. (1988). The neurobiology of aging: Does it predispose to depression? *Neurobiol. Aging 9*:101-117.
46. Maas, J. W. (1978). Clinical and biochemical heterogeneity of depressive disorders. *Ann. Intern. Med. 88*:556-563.
47. Charney, D. S., Menkes, D. B., and Heninger, G. R. (1981). Receptor sensitivity and the mechanism of action of antidepressant treatment implications for the etiology and therapy of depression. *Arch. Gen. Psychiatry 38*:1160-1180.
48. Veith, R. C., Bielski, R. J., Bloom, V., Fawcett, J., Narasimhachari, N., and Friedel, R. O. (1983). Urinary MHPG excretion during treatment with desipramine and amitriptyline: Prediction of response, effect of treatment and methodological hazards. *J. Clin. Psychopharmacol. 3*:18-27.
49. Arana, G. W. and Baldassarini, R. J. (1986). The dexamethasone suppression test for diagnosis and prognosis in psychiatry. *Arch. Gen. Psychiatry 42*:1193-1204.
50. Fawcett, J., Maas, J. W., and Dekirmenjian, H. (1972). Depression and MHPG excretion: Response to dextroamphetamine and tricyclic antidepressants. *Arch. Gen. Psychiatry 26*:246-251.
51. Quitkin, F., Rifkin, A., and Klein, D. F. (1978). Imipramine response in deluded depressive patients. *Am. J. Psychiatry 135*:806-811.

52. Nelson, J. C. and Bowers, M. G., Jr. (1978). Delusional unipolar depression. *Arch. Gen. Psychiatry 35:1321-1328.*
53. Myers, B. S., Kalayam, B., and Mei-Tal, V. (1984). Late-onset delusional depression: A distinct clinical entity? *J. Clin. Psychiatry 45*:347-349.
54. Meyers, B. S., Greenberg, R., and Mei-Tal, V. (1985). Delusional depression in the elderly. In *Treatment of Affective Disorders in the Elderly.* Edited by C. A. Shamoian. Washington, D.C., American Psychiatric Press, pp. 17-28.
55. Baldassarini, R. (1985). Clinical and epidemiologic aspects of tardive dyskinesia. *J. Clin. Psychiatry 46* (Sect. 2):8-13.
56. de Montigny, C., Cournoyer, G., Morissette, R., Langlois, R., and Caille, G. (1983). Lithium carbonate addition in tricyclic antidepressant-resistant unipolar depression. Correlations with the neurobiologic actions of tricyclic antidepressant drugs and lithium ion on the serotonin system. *Arch. Gen. Psychiatry 40*:1327-1334.
57. Heninger, G. R., Charney, D. S., and Sternberg, D. E. (1983). Lithium carbonate augmentation of antidepressant treatment. *Arch. Gen. Psychiatry 40*: 1335-1342.
58. Scher, M., Krieger, J. N., and Juergens, S. (1984). Trazodone and priapism. *Am. J. Psychiatry 140*:1362-1363.
59. Janowski, D., Curtis, G., Zisook, S., Kahn, K., Resovsky, K., and LeWinter, M. (1983). Ventricular arrhythmias possibly aggravated by trazodone. *Am. J. Psychiatry 140*:796-797.
60. Wernicke, J. F. (1985). The side effect profile and safety of fluoxetine. *J. Clin. Psychiatry 46*(3, Sect. 2):59-67.
61. Fuller, R. W. and Wong, D. T. (1987). Serotonin reuptake blockers in vitro and in vivo. *J. Clin. Psychopharmacol. 7*:36S-43S.
62. Soroko, F. and Maxwell, R. A. (1983). The pharmacological basis for therapeutic interest in bupropion. *J. Clin. Psychiatry 44*(Sect. 2):67-73.
63. Roose, S. P., Glassman, A., Siris, S. G., Walsh, B. T., Bruno, R. L., and Wright, L. B. (1981). Comparison of imipramine- and nortriptyline-induced orthostatic hypotension: A meaningful difference. *J. Clin. Psychopharmacol. 1*:316-319.
64. Glassman, A. H. and Bigger, J. T., Jr. (1981). Cardiovascular effects of therapeutic doses of the tricyclic antidepressants. *Arch. Gen. Psychiatry 38*:815-820.
65. Veith, R. C., Bloom, V., Bielski, R., and Friedel, R. O. (1982). The effects of comparable plasma concentrations of desipramine and amitriptyline. *J. Clin. Psychopharmacol. 2*:394-398.
66. Giardina, E. V., Barnard, T., Johnson, L., Saroff, A. L., Bigger, J. T., and Louie, M. (1986). The antiarrhythmic effect of nortriptyline in cardiac patients with ventricular premature depolarizations. *J. Am. Coll. Cardiol. 7*:1361-1369.
67. Glassman, A. H., Giardina, E. V., Perel, J. M., and Davies, M. (1979). Clinical characteristics of imipramine-induced orthostatic hypotension. *Lancet 1*:468-472.
68. Glassman, A. H., Johnson, L. L., Giardina, E. G. V., Walsh, B. T., Roos, S. P., Cooper, T. B., and Bigger, J. T., Jr. (1983). The use of imipramine in depressed patients with congestive heart failure. *JAMA 250*:1997-2001.
69. Raeder, E. A., Zinsli, M., and Burckhardt, D. (1979). Effect of maprotiline on cardiac arrhythmias. *B. Med. J. 2*:102.

70. Steinberg, M. I., Smallwood, J. K., Holland, D. R., Bymaster, F. P., and Bemis, K. G. (1986). Hemodynamic and electrocardiographic effects of fluoxetine and its major metabolite, norfluoxetine, in anesthetized dogs. *Toxicol. Appl. Pharmacol. 82*:70-79.
71. Veith, R. C. (1985). Cardiovascular effects of the antidepressants in treating the elderly patient. In *Treatment of Affective Disorders in the Elderly*. Edited by C. A. Shamoian. Washington, D.C., American Psychiatric Press, pp. 39-50.
72. Roose, S. P., Glassman, A. H., Giardina, E. G. V., Walsh, B. T., Woodrin, S., and Bigger, J. T. (1987). Tricyclic antidepressants in depressed patients with cardiac conduction disease. *Arch. Gen. Psychiatry. 44*:273-27x.
73. Robinson, D. S., Nies, A., Corcella, J., Cooper, T. B., Spencer, C., and Keefover, R. (1982). Cardiovascular effects of phenelzine and amitriptyline in depressed outpatients. *J. Clin. Psychiatry 43*:8-15.
74. Blumenthal, M. D. and Davie, J. W. (1980). Dizziness and falling in elderly psychiatric outpatients. *Am. J. Psychiatry 137*:203-206.
75. Fisch, C. (1985). Effect of fluoxetine on the electrocardiogram. *J. Clin. Psychiatry 46*(3, Sect. 2):42-44.
76. Farid, F. F., Wenger, T., Tsai, S. Y., Singh, B. N., and Stern, W. C. (1983). Use of bupropion in patients who exhibit orthostatic hypotension on tricyclic antidepressants. *J. Clin. Psychiatry 44*:170-173.
77. Davidson, J. R. T., Miller, R. D., Turnbull, C. D., and Sullivan, J. L. (1982). Atypical depression. *Arch. Gen. Psychiatry 39*:527-534.
78. Ashford, W. and Ford, C. V. (1979). Use of MAO inhibitors in elderly patients. *Am. J. Psychiatry 136*:1466-1467.
79. Robinson, D. S., Nies, A., Ravaris, C. L., Ives, J. O., and Bartlett, D. (1978). Clinical pharmacology of phenelzine. *Arch. Gen. Psychiatry 35*:629-635.
80. Chiarello, R. J. and Cole. J. O. (1987). The use of psychostimulants in general psychiatry. A reconsideration. *Arch. Gen. Psychiatry 44*:286-295.
81. Woods, S. W. (1986). Psychostimulant treatment of depressive disorders secondary to medical illness. *J. Clin. Psychiatry 47*:12-15.
82. Askinazi, C., Weintraub, R. J., and Karamouz, N. (1986). Elderly depressed females as a possible subgroup of patients responsive to methylphenidate. *J. Clin. Psychiatry 47*:467-469.
83. Kaplitz, S. E. (1975). Withdrawn, apathetic geriatric patients responsive to methylphenidate. *J. Am. Geriatr. Soc. 23*:271-276.
84. Katon, W. and Raskind, M. (1980). Treatment of depression in the medically ill elderly with methylphenidate. *Am. J. Psychiatry 137*:963-965.

17

Treatment of Depression in the Frail Elderly

IRA KATZ and SHARON M. CURLIK
Medical College of Pennsylvania, Philadelphia Geriatric Center
Philadelphia, Pennsylvania

PATRICIA PARMELEE
Philadelphia Geriatric Center
Philadelphia, Pennsylvania

GEORGE M. SIMPSON
Medical College of Pennsylvania/Eastern Pennsylvania Psychiatric Institute
Philadelphia, Pennsylvania

DEFINITION OF THE PROBLEM

The treatment of depression is increasingly recognized as a critical component of care for the elderly. Of necessity, most of the research on depression in the elderly has been conducted on those patients who can be studied with the greatest rigor: that is, those meeting DSM-III diagnostic criteria for major depression and those for whom treatment response is not complicated by medical illness. Little is known about depression as manifest in the frail aged—in those elderly patients for whom depression coexists with chronic medical illness and functional disability. Coexisting illnesses, dependence, and multiple sources of disability, all require that psychiatrists modify their approach to diagnosis and treatment. This chapter is written at a time when we are keenly aware of gaps in our knowledge. We hope it can serve to focus attention on the problem and to provide both conceptual and pragmatic guidelines for the treatment of these patients.

The depressive disorders of late life are heterogeneous in phenomenology and severity. Blazer and Williams (1) estimated that nearly 15% of the elderly living in the community have a significant degree of dysphoria. Of these, 3.7% have a major depression (1.8% with primary depression; 1.9% with depression secondary to another psychiatric disorder), 6.5% have a depression associated with a significant medical disorder, and 4.5% have dysphoria alone. The high prevalence of depressive symptoms confirms Gurland's estimate that 18% of the elderly have a "pervasive depression" (2). The low prevalence of primary major depression in the elderly has been confirmed by the more recent Epidemiological Catchment Area Study that estimated the prevalence of major depression as 0.1-0.5% for men and 1.0-1.6% for women (3). However, studies of patients seen in settings in which they are receiving medical care demonstrate higher rates of depression (4-6). Unfortunately, depression in these settings is difficult to characterize. Depressive symptoms are regularly associated with chronic illness and functional disability, and it can be difficult to distinguish between somatic or vegetative symptoms of depression and related symptoms of chronic medical or neurological disease.

There have been systematic pharmacologic treatment studies of depression in patients with cerebrovascular, cardiac, and neurologic diseases, as well as in patients hospitalized on rehabilitation units for other illnesses (7-15). These reports demonstrate that, despite the diagnostic problems, depressions in medically ill patients do respond to standard treatment. However, the literature is not uniformly optimistic about treatment response in elderly patients with chronic illnesses, and several naturalistic studies suggest that the outcome of treatment is less favorable in those with physical illness (4, 16-18). Both the severity of illness at the initiation of treatment and the onset of new illness during follow-up may be associated with a poor outcome. The ambiguity of diagnosis and treatment responses is coupled with concerns about the greater vulnerability of these patients to adverse effects from antidepressant treatment. The stakes involved in treating depression in the frail elderly are high. At best, treatment of depression can make the difference between continued independent living and institutional placement. However, further research is necessary to determine when treatment is likely to be successful and when therapeutic restraint is more appropriate because response is unlikely, or because the risks of treatment are unacceptably high.

DEPRESSION IN AGED PATIENTS IN AN INSTITUTION

Available studies document a high prevalence of depressive symptoms and specific depressive disorders among nursing home residents (19-22): the prevalence of psychiatric disorders in congregate housing facilities has not been studied as extensively. To better understand these problems, we investigated depression among elderly patients who live in the residential care setting, both in a nursing home and congregate housing apartments. Table 1 outlines findings on the prevalence of psychiatric disorders in these settings.

Depression in the residential care setting occurs both as a primary disorder and as a secondary disorder in the presence of a concomitant medical or dementing disease. In our sample, approximately 23% of nursing home patients with dementia had clinically significant depression. In congregate housing, patients are usually healthier and more functional. Approximately 57% of those assessed in the congregate apartments received no psychiatric diagnosis

Table 1 Psychiatric Diagnoses in the Institutional Aged

Diagnosis	N	%	% (excluding pending)
Normal	290	30.1	31.9
Dementia			
uncomplicated	250	26.0	27.5
with affective/behavioral symptoms	133	15.7	16.5
Major depression	68	7.1	7.5
Other depression	104	10.8	11.4
Other disorders	43	4.5	4.7
Pending clinical diagnosis	53	5.5	—
Total	941		

Diagnoses were established by consensus in a clinical conference after independent evaluation by both a geriatric psychiatrist and clinical psychologist. "Normals" include those without demonstrable symptoms at screening and those without current diagnoses by clinical evaluation.

Table 2 Association Between Depression and Disability in the Institutional Aged

	Disability (PSMS)		
	Euthymic	Dysphoric	Depressed
Apartments	8.89	10.04	10.19
	(N = 121)	(N = 25)	(N = 17)
Nursing home	12.60	14.46	14.39
	(N = 25)	(N = 13)	(N = 18)

Affective status was established by clinical assessment. Disability was estimated using the Physical Self Maintenance Scale (Lawton, M. P. and Brody, E. P. (1969). *Gerontologist 9*:179-188). The severity of physical illness was estimated by physician ratings using the Cumulative Illness Rating Scale (Linn, B. S., Linn, M. W., and Gurel, L. (1968). *J. Am. Geriatr. Soc. 16*:622-626). The relationship between depression and disability remained significant ($F = 9.19$; $p < 10^{3}$) even after controlling for site of residence and severity of physical illness.

versus only 11% of those in a nursing home ($p < 0.0001$). Nursing home residents differed from those in the apartments in the prevalence of dementia (77% versus 26%), although the prevalence of major depression was comparable in the two settings. In the institutional setting—both nursing home and congregate housing—depression and dysphoria are associated with increased disability and functional impairment (Table 2). However, these data cannot distinguish between depression as a cause or as a result of disability. Disentangling this issue has become a major concern for researchers and clinicians alike. The research investigator and the clinician face similar problems; for both, evaluation of patients over time is necessary to determine the extent to which depression is a potentially reversible cause of disability.

CLINICAL MANAGEMENT OF DEPRESSION IN THE FRAIL ELDERLY

The frail elderly patients under discussion are in need of intensive psychiatric services. Although research on the interrelationships between depression, chronic illness, and disability are necessary, clinicians cannot defer working with these patients until the relevant problems are answered definitively. This discussion of pragmatic issues is presented to provide a rationale for work with these patients now.

Problems of Access

Most elderly patients with depression do not seek treatment from psychiatry (23). They are more likely to seek help from medical professionals. Therefore, the burden for recognizing psychopathology and referring patients for psychiatric evaluation falls upon the primary care physician. However, these physicians commonly underdiagnose depression (24). Screening programs using standardized rating scales for depression, such as the Geriatric Depression Scale of Yesavage et al. (25) could facilitate case identification.

Depression associated with acute medical illness may remit when the somatic illness improves (26). Although patients with depression are frequently identified during hospitalization for medical illness, initiation of drug treatment during hospitalization is best reserved for times when the depression is severe, when it clearly predates the medical illness or when it may have contributed to it. In other cases, it is best deferred until after a period of convalescence.

Combining Psychiatric Treatment and Rehabilitation

The importance of the recognition and treatment of depression in patients with chronic illness and disability is stressed because it is treatable, even when the underlying medical or neurological disease is irreversible. Treatment of depression with pharmacotherapy or psychotherapy, or both, should be only one of several approaches to minimizing disability, including management of sensory impairment or chronic pain; use of appropriate prosthetic devices and mechanical aides to improve ambulation and selfcare; and environmental manipulations to increase autonomy and independence. Physical therapy, occupational therapy, and therapeutic activities all can be of benefit. These issues of combined treatment echo the dialogue within psychiatry relative to combining psychotherapy and drug treatment. For some patients, treatment of depression is necessary before other approaches at rehabilitation can proceed; for others, depression may remit as a result of participation in a rehabilitation program and the alleviation of disability. In general, however, it is reasonable that psychiatric treatment and other approaches to minimizing disability should proceed in parallel.

Whom to Treat

The somatic symptoms of depression (fatigability, sleep disturbance, appetite disturbance, complaints or evidence of impaired concentration or cognitive impairment, and psychomotor retardation or agitation) best predict the need for antidepressant medication (27). However, in the presence of concomitant medical or neurological disease (28,29) these symptoms can be unreliable as indicators of specific depressive disorders. The best studied examples of this problem may be cases in which depression coexists with cognitive impairment. Depression can cause substantial reversible cognitive impairment that may mimic symptoms of dementia. Much work has been devoted to distinguishing between this reversible dementia syndrome of depression (or "pseudodementia") and the irreversible dementing disorders. The studies of Reiffler and co-workers represent a significant advance in the clinical approach to this problem. They noted that co-existing (major) depression and cognitive impairment could be due to either primary depression, with reversible cognitive impairment, or to primary dementia, with a secondary depression (30-32). Treatment must be considered for either. In the former, treatment of the depression can reverse the cognitive impairment; in the latter, it can alleviate a component of the patients disability with distress, even if the underlying dementia is irreversible.

A similar approach can be applied to patients with other coexisting medical disorders. When depressive symptoms and bradykinesia persist after what apparently is adequate treatment for parkinsonism, an empirical trial of antidepressant medication may be necessary to distinguish whether or not a major depression is a reversible component of the disability. The same holds true for fatigability in patients with cardiac or pulmonary disease, and pain or motor disability in patients with arthritis. The presence of other causes for either symptoms or disability should not decrease one's threshold for the recognition and treatment of depression. At present, the best approach to diagnosis requires the physician to factor the symptoms, using clinical judgment, to estimate what component of the symptoms can be explained by medical illness and what component may be due to depression. When it is difficult to decide whether symptoms result from depression or a coexisting chronic illness, an empirical treatment with antidepressant therapy may be indicated to ensure that a treatable source of disability is not overlooked.

Initiation of Treatment: Consolidation of the Treatment Team

Treatment of the elderly depressed patient requires that the psychiatrist freely communicate with the patient's primary physician to obtain additional diagnostic evaluations, to rule out treatable causes of dementia, to determine whether chronic medical or neurological illnesses are optimally treated, and to identify any drugs that may be contributing to depressive symptoms or that may interact with antidepressant medication.

Once a decision to institute therapy with antidepressant medications is made, the primary care physician and the psychiatrist should discuss the choice of agents and the dosage schedule. Patients receiving antidepressant medications require individualized monitoring for early signs of adverse effects. For example, patients with even mild symptoms of dementia who receive anticholinergic agents may be at increased risk for deterioration of their cognitive state. Those with cardiovascular disease are at increased risk for the occurrence of orthostatic hypotension, low blood pressure and falls, cardiac arrhythmias, and cerebrovascular accidents. Clinical management should include regularly scheduled monitoring of blood pressure (with orthostatic changes), electrocardiograms (ECG), cognitive status, autonomic symptoms, and subjective side effects, as well as blood levels of antidepressants (when available). Patients with other disorders may require additional monitoring; for example, those with glaucoma may require measurement of intraocular pressure. The psychiatrist and the primary care physician should jointly determine who is best able to monitor adverse effects and conduct dosage adjustments. When appropriate, ancillary services, such as visiting nurses, should be considered, especially when transportation is a problem. The patient, and the family (or other caregivers), should be informed about potential adverse effects of the medications and procedures to follow when concerned about side effects.

Evaluating Adverse Effects

Physicians who prescribe medications for frail elderly patients should determine if any medical symptoms that may be similar to adverse drug effects are present before drug treatment is initiated. In elderly patients, when symptoms occur during the course of treatment, it is often difficult to determine whether an adverse medical event is related to a specific medication (or drug interaction) or whether it is an independent, intercurrent illness. The initial response to adverse events must be a dose reduction of all agents that could potentially contribute to the symptoms. Next, a careful clinical and laboratory search should be made for findings that suggest other causes. If other causes are found, medication may be reinstituted, especially if the drug is of known benefit to the individual patient.

Evaluation of Nonresponders to Antidepressant Therapy

For those patients who do not respond to treatment with antidepressant medication, an initial step must be a reevaluation of both the adequacy of treatment and the diagnosis. The most common cause of a therapeutic response failure is "inadequate" treatment. Although problems related to overmedication of the elderly have been discussed in great detail, it is also important to emphasize the risks of undermedication and inadequate treatment.

When patients with a definite diagnosis of major depression do not respond to an adequate course of treatment, other types of treatment must be considered, including the addition of lithium to the medication regimen, a different antidepressant, or electroconvulsive therapy. The situation is more difficult when the diagnosis is in doubt and treatment has been empirically initiated to determine whether depression is making a significant contribution to disability.

Evaluation of Partial Responses

The result of antidepressant treatment in younger adults with primary depression is generally bimodal, and if patients do respond to treatment, they exhibit essentially complete remission of symptoms (32). Partial responses may occur more frequently in elderly patients (33). It is often unclear if residual symptoms result from a partial remission of the depression or from symptoms of a coexisting medical illness. When evaluating such partial responses, the adequacy of the treatment in terms of dosage, treatment duration, and the possible confounding effect of adverse drug effects should be reviewed.

Maintenance Treatment

With the frail elderly, as with other patients, it is possible to conceptualize three phases of treatment: an active phase when depressive symptoms are being brought under control, a continuation phase (from 6-12 months) to prevent relapse, and a maintenance phase (often indefinitely) for specific patients at risk for recurrent depression. Recent data suggest that maintenance therapy may commonly be necessary in the elderly (16,34-37). Estimation of the risk/benefit ratios of maintenance treatment requires input from all physicians involved in the patient's care; the weighing of alternatives requires additional input from the patient and family caregivers.

CHOICE OF ANTIDEPRESSANT TREATMENT

Choice of an Antidepressant Medication

Nortriptyline has several properties which suggest that it may be a useful first-line drug for the treatment of depression in the frail elderly. Its clinical pharmacology has been intensively studied for more than 20 years, and it is probably the best understood of the tricyclic antidepressants. Adequate treatment with nortriptyline can be defined in terms of plasma levels of the drug (between 50 and 150 ng/mL) and duration of treatment (4-6 weeks at adequate blood levels). A knowledge of these parameters allows optimization of the treatment response as well as identification of those patients for whom the drug's side effects make an adequate trial impossible. Most importantly, this knowledge enables the clinician to operationally define when a patient is nonresponsive and to recognize when reevaluation of the diagnosis or modification of the treatment plan is necessary (22,38,39). Nortriptyline does have some anticholinergic and quinidine-like activity. It may cause orthostatic hypotension. Nevertheless, it is a reasonable first-choice drug for the frail elderly patient. Desipramine also may be considered. It has the advantage of lower anticholinergic activity than nortriptyline; however, plasma level-response correlations are not as firmly established as are those of nortriptyline (40-42).

Other antidepressants commonly used in the frail elderly include doxepin, trazadone, maprotiline, and now fluoxetine. Use of amoxapine is complicated by its neuroleptic activity and potential for tardive dyskinesia. Other agents that should probably be avoided in this population include amitriptyline (owing to anticholinergic side effects), imipramine (owing to excessive symptomatic orthostatic hypotension and disturbances of cardiac conduction), and protriptyline (an agent whose side effect profile and exceptionally long half-life make dose adjustment difficult). Some of the newest of the antidepressants (e.g., fluoxetine) have pharmacological properties that may make them particularly useful in the frail elderly. However, when alternatives exist, the use of new medications in older individuals should probably be avoided. In elderly patients with increased vulnerability to adverse effects, the use of newly approved medications should be deferred until further experience has been accumulated in younger patient groups.

Monoamine oxidase inhibitors (MAOIs) can be used safely and effectively in the elderly, even in patients who have not responded to adequate treatment with tricyclic antidepressants (43). When considering the use of MAOIs in patients with chronic illness and disability, one should consider drug interactions with medications that the patient is currently taking, as well as potential interactions with medications that may be necessary if the patient's medical state deteriorates. For example, the patient with chronic obstructive pulmonary disease may require both adrenergic agonists and phosphodiesterase inhibitors, agents that could interact with the MAOIs. (For a more detailed discussion of MAOIs, see Chapter 6.)

Dose Requirements and Pharmacokinetic Parameters of Tricyclic Antidepressants

A provocative paper by Lakshmanan et al. (8) reported a significant drug-placebo difference in a double-blind placebo-controlled study of low doses of doxepin for treatment of depression occurring in an inpatient rehabilitation unit. However, the use of low doses of tricyclic antidepressants for geriatric patients requires further clarification. Treatment should always be started at low drug doses; however, a lack of response to such doses does not imply treatment-resistance in the elderly, and the antidepressant dosage should be titrated upward (as tolerated) until the patient has received an adequate course of therapy.

The pharmacokinetic metabolism of nortriptyline in the aged has been studied by several investigators. Early studies reported by Braithwaite found a significant correlation between age and nortriptyline half-life (44). However, several, more recent studies, found no significant relationship between young and elderly patients (39,45-49). The patient populations for these studies have been primarily from those in their 60s and 70s. Studies by Dawling on the kinetics of nortriptyline in a small group of patients (age average, 81) in an acute geriatric medical inpatients service suggested that a dose of 30 mg/day would be optimal (50). Our investigation of the pharmacokinetics of nortriptyline in a group of 22 elderly patients (mean age 84.6) living within institutions found that nortriptyline kinetics are linear and that the average "therapeutic" dose of nortriptyline in this population of frail elderly patients was approximately 50-80 mg/day, compatable with the dose requirements for younger adults (Fig. 1). Possibly, the dose requirements suggested by Dawling were a reflection of acute medical illness, rather than age or chronic disease. Age-related differences in nortriptyline metabolism appear to be small and of minimal clinical significance, in contrast with the tertiary amine tricyclics for which highly salient effects of aging have been reported (51,52).

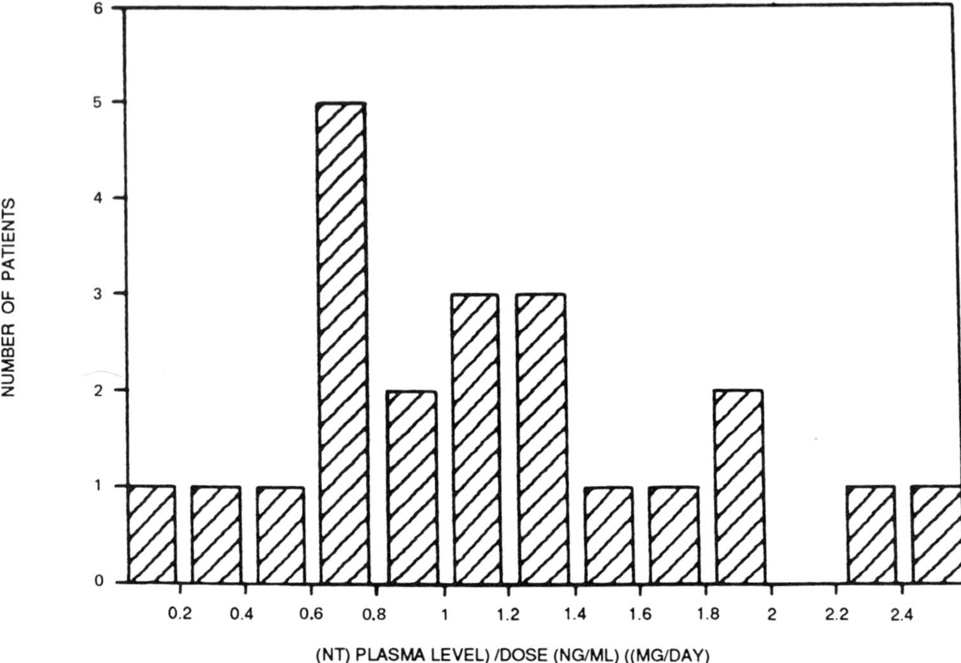

Figure 1 The distribution ratio (nortriptyline plasma level/dose) at steady-state is for a sample of 22 patients, average age 84. Mean = 1.19; SD = 0.62. The plasma level/dose ratio for an individual is a measure of that individuals absorption, distribution, and metabolism of nortriptyline. The amount of drug required to achieve a plasma level of 100 ng/ML is 100/(plasma level/dose).

Early identification of slow metabolizers by using pre-steady-state measurements for dose prediction (see Chapter 5) can identify patients who require smaller doses and slower dose increments. Measurement of plasma levels 24 hr after an initial test dose can predict steady-state plasma levels, an approach that can be extended to the elderly (53). Schneider et al. evaluated the relationship between plasma levels 24 hr after an initial 25-mg test dose and plasma levels observed at steady-state during clinical treatment (45); the correlation coefficient at a dose of 50 mg/day was 0.83; this test dose procedure can identify the slow (and rapid) metabolizers. The 25-mg test dose procedure and the relationship between test dose and steady-state levels remained valid in our population, even though the patients were approximately a generation older than those of previous investigators.

Another approach is the use of "steady-state" blood levels as a guide to dose adjustment. Even in the very old, steady-state nortriptyline blood levels are achieved within 5-7 days. The linearity of nortriptyline kinetics implies that increments in plasma level will be proportionate to increments in dose. The problem here is the delay in identifying slow drug metabolizers. Accordingly, starting doses should be chosen more cautiously.

It has also been observed that the 10-hydroxylated metabolites of nortriptyline are pharmacologically active and that they may contribute to both therapeutic and adverse effects. Accumulation of these metabolites may be greater in the elderly (54,55), and their concentrations should be measured (when available) in elderly patients treated with nortriptyline.

Concomitant Treatment

The use of neuroleptic drugs, in addition to tricyclic antidepressants, may be necessary in treating elderly patients with delusional depression and in those with severe agitation. It is prudent to minimize central anticholinergic, peripheral autonomic, and cardiac effects, by use of high-potency neuroleptics. Given the current state of knowledge, the neuroleptics should be considered adjunctive treatment useful for the immediate control of symptoms. The neuroleptics should be discontinued after the depression and the target behavior have been controlled.

Similarly, benzodiazepines may be necessary to control anxiety or sleep disturbance during the initial phases of antidepressant treatment; however, the use of long-acting benzodiazepines should be avoided. Again, these agents should be discontinued as soon as possible. Although there are fixed-dose products that combine either neuroleptics or benzodiazepines with antidepressants, these have no place in the psychopharmacologic treatment of the elderly.

Methylphenidate

Methylphenidate is an indirect catecholamine agonist. Although the drug has been investigated for use in the treatment of psychiatric disorders for over 30 years, it is currently approved only for use in the treatment of attention deficit disorder and of narcolepsy. There have been recurrent reports suggesting its usefulness in the treatment of other disorders (including depression, anergia, apathy, and withdrawal); however, such indications have not been established. Early studies of its efficacy as an antidepressant, both positive and negative, were flawed by limitations in design, inadequate diagnoses, heterogeneous patient populations, and lack of quantitative outcome measures. (For a more detailed discussion, see Chapter 9.)

Even though methylphenidate affects information processing in the normal elderly (56), it is not helpful in treating the cognitive deterioration of Alzheimer's disease (57,58). However, beneficial effects have been suggested in the treatment of secondary symptoms of dementia, such as depression, apathy, and withdrawal. In a well-designed, placebo-controlled, double-blind study of methylphenidate for treatment of "institutional chronically ill senile patients," with symptoms that included lack of interest and motivation; lowered self-esteem, confidence, and dignity; and listlessness, Kaplitz (59) found improvement and significant drug-placebo differences for several affective and behavioral measurements.

There has been a recent resurgence of interest in the use of methylphenidate for treatment of depression in the elderly. However, the results of controlled studies on adult populations have been ambiguous. Nevertheless, a series of case reports and retrospective record reviews have suggested that methylphenidate may have a specific value for treatment of depression in older patients with medical or neurological illness (60-67). The potential importance of this is suggested by Pritchard and Mykyta, whose results from an open investigation of methylphenidate, in patients for whom apathy interfered with treatment in an inpatient rehabilitation setting, suggested that treatment could improve the potential for discharge to the community (68).

Although plasma level-response correlations or other predictors of therapeutic outcome are not available for methylphenidate, there are suggestions that responses can occur after only a few days. Thus, a therapeutic trial can be conducted with methylphenidate within a time frame that may be accessible in an inpatient medical or rehabilitation setting. Even though methylphenidate may have a place in the psychopharmacologic treatment of the frail elderly, clinicians should, nevertheless, approach this agent with caution, realizing that little is known about its long-term use or the need for continuation or maintenance treatment in the elderly.

SUMMARY: THE ROLE OF THE GERIATRIC PSYCHIATRIST

The initial focus of psychiatric intervention in the frail elderly patient should be directed toward decreasing overall disability. Ensuring that depression has been included as a cause of disability may frequently require empirical trials of antidepressant medication. Moreover, psychiatric treatment may serve as a stage of "passage" for patients and their families, helping them determine how much of the elderly patient's capacity for self-care and instrumental activities is reversible. Geriatric psychiatrists, trained in both the medical and psychosocial domains, are appropriately the persons to coordinate the multidisciplinary approach necessary to search for other treatable sources of disability and to ensure adequate treatment for depression. This preparation also enables them to assist patients with irreversible disability and their families to minimize distress, to improve strategies for coping, and to facilitate adaptation.

ACKNOWLEDGMENTS

Research reported was supported by grants MH40830 and MH41489 from the National Institute of Mental Health and by research support from the Office of Mental Health of the Commonwealth of Pennsylvania. The authors gratefully acknowledge the editorial assistance of Ms. Janice Wright.

REFERENCES

1. Blazer, D. and Williams, C. D. (1980). Epidemiology of dysphoria and depression in an elderly population. *Am. J. Psychiatry 137*:439-444.
2. Gurland, B. J., Copeland, J., Kuriansky, J., et al. (1983). *The Mind and Mood of Aging*. New York, Haworth Press.
3. Myers, J. K., Weissman, M. M., Tischler, G. L., et al. (1984). Six month prevalence of psychiatric disorders in the community. *Arch. Gen. Psychiatry 41*:959-967.
4. Kukall, W. A., Koepsell, T. D., Inui, T. S., Borson, S., Okimoto, J., Raskind, M. A., and Gale, J. L. (1986). Depression and physical illness among elderly general medical clinic patients. *J. Affect. Disord. 10*:153-162.
5. Okimoto, J. T., Barnes, R. F., Veith, R. C., Raskind, M. A., Inui, T. S., and Carter, W. B. (1982). Screening for depression in geriatric medical patients. *Am. J. Psychiatry 139*:799-802.
6. Borson, S., Barnes, R. A., Kukall, W. A., Okimoto, J. T., Veith, R. C., Inui, T. S., Carter, W., and Raskind, M. A. (1986). Symptomatic depression in elderly medical out-patients. Prevalence, demography and health service utilization. *J. Am. Geriatr. Soc. 34*:341-347.
7. Lipsey, J. R., Robinson, R. G., Pearlson, G. D., et al. (1984). Nortriptyline treatment of post stroke depression: A double-blind study. *Lancet 1*:297-300.
8. Lakshmanan, M., Mion, L. C., and Frangley, J. D. (1986). Effective low dose tricyclic antidepressant treatment for depressed geriatric rehabilitation patients: A double blind study. *J. Am. Geriatr. Soc. 34*:421-426.
9. Anderson, J., Aabro, E., Gulmann, N., et al. (1980). Anti-depressive treatment in Parkinson's disease. A controlled trial of the effect of nortriptyline in patients with Parkinson's disease treated with L-dopa. *Acta. Neurol. Scand. 62*:210-219.
10. Veith, R. C., Raskind, M. A., Caldwell, J. H., et al. (1982). Cardiovascular effects of tricyclic antidepressants in depressed patients with chronic heart disease. *N. Engl. J. Med. 306*:954-959.
11. Reynolds, C. F., Perel, J. M., Kupfer, D. J., Zimmer, B., Stack, J. A., and Hoch, C. C. (1987). Open-trial response to antidepressant treatment in elderly patients with mixed depression and cognitive impairment. *Psychiatry Res. 21*:111-122.
12. Reifler, B. V., Larson, E., Terri, L., and Poulsen, M. (1986). Dementia of the Alzheimer's type and depression. *J. Am. Geriatr. Soc. 34*:855-859.
13. Tariot, P. N., Cohen, R. M., Sunderland, T., et al. (1987). L-Deprenyl in Alzheimer's disease. *Arch. Gen. Psychiatry 44*:427-433.

14. Jenike, M. A. (1985). Monoamine oxidase inhibitors as treatment for depressed patients with primary degenerative dementia (Alzheimer's disease). *Am. J. Psychiatry 142*:763-764.
15. Sumergrad, P. (1985). Depression in Binswagner's encephalopathy responsive to tranylcypromine: Case report. *J. Clin. Psychiatry 46*:69-70.
16. Murphy, E. (1983). The prognosis of depression in old age. *Br. J. Psychiatry 142*: 111-119.
17. Cole, M. G. (1985). The course of elderly depressed out-patients. *Can. J. Psychiatry 30*:217-220.
18. Post, F. (1972). The management and nature of depressive illnesses in late life: A follow-through study. *J. Affect. Disord. 1*(suppl.):S41-S45.
19. Hyer, L., and Blazer, D. (1982). Depression in long term care facilities, In *Depression in Late Life*. Edited by D. Blazer. St. Louis, C. V. Mosby, pp. 268-295.
20. Rovner, B. W., Kafonek, S., Filipp, L., et al. (1986). Prevalence of mental illness in a community nursing home. *Am. J. Psychiatry 143*:1446-1449.
21. Snowden, J. and Donnelly, N. (1986). A study of depression in nursing homes. *J. Psychiatry Res. 20*:327-333.
22. Katz, I. R., Curlik, S., and Lesher, E. L. (1988). Use of antidepressants in the frail elderly: When, why and how. *Clin. Geriatr. Med. 4*:203-222.
23. Weissman, M. M. and Myers, J. K. (1979). Depression in the elderly: Research directions in psychopathology, epidemiology and treatment. *J. Geriatr. Psychiatry 12*:187-201.
24. Nielson, A. C. III and Williams, T. A. (1980). Depression in ambulatory medical patients: Prevalence by self-report questionnaire and recognition by nonpsychiatric physicians. *Arch. Gen. Psychiatry 37*:999-1004.
25. Yesavage, J. A., Brink, T. L., Rose, T. L. et al. (1983). The Geriatric Depression Rating Scale: Comparison with other self-report and psychiatric rating scales. In *Assessment in Geriatric Psychopharmacology*. Edited by T. Crook, S. Ferris, and R. Bartus. New Canaan, Conn. Mark Powley Associates, pp. 153.
26. Moffic, H. S., and Paykel, E. S. (1985). Depression in medical in-patients. *Br. J. Psychiatr. Res. 20*:327-333.
27. Bielski, R. J. and Friedel, R. O. (1976). Prediction of tricyclic antidepressant response: A critical review. *Arch. Gen. Psychiatry 33*:1479-1489.
28. Steuer, J., Bank, L., Olsen, E. J., and Jarvick, L. F. (1980). Depression, physical health and somatic complaints in the elderly: A study of the Zung Self-Rating Depression Scale. *J. Gerontol. 35*:683-688.
29. Gurland, B. J., Dean, L. L., and Cross, P. S. (1983). The effects of depression on individual social functioning in the elderly. In *Depression and Aging*. Edited by L. D. Breslau and M. R. Haug. New York, Springer Publishing, p. 256.
30. Reifler, B. V. (1982). Arguments for abandoning the term pseudodementia. *J. Am. Geriatr. Soc. 30*:665-668.
31. Reifler, B. V. (1986). Mixed cognitive-affective disturbances in the elderly: A new classification. *J. Clin. Psychiatry 47*:354-356.
32. Hamilton, M. (1982). The effect of treatment on the melancholias (depression). *Br. J. Psychiatry 140*:223-230.

33. Plotkin, D. A., Gerson, S. C., and Jarvik, L. F. (1987). Antidepressant drug treatment in the elderly. In *Psychopharmacology, The Third Generation of Progress.* New York, Raven Press.
34. Murphy, E. (1986). *Affective Disorders in the Elderly.* New York, Churchill-Livingston.
35. Post, F. (1985). Psychotherapy, electroconvulsive treatments and long-term management of elderly depressives. *J. Affect. Disord.* *1*(suppl.):S41-S45.
36. Cook, B. L., Helms, P. M., Smith, R. E., and Tsai, M. (1986). Unipolar depression in the elderly: Reoccurrence on discontinuation of tricyclic antidepressants. *J. Affect. Disord.* *10*:91-94.
37. Squillace, K., Post, R. M., Savard, R., and Erwin-Gorman, M. (1984). Life charting of the longitudinal course of recurrent affective illness. In *Neurobiology of Mood Disorders.* Edited by R. M. Post and J. L. Bullenger. Baltimore, Williams & Wilkins, pp. 38-59.
38. Rubin, E. H., Biggs, J. J., and Preskorn, S. H. (1985). Nortriptyline pharmacokinetics and plasma levels: Implications for clinical practice. *J. Clin. Psychiatry* *46*:10-16.
39. Kumar, V., Smith, R. C., Reed, K., and Leelavathi, D. E. (1987). Plasma levels and effects of nortriptyline in geriatric depressed patients. *Acta Psychiatr. Scand.* *75*:20-28.
40. Nelson, J. C., Jatlow, P. I., and Mazure, E. (1985). Desipramine plasma levels and response in elderly melancholic patients. *J. Clin. Psychopharmacol.* *5*:217-220.
41. Kutcher, S. P., Shulman, K. I., and Reed, K. (1986). Desipramine plasma concentration and therapeutic response in elderly depressives: A naturalistic pilot study. *Can. J. Psychiatry* *31*:752-754.
42. Cutler, N. R., Zavadil, A. P., Eisdorfer, C., Ross, R. J., and Potter, W. Z. (1981). Concentrations of desipramine in elderly women. *Am. J. Psychiatry* *138*:1235-1237.
43. Georgotas, A., Friedman, E., McCarthy, M., Mann, J., Krakowski, M., Siegel, R., and Ferris, S. (1983). Resistant geriatric depressions and therapeutic response to monoamine oxidase inhibitors. *Biol. Psychiatry* *18*:195-205.
44. Braithwaite, R., Montgomery, S., and Dawling, S. (1978). Nortriptyline in depressed patients with high plasma levels. *Clin. Pharmacol. Ther.* *23*:303-308.
45. Schneider, L. S., Cooper, T. B., Staples, F. R., and Sloane, R. B. (1987). Prediction of individual dosage of nortriptyline in depressed elderly outpatients. *J. Clin. Psychopharmacol.* *7*:311-314.
46. Smith, R. C., Reed, K., and Leelavathi, D. E. (1980). Pharmacokinetics and the effects of nortriptyline in geriatric depressed patients. *Psychopharmacol. Bull.* *16*:54-57.
47. Georgotas, A., McCue, R. E., Hapworth, W., Friedman, E., Kim, O. M., Welkowitz, J., and Cooper, T. B. (1986). Comparative efficacy and safety of MAOI's vs. TCA's in treating depressed elderly. *Biol. Psychiatry* *21*:1155-1166.
48. Sorenson, B., Kragh-Sorenson, P., Larsen, N., and Hvidberg, E. F., (1978). Practical significance of nortriptyline plasma control. A prospective evaluation under routine conditions in endogenous depression. *Psychopharmacology* *59*:35-39.

49. Turbott, J., Norman, T. R., Burrows, G. D., et al. (1980). Pharmacokinetics of a nortriptyline in elderly volunteers. *Commun. Psychopharmacol. 4*:225-231.
50. Dawling, S., Crome, P., and Hyer, E. J. (1981). Nortriptyline therapy in elderly patients: Dosage prediction from plasma concentration at 24 hours after a single 50 mg dose. *Br. J. Psychiatry 139*:413-419.
51. Nies, A., Robinson, D. S., Friedman, M. J., Green, R., Cooper, T. B., Ravaris, C. L., and Ives, J. O. (1977). Relationship between age and tricyclic antidepressant plasma levels. *Am. J. Psychiatry 134*:790-793.
52. Preskorn, S. H. (1986). Tricyclic antidepressant plasma level monitoring. An improvement over the dose-response approach. *J. Clin. Psychiatry 47* (suppl.): 24-30.
53. Cooper, T. and Simpson, G. M. (1978). Prediction of individual dosage of nortriptyline. *Am. J. Psychiatry 135*:333-335.
54. Bertilsson, L., Mellstrom, B., and Sjoqvist, F. (1979). Pronounced inhibition or noradrenalin uptake by 10-hydroxy-metabolites of nortriptyline. *Life Sci. 25*: 1285-1292.
55. Young, R. C., Alexopoulos, G. S., Shamoian, C. A., Dhar, A. K., and Kutt, H. Plasma 10-hydroxy-nortriptyline in elderly depressed patients. *Clin. Pharmacol. Ther. 35*:540-544.
56. Halliday, R., Callaway, E., Naylor, H., et al. (1986). The effects of stimulant drugs on information processing in elderly adults. *J. Gerontol. 41*:748-757.
57. Crook, T., Ferris, S., Sathananthan, G., et al. (1977). The effect of methylphenidate on test performance in the cognitively impaired aged. *Psychopharmacology 52*:251-255.
58. Crook, T. (1979). Central nervous system stimulants: Appraisal of the use in geropsychiatric patients. *J. Am. Geriatr. Soc. 27*:476-477.
59. Kaplitz, S. E. (1975). Withdrawn, apathetic geriatric patients responsive to methylphenidate. *J. Am. Geriatr. Soc. 23*:271-276.
60. Katon, W. and Raskind, M. (1980). Treatment of depression in the medically ill elderly with methylphenidate. *Am. J. Psychiatry 137*:963-965.
61. Kaufmann, M. W., Murray, G. B., and Cassem, N. H. (1982). Use of psychostimulants in medically ill depressed patients. *Psychosomatics 23*:817-819.
62. Kaufmann, M. W., Cassem, N. H., Murray, G. B., et al. (1984). Use of psychostimulants in medically ill patients with neurological disease and major depression. *Can. J. Psychiatry 29*:46-49.
63. Kaufmann, M. W., Cassem, N., and Murray, G. (1984). The use of methylphenidate in depressed patients after cardiac surgery. *J. Clin. Psychiatry 45*: 82-84.
64. Fisch, R. Z. (1985-86). Methylphenidate for medical in-patients. *Int. J. Psychiatry Med. 15*:75-79.
65. Askinazi, C., Weintraub, R. J., and Karamouz, N. (1986). Elderly dependant females as a possible subgroup of patients responsive to methylphenidate. *J. Clin. Psychiatry 47*:467-469.
66. Fernandez, F. and Adams, F. (1986). Methylphenidate treatment of patients with head and neck cancer. *Head Neck Surg. 8*:296-300.

67. Woods, S. W., Tesar, G. E., Murray, G. B., et al. (1986). Psychostimulant treatments of depressive disorders secondary to medical illness. *J. Clin. Psychiatry* *47*:12-15.
68. Pritchard, J. G. and Mykyta, L. J. (1975). Use of a combination of methylphenidate and oxprenolol in the management of physically disabled, apathetic, elderly patients: A pilot study. *Curr. Med. Res. Opin.* *3*:26-29.

18

Antidepressant Drug Use in Pediatric and Adolescent Patients with Affective Disorder

CARROLL W. HUGHES and SHELDON H. PRESKORN

St. Francis Regional Medical Center
University of Kansas School of Medicine
Wichita Veterans Administration Medical Center
Wichita, Kansas

INTRODUCTION

There have been significant strides made in the understanding of childhood and adolescent depression over the last decade. This contrasts with the historical position that major depressive disorder (MDD) did not occur in children and adolescents (1) or, if it did, then it was somehow different from adult MDD (2). Glazer referred to a "masked" depression in children that had many of the symptoms of the adult MDD (2), but was not equivalent to it. Glazer's opinion was based on the theory that children did not have sufficient superego development to develop an overt depressive syndrome. Fortunately, work on childhood and adolescent mood disorders has progressed since these views were expounded.

This chapter begins with a brief review of the recent research on childhood and adolescent depression and a summary of the descriptive profile of the depressed child and adolescent. Consideration is then given to various approaches for the diagnostic workup and assessment of the depressed child and adolescent, followed by a consideration of recent treatment strategies. These treatments include pharmacologic approaches (with optimum doses determined by plasma drug level monitoring) and psychotherapeutic approaches (alone or as supplementation to medication therapy). We conclude the chapter with a discussion of future goals of research and a summary of the existing understanding of mood disorders in children and adolescents.

Recent research is not in agreement with the earlier theories. Our data (3-9) and that of others (10,11) indicate that MDD does occur in children, as well as in adolescents (12,13) and is similar to MDD in adults in several ways. First, one often finds a persistent depressive mood, as well as the presence of vegetative signs and symptoms (including disturbances in sleep, appetite, and energy), impaired concentration and attention, and loss of interest in usual activities. Moreover, suicidal ideation does occur in childhood depression leading to both attempts and successful suicides. Second, depressed children often have a strong familial loading for affective illness. Third, the rate of nonsuppression in the dexamethasone suppression test (DST) is similar in children and in adults with MDD, and these children tend to be the most responsive to antidepressant treatment (14). Fourth, antidepressants are effective in some children with MDD, although the response rate may be lower than those seen in adults with this disorder. Furthermore, the minimum plasma drug concentration necessary for antidepressant response is similar in children and adults with MDD.

DESCRIPTIVE PROFILE

The pattern of affective disorder and suicidal ideation has been found to be substantial in childhood depression (15). Recent research indicates that most suicides occur in the context of depression (16). According to 1986 statistics for the United States, suicide before the age of 12 appears to be rare. However, the rate rises rapidly to 8:1 million at ages 10-14 (up from 0.06:1 million below the age of 10), and a 1000-fold increase is seen for ages 15-19 (76:1 million) (17). Clearly, the child or adolescent with a mood disorder is at substantial risk for suicide in comparison with normal children (18-20).

The impact of MDD on the child's ability to adapt as a productive member of society remains to be examined. Several recent works have emphasized the need for studies of developmental continuities in depressed children (13, 17,21-23). For example, does the occurrence of depression in childhood have implications for personality development (e.g., relationship to conduct disorder)? Do depressed children become depressed adolescents or depressed adults? Conduct disorder, in particular, is of interest because its symptoms overlap with those of mood disorders, and because the two disorders frequently occur together. Our initial research found that approximately 40% of the children also had a diagnosis of conduct disorder. Puig-Antich et al. observed a similar prevalence of conduct disorder (37%) in their depressed children (24,25). An important question is which syndrome predominates in later life: depressive disorder of conduct-antisocial disorder? Does treatment of the childhood depressive episode have long-term effects on the conduct disorder and its sequelae (e.g., alcohol and drug abuse), personality development, and social adjustment? Puig-Antich found that 70% of the conduct disorders disappeared when the depressive symptoms improved, although longitudinal data in their study was limited. Interestingly, the onset of a second depressive episode was often preceded by a return of conduct disorder behavior, and similar findings have been observed with conduct-related problems associated with suicidal and depressed adolescents (13,26,27).

Anxiety symptoms have also been associated with childhood mood disorders (28). For example, school refusal, phobias, and anxiety were greater among depressed compared with the nondepressed children with psychiatric disorders (29). Similarly, Kovacs et al. observed anxiety symptoms in approximately 33% of children with MDD, and Puig-Antich reported that up to 59% of his subjects had separation anxiety (11).

Several investigators have described important features in children and adolescents that meet DSM-III and DSM-III-R criteria for MDD. For example, male/female ratio is about 2-3:1 in children aged 6 to 12. This ratio begins to diminished in early puberty, and by about 14 years, more females than males have a diagnosis of mood disorder.

All races appear to be equally represented, as are all socioeconomic classes, and distribution differences in many studies appear to reflect racial-socioeconomic proportions consistent with their respective catchment areas. Similarly, all ages are represented; however, there is a particularly noticeable increase at puberty. This finding, together with the shift in the male/female ratio, suggests the possibility that sex hormones may be important in the expression of the disorder.

Marital discord is not uncommon in the parents of depressed children and adolescents. The majority (68%) of parents of the children in our studies were remarried, separated, divorced, or single. Furthermore, we found that a death in the family was not uncommon (13%) and, consequently, indices of psychosocial stress for these individuals tended to be fairly high.

A large percentage of the mothers (39%) were currently depressed and required treatment. Many of the mothers met criteria for a lifetime diagnosis of MDD (even if they were not currently depressed). A lesser, but still significant number of fathers had a diagnosis of MDD (30% lifetime, 10% currently depressed) or met criteria (55%) for some other lifetime psychiatric disorder (most commonly substance abuse or antisocial personality disorder).

In our studies, approximately 85% of the children had substantial school problems (e.g., learning disabilities, absenteeism, conduct problems, poor grades, and social withdrawal). However, although hyperactivity has frequently been associated with school problems in children, we excluded children who met criteria for both MDD and attention deficit disorder with hyperactivity. For example, the average scores on the Conner scale for hyperactivity was 26.9: to qualify for hyperactivity one would expect a score higher than 36 (30,31).

Finally, factor analysis of scores from several rating instruments used for our studies of mood disorders revealed many features common to adult MDD. The factors included vegetative-affect (e.g., appetite, sleep, and such); suicide-self-esteem issues; and behavioral changes on the part of the child. Other symptom clusters included noncompliance issues, guilt-low energy, and school problems. We found that children most often identified school problems, whereas the parent was more likely to report that the child was noncompliant. The clinician often identified feelings of guilt and low-energy levels as the most prominent symptoms of depression. In this regard, if "work" is substituted for "school," and "social withdrawal" is substituted for "noncompliance," then the symptom profile for the adult and childhood MDD become remarkably similar.

DIAGNOSTIC WORKUP

The typical diagnostic workup for childhood depression usually begins with a routine clinical interview that is based on the referral problem (e.g., school phobia). Frequently, the referral is not obviously for depression. Rather, parents are concerned about changes in behavior (irritability, anhedonia, withdrawal), poor school performance (school phobias, frequent absences, increased fighting, or noncompliance), running away, or possible substance abuse. Occasionally, the referral will include somatic complaints of headache, gastric distress, enuresis, or encopresis. Furthermore, it is very helpful to have a standardized school report form that can be sent to the child's teacher, because it is not uncommon for a depressed child to rate his or her performance below the level that the teacher rates it.

Under ideal circumstances, the initial intake interview is supplemented with a structured interview, such as the Diagnostic Interview for Children and Adolescents (DICA) (32,33). Trained nursing, social work, or psychology staff can administer these interviews. The DICA results in a structured review of all major psychiatric disorders and is keyed to the DSM-III-R. The DICA has other advantages, such as separate parent and child-adolescent forms, whereby the child often reveals information of which the parent is unaware.

Additional instruments are available that help the clinician determine the severity of the affective disorder, such as the Childhood Depression Inventory (23) which is a 27-item self-rated depression inventory. The instrument is easily scored and provides the clinician with a quantitative sense of the severity of the depression. In our work, we also employ a Clinical Global

Impression (CGI) rating, which assess global symptom severity (35) and can be repeated over the course of treatment to monitor improvement. Such instruments can become a part of the patient's record and help document clinical response or provide a useful reference for subsequent depressive episodes. Finally, a rating scale used more commonly in research studies is the Children's Depressive Rating Scale-Revised (CDRS-R) (36), which is comparable with the Hamilton Depression Rating Scale for adults (37) that scores symptom severity based upon 17 symptoms.

Other standard assessments include a physical examination, blood chemistries and thyroid function tests, Conner's scale for hyperactivity (30,31), a school report and, when indicated, psychological testing. Children with an organic brain disease, attention deficit disorder, an IQ <70 on the Wechsler Intelligence Scale for Children-Revised (38), psychotic symptoms, or unstable medical conditions will require special consideration before beginning treatment for MDD.

When we conducted a structured diagnostic interview with the depressed child and the parent, we found that most children and adolescents met DSM-III-R criteria for major adult affective disorder and also had a diagnosis of conduct disorder or anxiety disorder. Most had a moderate to severe rating of depression, and 85% experienced some difficulty in school as reflected in attendance, performance, or ability to socialize. Furthermore, most children experienced a symptom profile similar to the depressed adult, including feelings of hopelessness, sadness, despair; depressed or irritable mood; low energy; appetite loss; disturbed sleep; and frequently, suicidal thoughts or actions.

The adolescent typically does not want to be hospitalized, even after a serious suicidal attempt, and he or she will deny and hide depressed feelings to prevent hospitalization. Interestingly, the symptoms of adolescent depression often do not include appetite changes or early-morning awakening. Rather, these patients describe hypersomnia with a dysphoric mood on wakening. Irritability, fatigue, anger, and psychomotor retardation are not uncommon for the first few hours of the day. Conduct problems, such as aggression, stealing, running away from home, and sexual promiscuity, are likely to complicate the picture and mislead the clinician away from a diagnosis of MDD. The parent most likely will focus on the change in their child's school performance or relationship with family members. Often, the child is more likely to report sleep disturbances and feeling like crying, whereas the parent will notice appetite changes. Of particular importance is that the parent is frequently unaware of the suicidal ideation until the child has carried out some self-destructive act. Furthermore, more subtle acts, such as running in front of cars, fire setting, wreckless driving, and excessive drinking, are often missed or misinterpreted by parents. If there is any suspicion of suicidal ideation by the patient, this possibility must be taken seriously and carefully explored. Hospitalization may be required to determine the severity of depression and diminish the substantial possibility of a self-destructive act.

Dexamethasone Suppression Test Studies

As a possible biological marker for depression in children, we examined cortisol response to dexamethasone (DST) in normal controls, depressed children, and those with other disorders (14,39,40). Children 12 and younger received 0.5 mg of dexamethasone orally, adolescents were given 1.0 mg, at 11:00 PM, and blood samples for cortisol were obtained at 8:00 AM and 4:00 PM the following day (41). Over 40% of children with MDD were DST nonsuppressors with 8:00 AM and 4:00 PM serum cortisol levels above 5 μg/dL. An additional 20% were so-called early escapers, indicating that they suppressed at 8:00 AM, but their cortisol levels at 4:00 PM were above 5 μg/dL. In contrast, the DST nonsuppression rates for normal (N = 18) and psychiatric controls (N = 50) were 0 and 15%, respectively. Moreover, the DST nonsuppressors showed the best response to imipramine and the poorest response to placebo treatment. Overall, the results for DST in children were similar to those previously found for adults (42). Furthermore, we have observed the best response rate to imipramine treatment in DST-nonsuppressor children when plasma levels of imipramine and its metabolite, desipramine, exceeded 125 ng/mL.

To date, studies of hospitalized adolescents indicate that DST results are variable ranging from 30 to 70% (41,43-45), and false-positive results also tend to be higher in these patients than in adults (42). (For further details on the clinical utility of the DST.

TREATMENT

Most antidepressant medications have not received formal Food and Drug Administration (FDA) labeling for use with children or adolescents. Nevertheless, in terms of drug tolerance and pharmacokinetics, prepubescent children usually have efficient livers and can metabolize drugs rapidly with a greater tolerance to higher doses (mg/kg body weight) than adults. A few months before the onset of puberty there appears to be a transient decrease in drug metabolism, during which high circulating levels of sex hormones compete for hepatic enzyme sites (46). Consequently, at this critical time there can be rapid increases in plasma drug levels, without any change in dose or body weight (47). Therefore, it is advisable to periodically monitor plasma drug levels together with Tanner stages of development as the child approaches puberty.

With onset of puberty, drug metabolism begins to resemble that seen in young adults. Because these adolescents can have far less adipose tissue than mature adults, drug concentration can build up more rapidly, compared with that in adults. Therefore, the physician should begin with low doses and gradually increase the dose to that of adult levels, adjusting for weight in adolescents. A more rapid dose titration may be required in severe cases or when close inpatient monitoring is feasible.

The most efficient way to determine the appropriate antidepressant dose for a given patient is to use therapeutic drug monitoring (TDM). We recommend that the clinician start at 2.5 mg/kg body weight or 75 mg of imipramine (IMI) at bedtime (in a 30-kg child). After 1 week on this regimen, 90% of children will have achieved steady-state plasma drug levels, meaning that their plasma concentration will remain constant over time if the dose is constant. A plasma sample is then drawn 10-12 hr after the last medication dose, and the resulting value will indicate the steady-state IMI (or other antidepressant) blood level. Because most tricyclic antidepressants follow linear pharmacokinetics in children and adolescents, the clinician can change the oral dose to raise or lower the plasma drug level to achieve an optimal range of 125-250 ng/mL. The steady-state TDM approach does not require repeated monitoring unless (1) noncompliance is suspected, (2) there is a significant change in the patient's physical status, or (3) a concomitant medication is added that might influence the antidepressant metabolism (e.g., an anticonvulsant, an analeptic such as methylphenidate, or a neuroleptic agent). Therapeutic drug monitoring represents a substantial advance over the old approach of dosage titration based on clinical indicators and ensures optimum response with less likelihood of toxicity.

To date, there have been no longitudinal studies examining potential consequences of long-term medication treatment on brain function, behavior, or physical health in adult life. Hence, the decision to initiate long-term treatment with medication in a child should be based upon the cost/benefit ratio of treating a serious mood disorder versus potential unknown future risks. Clearly, the case can be made that the child or adolescent at significant risk for suicide merits pharmacologic intervention if psychotherapy or family counseling has not been effective within 4-6 weeks. If there is no response to therapeutic concentrations of IMI (or another antidepressant) within 4-6 weeks at therapeutic plasma levels, then the drug should be gradually discontinued. If neither psychotherapy nor IMI is effective, one option is to switch to another type of antidepressant such as fluoxetine, bupropion, trazodone, or a monoamine oxidase inhibitor realizing that none of these medications have been formally labelled for use in children or adolescents and that their use requires a careful assessment of the relative potential risks versus benefits. This latter option requires even greater caution because optimum doses of these compounds are not known, and the risk of adverse effects is less well studied.

Studies with Imipramine

Although there is an increasing literature on childhood and adolescent depression (10-13,17,21-22,48), less information is available on controlled trials of antidepressants in children (3-9,25,49). Our studies with IMI have progressed in stages from assessing interindividual variability in drug levels and the relationship between drug concentration in plasma and antidepressant response and adverse effects to a classic double-blind drug versus placebo study. Based on our work we have reached the following conclusions: First, IMI is more effective than placebo in the treatment of MDD in children, and the drug response rate can approach 70% when plasma drug levels are taken into account. In contrast, the placebo response rate is less than 30%. Second, the time course for antidepressant response to IMI is similar to that observed in adults treated with this agent. Within 3 weeks of initiating therapy, an antidepressant response is often observed, as long as the plasma drug level is within the therapeutic range. Third, the minimum plasma IMI level necessary for antidepressant response in children in remarkably similar to that observed in adults. Finally, patients who are DST nonsuppressors show the best response to IMI and the poorest response to placebo.

Therapeutic Plasma Drug Level Range

We have found that the ideal plasma IMI concentration necessary for antidepressant response in children is 125-250 ng/mL. Below 125 ng/mL, the drug response rate is reduced, and above 250 ng/mL, the response rate is also reduced and side effects increase (6). We also found a 10- to 20-fold difference in steady-state plasma levels of IMI and its metabolites in depressed children, taking the same dose of IMI. This variability in plasma drug concentration is unrelated to age, height, weight, or gender, and can lead to differences in drug concentrations, ranging from subtherapeutic to toxic. In fact, only 20-30% of children will be in the optimum range when receiving 75 mg of IMI daily, whereas 55-65% will have low plasma levels, and 15% will have excessively high plasma drug levels.

Antidepressant Doses

The FDA initially recommended an upper dosage limit of 2.5 mg/kg for IMI. However, a number of studies have now shown that dosages up to 5.0 mg/kg are required for clinical response. We have been able to substantiate the need for higher doses in children based upon the aforementioned variability in plasma drug levels. Therefore, our recommendation is to begin with a low dose and use TDM as a guide to dosage adjustment to maximize efficacy and minimize toxicity.

After achieving clinical response, treatment is usually continued up to 6 months to prevent relapse. Abrupt withdrawal of antidepressants is to be avoided and a slow taper over several weeks is preferable. If only 5-10 days are used to discontinue IMI, children may develop withdrawal symptoms of nausea, vomiting, drowsiness, decreased appetite, tearfulness, and headaches that may be mistaken for a return of depression.

Side Effects

The effects of tricyclic antidepressants on cardiac function is important when the dose exceeds 3 mg/kg, and electrocardiograms (ECG) should be obtained every 2 weeks if dosage is being increased. Significant slowing of cardiac conduction (PR interval over 0.20, QRS interval over 0.12) may require lowering the dose. If TDM is available to achieve optimum plasma concentrations of IMI plus desipramine (125-250 ng/mL), then close cardiac monitoring is less essential, unless there is preexisting cardiac disease.

The most common adverse side effects we have observed in children taking IMI are anticholinergic—dry mouth, blurred vision, and constipation. These are typically transient and diminish with time. In addition, some children will experience symptoms of orthostatic lightheadedness, which is thought to be the result of the antiadrenergic activity of the drug. Although most side effects are unwanted, there are several beneficial side effects of the drug, including sedation, which can result in better sleep, and an antienuretic effect for those patients with enuresis.

Tricyclic Antidepressant Toxicity

Serious toxic effects on the cardiovascular and central nervous systems can occur at high plasma drug levels. Cardiovascular toxicity is characterized by prolongation of intracardiac conduction, profound changes in blood pressure and heart rate, and sudden death. Central nervous system toxicity includes a confusional state, seizures, and coma. The toxic confusional state is particularly important to recognize as 3 out of 80 children (3.75%) treated by us developed an IMI-induced delirium. One was taking 75 mg and the other two over 100 mg. Their respective ages were 8, 9, and 10 years. With weights between 30 and 35 kg, their respective milligram per kilogram doses were 2.5-3.3 mg/kg. All had plasma levels above 450 ng/mL. In contrast, none of the other 76 children with plasma levels below 450 ng/mL developed a toxic confusional state. This syndrome was characterized by confusion, disorientation, impaired concentration-attention, sedation, social withdrawal, and psychotic symptoms (i.e., hallucinations, delusion, and thought disorder). It developed insidiously over 7 to 10 days and was not associated with substantial peripheral anticholinergic side effects, in comparison with children who did not develop delirium.

Antidepressant overdose is a particularly serious problem for children and adolescents. A dose of 10 mg/kg can be highly toxic, and a dose above 20 mg/kg can be lethal. Patients with serious overdoses should be admitted to the hospital and continuous cardiac monitoring implemented for at least 24 hr. A substantial overdose can be complicated by convulsions, coma, and life-threatening cardiac arrhythmias. Hence, many clinicians will want to limit the amount of drug prescribed at any one time when initiating treatment or if the patient is behaviorally unstable.

BIPOLAR DISORDER IN CHILDREN

Bipolar disorders and pure mania are much less common in children or adolescents. Nevertheless, these disorders are being reported more frequently as the level of sophistication in diagnosis increases (50). Historically, bipolar disorder in children was usually misdiagnosed as schizophrenia. The misdiagnoses usually resulted from the presence of psychotic features, even though the characteristic features of mania were often present, including decreased need for sleep, grandiosity, overactivity, sexual promiscuity, and intermittent depressive symptoms.

It has been only recently that well-designed, systematic studies with lithium carbonate have been conducted in children, and results now indicate its efficacy in bipolar mood disorders in children and adolescents. When prescribing lithium to children and adolescents pretreatment values of electrolytes, serum creatinine, and thyroid function tests should be obtained. Lithium responsiveness in children appears to require blood levels (1.0-2.0 mEq/L) that are higher than those reported for adults (0.5-1.5 mEq/L). Similarly, therapeutic response appears to take longer in children (2-4 weeks) compared with adults (5-10 days).

AFTERCARE AND COURSE OF CHILDHOOD OR ADOLESCENT MOOD DISORDER

Presently, the natural course of mood disorder in children is not well understood. Poznanski et al. (36) reported that almost 50% of depressed children still had symptoms after 5 years follow-up. Kovacs et al. (11) in a systematic, longitudinal study of depressed children reported that the average length of a depression was 9 months, and that few depressive disorders spontaneously remitted within 3 months, but most had done so by 18 months. They also found that multiple depressive episodes could be expected and that a subgroup of children would continue to have chronic, nonremitting MDD. Poznanski (51) suggests that some children develop a dysthymic disorder that eventually becomes MDD. Interestingly, several recent studies have suggested that children's moods are particularly influenced by a depressive episode in a parent, and that treatment of the parent can often have a stabilizing effect on the child's environment. Similarly, psychopharmacologic intervention can enhance the child's response to psychotherapy as well as psychosocial adjustment in terms of school work and socialization with peers.

Several studies have suggested that children with psychiatric disorders in childhood are at significant risk for serious psychopathology and social maladjustment in adulthood. For example, Dahl followed 146 male and 172 female patients for 20 years past their initial admission to child psychiatric units in Denmark (52) and found that 33% of the women and 27% of the men had also been hospitalized as an adult. However, Robin's follow-up study at the St. Louis Child Guidance Clinic indicated that a diagnosis in childhood did not necessarily predict a diagnosis in adulthood (53). By contrast, a more recent study by Akiskal et al. (10) of the children of manic-depressives found that 19 of 24 children suffering from an acute depressive episode had recurrences later in life. Although recurrent depressive episodes were the most common, six children went on to experience a manic psychosis. Significantly, 37.5% of the 24 patients had become bipolar within 3 years.

In summary, there is a lack of well-controlled follow-up studies of patients with childhood depression. Case studies of children with depression leave us with the impression that these patients are at substantial risk for having psychopathology in adolescence and adulthood. Clearly, well-designed follow-up studies are needed.

CONCLUSIONS

The findings from these studies are important for the following reasons: The existence of childhood depression has been questioned by many clinicians, and in the mid-1970s, its existence was considered impossible based upon some psychodynamic constructs. However, data gathering by us and others now indicate that MDD in children does indeed exist and is similar to that of adults. Furthermore, in our controlled treatment studies children with MDD responded better to IMI therapy than nonpharmacologic interventions.

Given the seriousness of acute depression in children and its potential long-term psychiatric problems, it is important for clinicians to diagnose, and aggressively treat, childhood affective disorders. Children represent our light for the future, and every effort should be made to preserve their psychological good health.

ACKNOWLEDGMENTS

For all of their help and contributions over the years to these studies of childhood mood disorders, the authors thank the following: E. Weller, P. Layborne, S. Shupe, K. Bolte, E. Penick, F. Jones, S. Bupp, M. Cantwell, H. Croskell, J. Schwartzman, R. Weller, M. Croskell, M. Fristad, R. Glotzbach, L. Keeler, R. Kumar, D. Mac, S. McConnell, M. Teare, S. Tucker, R. Hassanein, E. Brown, M. Bober, M. McGowan, and A. Lumary. The authors particularly thank Linda K. Hughes, for her careful editorial review of this manuscript.

REFERENCES

1. Rie, H. D. (1966). Depression in childhood: A survey of some pertinent contributions. *J. Am. Acad. Child Adolesc. Psychiatry 5*:653-686.
2. Glaser, K. (1968). Masked depression in children and adolescents. *Annu. Prog. Child Psychiatry Child Dev. 1*:345-355.
3. Hughes, C. W., Preskorn, S. H., Weller, E., Weller, R., and Hassanein, R. (1988). Imipramine vs. placebo studies of childhood depression: Baseline predictors of response to treatment and factor analysis of presenting symptoms. *Psychopharmacol. Bull. 24*:275-279.
4. Preskorn, S. H., Weller, E., Hughes, C. W., Weller, R., and Bolte, K. (1987). Depression in prepubertal children: Dexamethasone nonsuppression predicts differential response to imipramine vs. placebo. *Psychopharmacol. Bull. 23*: 128-133.
5. Preskorn, S. H., Weller, E., Weller, R., and Glotzbach, E. (1983). Plasma levels of imipramine and adverse effects in children. *Am. J. Psychiatry 140*:1332-1335.
6. Preskorn, S. H., Weller, E., Hughes, C. W., and Weller, R. (1986). Plasma monitoring of tricyclic antidepressants: Defining the therapeutic range for imipramine in children. *Clin. Neuropharmacol. 9*(suppl. 4):265-268.
7. Preskorn, S. H., Weller, E., and Weller, R. (1982). Depression in children: Relationship between plasma imipramine levels and response. *J. Clin. Psychiatry 42*:450-453.
8. Preskorn, S. H., Weller, E., Hughes, C. W., and Weller, R. (1988). Depression in children: Defining the therapeutic range for imipramine. In *New Directions in Affective Disorders.* Edited by B. Lerer and S. Gershon, New York, Springer-Verlag.
9. Preskorn, S. H., Weller, E., Hughes, C. W., and Weller, R. (1988). Depression in children: Concentration-dependent CNS toxicity of tricyclic antidepressants. *Psychopharmacol. Bull. 24*:140-142.
10. Akiskal, H. D., Downs, J., Jordan, P., Watson, S., Daugherty, D., and Pruitt, D. B. (1985). Affective disorders in referred children and younger siblings of manic-depressives. *Arch. Gen. Psychiatry 42*:996-1003.
11. Kovacs, M., Feinberg, T. L., Crouse-Novak, M. A., Paulauska, S., and Finkelstein, R. (1984). Depressive disorders in childhood. I. A longtidudinal pro-

spective study of characteristics and recovery. *Arch. Gen. Psychiatry 41*:229-239.
12. Friedman, R. C., Hurt, S. W., Clarkin, J. F., Corn, R., and Aronoff, M. S. (1983). Symptoms of depression among adolescents and young adults. *J. Affect. Disord. 5*:37-43.
13. Mitchell, J., McCauley, E., Burke, P. M., and Moss, S. J. (1988). Phenomenology of depression in children and adolescents. *J. Am. Acad. Child Adolesc. Psychiatry 27*:12-20.
14. Weller, E., Weller, R., Fristad, M., Preskorn, S. H., and Teare, M. (1985). The dexamethasone suppression test in prepubertal depressed children. *J. Clin. Psychiatry 46*:511-513.
15. Andreasen, N. C., Endicott, J., Spitzer, R. L., and Winokur, G. (1977). Family history method using diagnostic criteria. *Arch. Gen. Psychiatry 34*:1229-1233.
16. Barraclough, B., Bunch, J., Nelson, B., and Sainsbury, P. (1974). A hundred cases of suicide: Clinical aspects. *Br. J. Psychiatry 125*:355-373.
17. Rutter, M., Izard, C. E., and Read, P. B. (1986). *Depression in Young People.* New York, Guilford Press.
18. Cantor, P. (1983). Depression and suicide in children. In *Handbook of Clinical Child Psychology.* Edited by E. C. Walker and M. C. Roberts. New York, Wiley-Interscience.
19. Kosky, R. (1983). Childhood suicidal behavior. *J. Child Psychol. Psychiatry 24*:457-468.
20. Sheras, P. L. (1983). Suicide in adolescence. In *Handbook of Clinical Child Psychology.* Edited by C. E. Walker and M. C. Roberts. New York, Wiley-Interscience.
21. Cantwell, D. P. and Carlson, G. A. (1983). *Affective Disorders in Childhood and Adolescence: An Update.* New York, Spectrum Publications.
22. Kashani, J. H., Hoeper, E. W., Beck, N. C., Corcoran, C. M., Fallahi, C., McAllister, J., Rosenberg, T., and Reid, J. C. (1987). Personality, psychiatric disorders, and parental attitude among a community sample of adolescents. *J. Am. Acad. Child Adolesc. Psychiatry 26*:879-885.
23. Puig-Antich, J. and Rabinovich, H. (1986). Relationship between affective and anxiety disorders in childhood. In *Anxiety Disorders of Childhood.* Edited by R. G. Helman, New York, Guilford Press.
24. Puig-Antich, J., Blau, S., Marx, N., Greenhill, L. L., and Chambers, W. (1978). Prepubertal major depressive disorder. A pilot study. *J. Am. Acad. Child Adolesc. Psychiatry 17*:695-707.
25. Puig-Antich, J. (1982). Major depression and conduct disorder in prepuberty. *J. Am. Acad. Child Psychiatry 21*:118-128.
26. Shaffer, D. and Fisher, P. (1981). The epidemiology of suicide in children and young adolescents. *J. Am. Acad. Child Psychiatry 20*:545-565.
27. Marriage, K., Fine, S., Moretti, M., and Haley, G. (1986). Relationship between depression and conduct disorder in children and adolescents. *J. Am. Acad. Child Adol. Psychiatry 25*:687-691.
28. Hershberg, S. G., Carlson, G. A., Cantwell, D. P., and Strober, M. (1982). Anxiety and depressive disorders in psychiatrically disturbed children. *J. Clin. Psychiatry 43*:358-361.

29. Pearce, J. B. (1978). The recognition of depressive disorder in children. *J. R. Soc. Med. 71*:494.
30. Conners, C. K. (1969). A teacher rating scale for use in drug studies with children. *Am. J. Psychiatry 126*:152-156.
31. Conners, C. K. (1970). Symptom patterns in hyperkinetic, neurotic and normal children. *Child Dev. 41*:667-682.
32. Orvaschel, H. (1985). Psychiatric interviews suitable for use in research with children and adolescents. *Psychopharmacol. Bull. 21*:979-989.
33. Reich, W., Herjanic, B., Welner, Z., and Gnadhy, P. R. (1982). Development of a structured psychiatric interview for children: Agreement on diagnosis comparing child and parent interviews. *J. Abnorm. Child Psychol. 10*:325-336.
34. Kovacs, M. (1982). Rating scales to assess depression in school-aged children. *Acta Paedopsychiatr. 46*:305-315.
35. Guy, W., ed. (1976). *ECDEU Assessment Manual for Psychopharmacology, Revised,* DHEW Pub. No. (ADM)76-338. Rockville, Md, National Institute of Mental Health.
36. Pozanski, E., Krahenbuhl, V., and Zrull, J. (1976). Childhood depression. *J. Am. Acad. Child Psychiatry 15*:491-501.
37. Hamilton, M. (1960). A rating scale for depression. *J. Neurol. Neurosurg. Psychiatry 23*:56-62.
38. Wechsler, D. (1974). *Wechsler Intelligence Scale for Children—Revised.* New York, Psychological Corp.
39. Weller, E., Weller, R., Fristad, M., and Preskorn, S. H. (1984). The dexamethasone suppression test in hospitalized prepubertal depressed children. *Am. J. Psychiatry 141*:290-291.
40. Weller, R., Weller, E., Fristad, M., Cantwell, M., and Preskorn, S. H. (1985). *Am. J. Psychiatry 142*:1370-1372.
41. Khan, A. U. (1987). Biochemical profile of depressed adolescents. *J. Am. Acad. Child Adolesc. Psychiatry 26*:873-878.
42. Carroll, B. J., Feinberg, M., and Greden, J. F. (1981). A specific laboratory test for the diagnosis of melancholia. *Arch. Gen. Psychiatry 38*:15-22.
43. Extein, I., Rosenberg, G., and Pottash, A. L. (1982). Dexamethasone suppression test in depressed adolescents. *Am. J. Psychiatry 139*:1617-1619.
44. Hsu, L., Molcan, K., and Cashman, M. (1983). The dexamethasone suppression test in adolescent depression. *J. Am. Acad. Child Adol. Psychiatry 22*:470-473.
45. Robbins, D. R. and Alessi, N. (1985). Suicide and dexamethasone suppression tests in adolescence. *Biol. Psychiatry 20*:94-119.
46. Popper, C. W. (1985). Child and adolescent psychopharmacology. In *Psychiatry.* Edited by J. O. Cavenar, R. Michels, S. B. Guze, and J. E. Helzer. Philadelphia, J.B. Lippincott.
47. Pippinger, C. E. (1980). Rationale and clinical application of therapeutic drug monitoring. *Pediatr. Clin. North Am. 27*:891-925.
48. Andreasen, N. C., Rice, J., Endicott, J., Coryell, W., Grove, W. M., and Reich, T. (1987). Familial rates of affective disorder. *Arch. Gen. Psychiatry 44*:461-469.

49. Petti, T. A. and Law, W. (1982). Imipramine treatment of depressed children: A double-blind study. *J. Clin. Psychopharmacol. 2*:107-109.
50. Mayo, J., O'Connel, R., and O'Brian, J. (1979). Families of manic-depressive patients: Effect of treatment. *Am. J. Psychiatry 136*:1535.
51. Poznanski, E. O. (1985). Affective disorders. In *Psychiatry.* Edited by J. O. Cavenar, R. Michels, S. B. Guze, and J. E. Helzer. Philadelphia, J.B. Lippincott.
52. Dahl, V. (1971). A follow-up study of child psychiatric clientele with special regard to manic depressive psychosis. In *Depressive States in Childhood and Adolescence.* Edited by A. L. Annell. Stockholm, Almquist and Wiksell, pp. 534-541.
53. Robins, L. N. (1966). *Deviant Children Grown Up: A Sociological and Psychiatric Study of Antisocial Personality.* Baltimore, Williams & Wilkins.

19

Antidepressant Medications During Pregnancy and Lactation:

Fetal Teratogenic and Toxic Effects

JOSEPHINE ELIA and GEORGE M. SIMPSON

Medical College of Pennsylvania/Eastern Pennsylvania Psychiatric Institute
Philadelphia, Pennsylvania

INTRODUCTION

Depression and Pregnancy

For centuries clinicians have observed an increased incidence of psychiatric illness in women during pregnancy and in the puerperium. The major psychiatric disorders tend to have an onset shortly after delivery, rather than at other stages of the childbearing process, whereas less disabling symptoms, such as dysphoria, anxiety, lack of energy, difficulty concentrating, and others, are found to have a higher incidence during pregnancy as well as in the postpartum period. Marcé (1) differentiated the clinical features of prepartum and postpartum mental illness 4 centuries ago and found that disorders occurring after childbirth were clinically distinct from other psychiatric disorders of that period.

Pugh et al. (2) studied admissions of women of childbearing age to public mental hospitals in Massachussets and found that, although the admission rate was below expectations throughout pregnancy, it rose several times the expected rate in the first 3 months after delivery.

Kendell et al. (3) identified all the women in the Camberwell catchment area who gave birth in 1970 and checked the case registry for any psychiatric consultation and admission in the 2 years before or after childbirth. Additionally, the distribution of psychiatric contacts was studied in both fathers and mothers. No variation in psychiatric contacts for fathers was observed. However, in mothers, the rates for both psychoses and depression were higher throughout this period and show a prominent peak in the 3 months immediately after childbirth.

Paffenbarger (4) reviewed medical records for all women, 15-44 years of age, who were inpatients on any psychiatric service in the Cincinnati hospital area, from 1940-1958. In this survey, 314 parapartum mental illness patients were identified: 72 with onset during pregnancy and 242 during the 6 months after delivery. These were compared with maternity patients who had delivered around the same date. Illnesses during pregnancy were evenly distributed by trimester, whereas illnesses after pregnancy clustered near the time of delivery. Moreover, there was a striking peak in the rate of mental illness in the first month after delivery. The low prepartum rate of disorders was interpreted to be the result of a protective effect of pregnancy, according to the authors.

This increased incidence of depression in the first few postpartum months was also reported by other investigators (5-8).

Less disabling psychiatric illnesses were investigated by Kumar (9) who found 6.0% of "neurotic" disturbances among primipara before pregnancy. The rate increased during pregnancy and in the postnatal period. Nilsson (7) reported a 17.7% rate of psychiatric symptoms during pregnancy in Sweden, and Cox (10) compared symptoms—such as fatigue, sleep disturbances, irritability, lack of concentration, anxiety, depression, and others—among pregnant Ugandan women with those in a nonpregnant, nonpuerperal group. He found an increased frequency of symptoms during pregnancy; however, for depressed mood, he found no statistical significance between the two groups.

Most of these studies indicate that women are more susceptible to minor psychiatric symptoms during pregnancy, but also that pregnancy provides some protection from the major disorders that peak shortly after delivery.

Even though medications are not usually indicated for minor disorders, they are essential for treating major psychiatric illness. A woman may be given an antidepressant during pregnancy and in the postpartum period for major depression. Panic disorders, obsessive compulsive disorders, and chronic pain also can require treatment during pregnancy. Many dermatological disorders respond to antidepressants, even in the absence of coexisting psychopathological conditions (11), further increasing the use of these medications and the exposure of women of childbearing age to their effects.

The next several sections will explore the physiological changes in pregnancy, placental transfer of antidepressants, and fetal and neonatal metabolism of these drugs. Animal and human teratogenic studies will be reviewed and the safety of using antidepressants during lactation will be investigated.

Because the highest prevalence of major depression and psychoses occurs right after delivery, this spectrum of postpartum disorders will be reviewed. Recommendations for the use of antidepressant medications during pregnancy and in the postpartum period will be made.

Maternal Physiology

Metabolic, endocrine, renal, and cardiac changes occur in pregnancy. Drug distribution becomes altered owing to the expansion of plasma volume (12) and a decrease in plasma protein concentration (13), both leading to decreased plasma concentrations and an increase in the metabolic half-life of medications. As only the free nonbound drug is pharmacologically active, changes in protein binding may have little biological or clinical significance (14).

Metabolism of antidepressants occurs mostly in the liver, and it involves the conversion of the parent compound into a more water-soluble metabolite that can be excreted by the kidneys. The hormonal milieu of pregnancy is thought to increase liver metabolic activity in humans (15) and, therefore, may increase the metabolism of antidepressants during pregnancy.

Renal blood flow almost doubles during pregnancy, and the glomerular filtration rate (GFR) also increases (16), which helps in the clearance of the metabolized drugs.

Delayed gastric emptying and increased intestinal transit time during pregnancy may lead to slower, but more complete, drug absorption and, thereby, higher serum drug levels (17).

Considering all of the foregoing factors, it appears that the increased volume distribution, the decreased plasma protein concentration, and the possible increased hepatic metabolism and increased renal clearance would result in the need for a higher dose of drug, whereas the increased half-life and increased absorption may reduce this requirement. However, these represent generalizations about antidepressants and there is, as yet, no clinical data to support these hypotheses. The physiological changes occurring during normal pregnancy are complex, and frequent blood level monitoring of tricyclic antidepressants is useful. Kerns (18) suggests that generally imipramine and other tertiary amine tricyclics that can cause hypotension should be avoided in favor of less hypotensive drugs. When complications such as edema develop, an even greater increase in extravascular volume occurs and, consequently, the volume in which drugs are distributed is increased (12). In preeclampsia or in the nephrotic syndrome, the total circulating albumin is reduced, causing saturation of binding sites and rises in the free-drug fraction (19). In these and other complicated cases, monitoring in the hospital may become necessary.

Placental Transfer of Antidepressants

Most psychotropic drugs cross the placenta. Their transfer occurs primarily by simple diffusion, depending upon the chemical properties of the drug, including molecular size, protein-binding affinity, polarity and lipid solubility, drug concentration, and duration of exposure (20). Nonionized, low-molecular-weight, lipid-soluble drugs are well absorbed.

Imipramine (21), desipramine (22,23), and nortriptyline (23) cross the placenta in animals. Amitriptyline and protriptyline did not cross sheep placental membrane (23).

Douglas and Hume (21) gave 20 rats in the third trimester of pregnancy an intramuscular injection of 10 mg/kg of imipramine and found that the concentrations of drug in the maternal plasma and fetal tissue were in equilibrium within 3 min. In a similar experiment with 10 mg/kg of desmethylimipramine (22), equilibration between the maternal and fetal system was reached within 1 min of the maternal intramuscular injection and remained constant throughout the 20 min of the experiment.

Van Petten (23) examined the maternal and fetal pressor response in sheep after the administration of a tricyclic antidepressant. By comparing maternal and fetal response he was able to determine which tricyclic crossed the placental barrier. The results showed that single doses of tricyclics did not produce prominent direct effects on the fetal cardiovascular activity. However, the pressor response to norepinephrine was potentiated in both mother and fetus when imipramine, desipramine, and nortriptyline were given to the mother. In contrast, amitriptyline and protriptyline produced norepinephrine potentiation in the mother, but not in the fetus, suggesting that these compounds did not cross the placenta.

In humans, case reports (24-27) of neonates who developed symptoms after maternal ingestion of imipramine or nortriptyline, definitively showed a placental transfer of these medications.

Drug Metabolism in the Fetus and Neonate

The human fetus can metabolize many foreign compounds. This extensive drug-metabolizing activity correlates with the presence of cytochrome P_{450} (28). The components of this microsomal drug oxidation system have been found in the human fetus, during the second trimester, in amounts of the same magnitude as in adult livers when calculated per gram of liver tissues in in vitro studies. The in vivo capability of function, however, is not known (29).

Excretion of most drugs, through the placental and fetal urine may be delayed. The purpose of drug metabolism is to render foreign compounds polar and more water-soluble. As a result, excretion into the urine is facilitated, whereas passage across tissue membranes, such as the placenta, is decreased.

Similar to the fetus, the neonate has proportionally less total serum protein for drug binding, less active hepatic degradative enzymes, and a lower glomerular filtration rate than the adult (19). The blood-brain barrier is still incomplete, and the immature central nervous system generally appears more sensitive to drug effects (20). Also, the neonate no longer exists in equilibrium with its mother through the placenta, and a drug concentrated in the fetus shortly before birth may have significantly prolonged postnatal effects.

Several symptoms secondary to maternal use of antidepressants have been reported in neonates (Table 1). Shearer (20) reported a case of urinary retention in an infant exposed to nortriptyline throughout pregnancy. Immature liver enzymes, as well as a possible genetic inability to metabolize the drug, was postulated. This case would not support the notion of a washout period for the fetus before delivery, since the bladder contained a large amount of urine, and it was hypothesized that the retention may have been occurring over a long period in utero.

Sjöqvist et al. (27) reported a case of a 20-year-old pregnant depressed woman who took 1.5-1.75 g of nortriptyline in an overdose. She became comatose and delivered a 3610-g infant, 20 hr after the ingestion. The newborn was conscious, with Apgar scores of 8 and 9 at 1 and 10 min, respectively. Its electrocardiogram (ECG) was abnormal with widened and split QRS complexes. These abnormalities persisted for 5 days, after which the ECG normalized. At birth, the maternal nortriptyline plasma level was 1 μg/mL, and the cord concentration was 0.43 μg/mL. At 12 and 24 hr after the ingestion, the infant plasma was 0.18 μg/mL. The half-life of the drug in the mother was calculated at 17 hr and in the neonate 56 hr. It is unclear whether the longer half-life is due to genetic factors or to immaturity of liver enzymes. No serious toxicity was seen in this newborn at a level of 0.2 mg/mL, although it is probable that the unbound fraction of nortriptyline was several times higher than that found in the adult. These observations support the idea that the newborn is not particularly sensitive to the action of nortriptyline.

Eggermont et al. (26) reported the case of a mother who received imipramine, amobarbital (Amytal), and methotrimeprazine (levomepromazine). In a second case, the mother received imipramine alone, and in a third case, clomipramine alone. The infants developed slowed and jerky movements, as well as seizures, marked respiratory and circulatory symptoms. The symptoms disappeared after the first week of life. The authors explain all of the symptoms by an increase in adrenergic activity and the anticholinergic side effects, and by the slower metabolism of the drugs in the newborn.

Table 1 Perinatal Complications

Author (Ref.)	Design	Medications	Results	Comments
Shearer et al. (24)	32-yr-old pregnant depressed woman treated with ECT before pregnancy and with nortriptyline 25 mg q.u.i.d. throughout pregnancy. The last dose was taken 12 hr before delivery.	Nortriptyline	Infant born with Apgar of 8, was lethargic at 10 hr of age and was treated with nalorphine. A large abdominal mass was found and urinary catherization produced 130 ml of urine with resolution of the mass at 18 hr of age. By 30 hr of age, the infant had not voided and required another catherization. Spontaneous urination occurred at 40 hr. Obstruction and reflux were ruled out.	Nortriptyline is metabolized by hydroxylation in the liver. The ability to metabolized the drug may be genetically determined. It is possible that this child manifested a toxic reaction to transplacental accumulation of nortriptyline because of immature liver enzyme function or a genetically determined inability to metabolize the drug. The urinary retation may have been long-standing in utero because the bladder contained a large quantity of urine. Urinary retention has not been reported as a side effect secondary to meperidine or nalorphine

Eggermont et al. (26)	Case reports of three pregnant mothers treated with different antidepressants during pregnancy.	Imipramine, amobarbital (Amytal), levomepromazine	This infant was cyanotic had mild respiratory distress, CHF, seizures in the first 5 days after birth. From the sixth day on, all symptoms disappeared.
		Imipramine	This infant was tachypnic, hypotonic, cyanotic, hypoactive. He had rhythmic jerks at the slightest stimulation. Symptoms also lasted for 6 days and then disappeared.
		Clomipramine	This infant had low Apgars, needed resuscitation. He also had tachycardia, tremors of the extremities, tonic and clonic movements, feeding difficulties, and laryngeal spasms. Symptoms disappeared gradually during the first week of life.

Table 1 (Continues)

Table 1 Continued

Author (Ref.)	Design	Medications	Results	Comments
Sjöqvist et al. (27)	20-yr-old depressed pregnant woman, treated with 25 mg t.i.d. of nortriptyline, overdosed on 1.5-1.75 g of the drug. Became comatose and delivered 20 hr after the ingestion.	Nortriptyline, diazepam	Newborn was conscious. Apgar scores were 8 and 9. ECG had widened and split QRS, which normalized in 5 days. Infant's plasma level was 0.18 μg/mL at 12 and 24 hr after birth. The half-life of the drug was three times as high as mother's.	
Webster (25)	Mother treated with desmethylimipramine throughout pregnancy	Desmethylimipramine	Labor and delivery were uncomplicated. Infant weighed 3.95 kg. At 24 hr of age, developed breathlessness, cyanosis, tachypnea, tachycardia, profuse sweating, irritability. The symptoms lasted for 10 days and then the child improved.	The author hypothesizes that the infant developed withdrawal symptoms.

Webster (25) treated a mother with desipramine during pregnancy. The infant was born after an uncomplicated delivery and developed breathlessness, cyanosis, tachypnea, tachycardia, profuse sweating, and irritability, lasting for 10 days, after which the child improved. These symptoms were attributed to the abrupt withdrawal from the antidepressants at birth.

TERATOGENICITY

No psychotropic drug has been proved safe for use during pregnancy, and all carry warnings by the Food and Drug Administration (FDA) (30). The effects of drugs on the human fetus are, in general, not even investigated before approval because of the restrictions of premarketing experimental studies. Data on teratogenicity are, in general, accumulated as a result of nonsystematic observations on pregnant patients who have inadvertently been given newly marketed drugs. Similar types of regulations exist in other countries with different degrees of postmarketing surveillance.

Proof of an individual drug's teratogenicity is difficult to establish. It may be more easily inferred if the defect produced is rare. However, the absence of reports of teratogenicity for a given drug does not imply safety. Data from animal studies may be either alarming or reassuring, but potential species difference precludes drawing conclusions about drug effects on the human fetus from such studies. A drug that reliably produces defects in animal species may not do so in humans. The converse is also true, and this was tragically demonstrated by the effects of thalidomide in infants, after preliminary animal studies revealed no teratogenic effects. Later studies showed thalidomide to have a strong species-specificity, and the typical limb malformations were produced in selected strains of white rabbits (31) and in monkeys (32).

During the first 2 weeks postconception, fertilization and implantation take place and dysmorphogenic substances will in general affect all cells, causing death of the embyro. From about 2-6 weeks postconception is the period of organogenesis, when the embryo shows extreme sensitivity to teratogens, the effect depending upon the time of exposure. The central nervous system, which continues its maturation throughout pregnancy and after birth, is vulnerable to teratogenic effects throughout gestation and in the postpartum period. Behavioral teratogenic studies that seem to be more sensitive to central nervous system changes are providing a critical tool in observing such effects. The following reviews cover teratogenic changes, anatomical as well as behavioral and physiological in animals. A review of case reports and studies of human teratogenicity follows.

Teratogenicity: Animal Studies

Guram et al. (33) reported gross abnormalities in hamsters treated with imipramine and amitriptyline. Both drugs caused gross anomalies that included exencephaly, cranioschisis, lower body atrophy, external liver, and others. The percentage of malformations was higher in the fetuses exposed to amitriptyline than in those exposed to imipramine; however, the percentage of resorptions was higher with imipramine. When given in combination with chlordiazepoxide, amitriptyline was teratogenic at a much lower dose.

Robson (34) observed three malformations with imipramine in 12 rabbits, and Harper (35) observed four malformations and higher resorption rates at the same dosage. Aeppli (36) found skeletal malformations in rabbits exposed prenatally to 2-hydroxy-imipramine.

Simpkins (37) reported an increase in infant mortality in rats treated with imipramine, as well as a decrease in birth weight and growth rate. He also noted an increased responsiveness of the β-adrenergic system in the aorta. Ali (38) observed that prenatal imipramine exposure in rats alters functional development of central adrenergic systems.

Gilani (39) exposed chick embryos and found that early injection in the eggs produced micromelia and hydrocephalia.

In contrast to the foregoing reports, Aeppli, Jelinek (40), and Oberholzer (41) found no anomalies in rats exposed to imipramine. Also, no anomalies were found in rabbits by Oberholzer. Hendrickx (42) likewise found no teratogenic effects in monkeys exposed acutely and chronically to imipramine while in utero. The abortion rate was higher than controls, and it was not related to dosage. At high levels maternal toxicity was also observed.

Simpkins (37) reported an increased infant mortality in rats exposed to doxepin during the first and second trimester. Exposure in the third trimester correlated with increased responsiveness of the β-adrenergic system in the aorta.

Preskorn (43) tested bupropion in rats, mice, and rabbits and found no teratogenic effects. A supernumerary 13th rib occurred in rabbits at all doses used, and this was considered to represent a skeletal variant which occurred spontaneously in high prevalence in this species. Two-generation reproduction and fertility studies were done with rats and F_1 and F_2 offspring showed no teratogenicity.

Poulson (44) investigated the effects of phenelzine and several of its derivatives in pregnant mice and found them to inhibit implantation. This effect was thought to be brought about by depressing the pituitary or hypothalamus.

Studies on animal teratogenicity are reviewed in Table 2.

Behavioral Teratogenicity

Animal studies (Table 3) clearly demonstrate that prenatal exposure to tricyclic antidepressants in therapeutic doses can produce behavioral changes that can persist. Rats exposed to imipramine in utero have less frequent ex-

Table 2 Teratogenicity of Antidepressants: Animal Studies

Authors (Ref.)	Design	Drugs	Results
Robson et al. (34)	Pregnant rabbits were given imipramine (30 mg/kg. sc).	Imipramine	Three malformations occurred in 12 treated cases.
Oberholzer (41)	Pregnant rats and rabbits were treated with imipramine (25-50 mg/kg, po).	Imipramine	No anomalies observed in offspring. Toxic effects in mothers who had higher doses were observed in the rats.
Harper et al. (35)	Pregnant rabbits were treated with imipramine (15 and 30 mg/kg, sc).	Imipramine	At the higher doses there were higher resorption rates, maternal toxicity, and four malformations.
Jelinek et al. (67)	Pregnant rats were treated with imipramine, amitriptyline (10-20 mg/kg, po).	Imipramine, amitriptyline	No anomalies observed in offspring.
Aeppli (36)	Pregnant rats were treated with imipramine, desmethylimipramine, and 2-OH-imipramine (40 mg/kg po).	Imipramine, desmethylimipramine, 2-OH imipramine	No anomalies observed in offspring.
	Pregnant rabbits were treated with 2-OH-imipramine (40 mg/kg, sc).	2-OH-imipramine	Skeletal anomalies observed in offspring.
DiCarlo et al. (1971)	Pregnant rats were treated with amitriptyline or butryptline, po.	Amitriptyline, butriptyline	Skeletal malformations were found in animals exposed to the amitriptyline.
Simpkins et al. (37)	Female rats were treated once daily for 7 days with doxepin (30 mg/kg) during 1st trimester or	Doxepin	Increased infant mortality.

Table 2 (Continues)

Table 2 Continued

Authors (Ref.)	Design	Drugs	Results
	2nd trimester or 3rd trimester		Increased infant mortality. Increased responsiveness of β-adrenergic system in the aorta.
	Female rats were treated with imipramine (30 mg/kg) during the 3rd trimester	Imipramine	Increased infant mortality. Decreased birth weight and growth rate of offspring. Increased responsiveness of β-adrenergic system in the aorta.
	(The doses of these tricyclics were chosen because they had been reported to be devoid of teratogenic effects.)		At doses of tricyclics that do not cause dysmorphic effects on the fetus, subtle alterations occur in selective adrenergic functions which can persist into adulthood of the rat.
Poulson and Robson (44)	White mice were given single daily SC injections of phenelzine on gestation days 1-6 at 25 mg/kg/day. The animals were given phenelzine derivatives during the other gestational days.	Phenelzine	Phenelzine and its derivative were effective in inhibiting implantation. They are thought to exert this activity by depressing the pituitary or hypothalamus.
Hendrickx (42)	Imipramine was administered po twice daily to 18 bonnet	Imipramine	No teratogenic effects were observed. Rate of absorption

	and 3 rhesus monkeys between gestation days 23 and 45 for 1-3 or 18-22 days at 1,2, and 10 times the recommended human dose.		higher than controls. Maternal toxicity occurred at the higher dose levels and the rate of abortion was higher than controls.
Gilani (39)	Chick embryos were treated with 0.01-0.16 mg of imipramine.	Imipramine	Early injection in the egg produced micromelia and hydrocephalia.
Guram et al. (33)	Pregnant hamsters were given a single IP dose of either imipramine or amitriptyline on gestation day 8. Dose range of imipramine used was 53-110 mg/kg. Dose range of amitriptyline used was 60-100 mg/kg.	Imipramine, amitriptyline	Imipramine produced 2.9-19.5% of malformations in the exposed fetuses. Amitriptyline produced 6.4-44.8% of malformations in the exposed fetuses. This study suggests that amitriptyline may be more teratogenic than imipramine in hamsters, whereas the percentage of fetal resorptions was higher with imipramine.
Guran et al. (1982)	Pregnant hamsters were given chlordiazepoxide in doses ranging between 280 and 3100 mg/kg on gestation day 8.	Chlordiazepoxide	Progressive increase in the level of maternal administration of the drug resulted in an increase in the percentage of fetal malformations which ranged from 3-55%.
	Pregnant hamsters were given amitriptyline in doses ranging between 60 and 100	Amitriptyline	Progressive increase in the level of maternal administration of the drug resulted

Table 2 (Continues)

Table 2 Continued

Authors (Ref.)	Design	Drugs	Results
	mg/kg on gestation day 8		in an increase in the percentage of fetal malformations which ranged from 5-44%.
	Pregnant hamsters were given a single injection of a combination of chlordiazepoxide-amitriptyline.	Chlordiazepoxide-amitriptyline	A dose-response relationship was found in which a maternal dose range of 13/33 mg/kg to 33/83 mg/kg of chlordiazepoxide-amitriptyline. produced 7-92% of fetal anomalies. CNS anomalies such as exencephaly, encephalocoele predominated. This study indicates that the teratogenic potential of the combined drugs is higher than that of either drug administered alone.
Tucker (1983)	Pregnant rats were given 150, 300, or 450 mg/kg/day of the drug during gestational days 6-15	Bupropion	No teratogenic effects observed.
	Pregnant rabbits were given 25, 50, 100, or 150 mg/kg/day of the drug during gestional days 6-18.	Bupropion	Offspring had an increased number of supernumerary 13th ribs (This occurred at all doses and was considered to represent a skeletal variant

		that occurred spontaneously in high incidence). There was also delayed ossification of the 5th phalanx which occurred only at very high doses.
Two-generation reproduction and fertility studies were done with male and female Long Evans rats that were given 100, 200, or 300 mg/kg/day of the drug for 6 and 15 days, respectively, before mating. Dosing of females continued throughout gestation and lactation.	Bupropion	F_1 offspring showed no teratogenicity. F_2 offspring showed no teratogenicity.

Table 3 Behavioral Teratogenicity: Antidepressants

Authors (Ref.)	Design	Drugs	Results
Werboff et al. (1951)	Prenatal administration of antidepressants to rats.	Isocarboxazid, iproniazid	Offspring were less susceptible to audiogenic seizures than controls.
Coyle (1975)	Pregnant rats were given 5 mg/kg oral doses of IMI on days 14-21 before mating until gestational day 19.	Imipramine	Behavior in an open field showed that exploratory responses were less frequent in the exposed offspring. Behavior in the spontaneous alternation tasks and a swimming maze did not differ from that of controls. The number of live offspring in the IMI group was significantly fewer than the control group, and the number of stillbirths was significantly higher than the control group.
Coyle and Singer (45)	Pregnant rats were given 5 mg/kg IMI po, before and throughout gestation. Pups were reared in different housing conditions. Behavior and brain histology were observed.	Imipramine	Pups reared in impoverished environment: Controls and experimental animals were equally poor in maze solving. Pups reared in enriched environment: IMI-exposed offspring were inferior to controls in maze solving. IMI-exposed offspring did not develop increased cortical thickness.
Echandia et al. (47)	Pregnant rats were given IMI, 3 mg/3 mg/kg/day, before mating and during gestation. A group of pups stayed with drug throughout lactation. A group of nonexposed in utero pups were given to drugged dams for lactation. A control group received no drug at any time.	Chlorimipramine	Behavioral differences were observed between the drug-exposed group and controls. These included a significant increase in digging and grooming, a decrease in exploration and social interactions in the drug-exposed group. These findings were more prominent among males than female pups. Chlorimipramine exposure dur-

			ing lactation had minor effects on behavior. No teratogenicity, decrease in body weight or increase in mortality occurred in the dosages used.
File et al. (1984)	Pregnant rats were given 7.5-15 mg/kg/day of the drug on gestational days 8-21. Behavioral tests were given to the offspring.	Clomipramine	Prenatal exposure increased the baseline of the acoustic startle in females only. In interaction tests of anxiety, males exposed to both dosages and females exposed to the lowest dosage, showed a similar profile to that seen after long-term administration of benzodiazepines in the adult.
Buelke-Sam et al. (1985)	Pregnant rats were given imipramine on gestational days 8-20 SC at doses of either 0, 5, or 10 mg/kg/day. Behavioral tests were conducted with the offspring.	Imipramine	Maternal weight gain during the dosing period was decreased by 20% in the high-dose group. There were no dose-related differences in the offspring body weight. Low-dose males turned significantly sooner in negative geotaxis testing, but more high-dose males successfully turned (84%) than did controls (61%). A significant reduction in auditory startle habituation amplitude was found in males from low-dose group. Locomotor activity before an amphetamine challenge was higher in IMI-exposed males. Low-dose males and high-dose females were more active following the challenge. Prenatal imipramine exposure appears to influence behavioral patterns in a manner dependent on sex and age as well as dose.

exploratory responses (45), decreased maze-solving capabilities, and decreased cortical thickness (46). Pups exposed to chlorimipramine in utero showed significant increase in digging and grooming, decreases in exploration, and fewer social interactions (47). Chlorimipramine exposure during lactation had minor effects on behavior (47). Early neonatal treatment of rats with monoamine oxidase inhibitor has resulted in nerve cell changes and decreased concentrations of norepinephrine and dopamine in the hypothalamus, reduced learning capacity, and diminished emotional reactivity in later life (48).

Receptor Changes Secondary to Prenatal Antidepressant Exposure

Most of the studies on antidepressants show a decrease in cortical β-adrenergic receptors in the exposed animals (49-51). Studies of other receptor changes secondary to prenatal antidepressant exposure are reviewed in Table 4.

Antidepressants: Human Studies

Several single case reports of maternal use of tricyclics during pregnancy and varied anomalies such as anophthalmia (52), absent fibula, hypoplastic tibia and foot (53), cardiac anomalies, lack of fusion of frontonasal processes (54) have been reported. In addition to these, McBride (55) reported a case of amelia associated with maternal use of imipramine during pregnancy. Two similar cases were subsequently reported. McBride's report aroused worldwide concern because it had been only a decade since a relatively rare birth defect, phocomelia, had reached epidemic proportions, later shown to be related to the administration of thalidomide.

The reports of these anomalies led to multiple studies designed to find any possible correlation between teratogenicity, mostly limb reduction, and antidepressants. Wilson (56), Rachelitski et al. (57), and Crombie et al. (58) showed no association between limb reductions and exposure to tricyclics in utero. The Australian Drug Evaluation Committee (59) investigated the cases of children born with limb reductions and found that the mothers had taken a variety of medications during pregnancy. Three of the seven mothers had not taken any antidepressants, and one of the mothers had taken nortriptyline at a time during the pregnancy when, on the basis of current knowledge of critical limb development, it would be unlikely to be relevant.

A retrospective study of cases of limb reduction by Banister et al. (60) showed that antidepressants had not been used by most of the mothers. However, one mother had taken amitriptyline during the first 12 weeks, and this infant was born with absent digits on one foot, a cerebral vascular abnormality, and hydrocephalus. Keunssberg and Knox (61) in a retrospective

Table 4 Receptors: Prenatal Antidepressant Exposure

Authors	Design	Drugs	Results
Tonge (1973)	Pregnant rats were given one of the two drugs in drinking water, before, during pregnancy, and until they were weaned on PND 21.	Imipramine, phencyclidine	Offspring were sacrificed at 3, 6, 9 mo. postweaning. NA, DA, and normetanephrine concentrations were measured in discrete areas of the brains. No statistical significant differences between catacholamine concentration in brain regions from rats of different ages were found.
Jason et al. (49)	Pregnant rats were given water or 15 mg/kg/day imipramine on GD 8-20 by oral intubation.	Imipramine	IMI-treated mothers gained significantly less weight during pregnancy, but the percentage giving birth, length of gestation, and litter size were all unaffected. Body weights of IMI-exposed offspring were significantly lower than controls until PND 14, and brain weights were lower until PND 30 IMI-exposed pups, had earlier eye opening, delayed surface righting reflex, and the development of negative geotaxis was altered. Hypothalamic NE and EPI levels

Table 4 (Continues)

Table 4 Continued

Authors	Design	Drugs	Results
			were unchanged in IMI-exposed pups at 7, 14, 30 days, whereas DA levels were unaffected at PND 7, 14, but were markedly lower than controls at PND 30. The number of cortical β-adrenergic receptors was decreased by 18.7% at PND 14, and by 9.1% on PND 30. Affinity for binding was increased at 30 days. Prenatal exposure to IMI produces behavioral and neurochemical consequences lasting well past cessation of drug exposure.
Ali et al. (35)	Pregnant rats were dosed SC on GD 8-20 with either 0, 5, or 10 mg/kg/day of IMI.	Imipramine	PND 1: male offspring from low-dose group showed a 65% reduction in β-adrenergic receptor binding and marked increase in brain EPI. PND 21: No consistant dose-related changes were found in binding. Cortical levels of EPI increased to 300% of control levels in low-dose males and high-dose females challenged with

			amphetamines. These same rats showed marked increase in locomotor activity following challenge.
De Ceballos et al. (50)	Pregnant rats were given SC distilled water or an antidepressant 10 mg/kg/day on GD 6 until delivery. On PND 25 pups were either tested behaviorally or killed. Controls were 25-day-old pups that were treated immediately before testing.	Chlorimipramine, iprindole, mianserin, nomifensine	No antidepressant drug had an overt effect on the number of pups born. Spontaneous locomotor activity was decreased after a single dose of antidepressant, and a significant decrease also occurred after prenatal exposure with CI-IMI, iprindole, and mianserin. Rats treated briefly with nomifensine had increased locomotor activity. Spontaneous locomotion was still increased, compared with controls, in the prenatally exposed animals to nomifensine. CI-IMI, iprindole, nomifensine enhanced the locomotor response to apomorphine. Acutely treated animals with mianserin decrease locomotion, but in utero mianserin did not modify the apomorphine-induced hyperactivity.

Table 4 (Continues)

Table 4 Continued

Authors	Design	Drugs	Results
			No changes in binding of [^{3}H]spiroperidol to striatal DA receptors after antidepressants were noted. However, the ability of DA to compete for these sites was significantly enhanced after prenatal exposure to all the antidepressants tested.
			This increase in agonist affinity for DA receptors may explain the long-lasting behavioral supersensitivity of DA receptors observed after extended treatment with typical or atypical antidepressants

De Ceballos et al. (51)	Pregnant rats were given SC distilled water or an antidepressant (10 mg/kg/day) on GD 6 until delivery. On PND 25, pups were either tested behaviorally or killed. Controls were 25-day-old pups that were treated immediately before testing.	Chlorimipramine, iprindole, mianserin, nomifensine	No antidepressant drug had an overt effect on the number of pups born. All antidepressants reduced the number of β-adrenoceptors in the prenatally exposed rats, CIMI, iprindole, mianserin decreased the density of 5-HT_2 receptors in prenatally exposed pups, whereas nomifensine increased it. Acute treatment of 25-day-old rats did not modify the characteristics of binding to β-adrenergic or 5-HT_2 receptors.
Simpkins et al. (37)	Pregnant rats treated with imipramine (30 mg/kg) during the 3rd trimester.	Imipramine	Increased responsiveness of β-adrenergic system in the aorta.

GD, gestational day; PND, postnatal day; NE, norepinephrine; IMI, imipramine; EPI, epinephrine; CI-IMI, chlorimipramine; DA, dopamine.

Table 5 Teratogenicity of Antidepressants: Human Studies

Authors	Design	Drugs	Results	Comment
Levy (1972)	Clinical observations of pregnant patients who were treated with tricyclics.	Tricyclics	No anomalies seen.	
Freeman (53)	Case report of a pregnant woman who had ingested amitriptyline during the first trimester.	Amitriptyline	Male infant with absent left fibula, hypoplastic tibia and foot.	Mother had also taken other medications during pregnancy
Crombie et al. (58)	Retrospective study of 8000 pregnancies lasting beyond 27 wk; 19 involved exposure to imipramine and 28 to amitriptyline.	Imipramine, amitriptyline	No abnormalities found in infants exposed to imipramine; 27 of the 28 exposed to amitriptyline were normal. One infant had swelling of the hands and feet at birth. At 2 yr of age was normal.	
Wilson (56)	Retrospective study of 120 cases involving reduction of limb deformities.	Antidepressants	None of the mothers had taken imipramine or related antidepressants.	
Sim (1972)	Case report of 81 patients who were given imipramine during pregnancy.	Imipramine	No fetal abnormalities occurred in these children.	
Banister et al. (60)	A retrospective study of 168 cases of congenital limb reductions born during 1969 to 1971.	Tricyclics	Of the 168 mothers, 25 had take tricyclics. In one case the mother had taken amitriptyline during the first 12 wk. This infant had absent digits on one foot, a cerebral	

			vascular abnormality, and hydrocephalus. This mother had also taken antibiotics for a UTI. In two cases, an unknown tranquilizer had been taken.	
Rochelifski et al. (57)	A retrospective study of 101 infants born with reduction deformities. Obstetricians and mothers were questioned and obstetrical records reviewed	Tricyclics	None of the infants with deformities were prenatally exposed to tricyclics	It is possible that there may have been underreporting of medications taken before obstetrical care was begun.
Keunssberg and Knox (61)	Retrospective study of 17 women who were prescribed imipramine within the first 10 wk of pregnancy.	Imipramine	14 of these had children; no abnormalities. One child had defective abdominal muscles and gut. One child had a diaphragmatic hernia. One fetus was aborted at 14 wk.	No conclusions can be drawn from these studies because the small number of subjects.
	13 women had been prescribed amitriptyline within the first 10 wk of pregnancy.	Amitriptyline	28 children were normal. One fetus aborted at 6 wk. One child was born with hypospadias.	
McBride (55) (1972)	Case reports of three mothers who had ingested imipramine during pregnancy.	Imipramine	Limb reduction in the infants.	

Table 5 (Continues)

Table 5 Continued

Authors	Design	Drugs	Results	Comment
Australian Drug Evaluation Committee (59)	Investigation of limb reduction cases	Tricyclics	They found that of seven mothers who had children with limb reductions, all had taken a variety of drugs during pregnancy. Three mothers had not taken any tricyclics during the pregnancy. One mother had taken nortriptyline at a time during the pregnancy when, on the basis of current knowledge of critical limb development, it would be unlikely to be relevant.	
Idanpaan-Heikkila and Saxon (62)	Retrospective study of tricyclic antidepressant use: 2784 cases of children with birth defects taken by the Finnish Register between 1967 and 1972 and an equal number of matched controls.	Tricyclics	Five malformed infants were born to women who had taken tricyclics during pregnancy; four had soft-tissue craniofacial or CNS anomalies, and one had multiple bone anomalies. Three of the women had taken imipramine and chlorapyramine (antihistamine) during the first trimester. In one case amitriptyline had been taken early in	Number of cases is small. Combination of drugs were involved.

Table 5 (Continues)

			the pregnancy, and in another case it had been taken during the last trimester. In the control group, one woman had ingested tricyclics.	
Rowe (1973)	Clinical observations of large numbers of child-bearing women receiving prescriptions for tricyclics in Australia. (1,169,708 prescriptions for antidepressants were written in a 9-mo period)	Tricyclics	Absence of any observable significant fetal malformations.	The absence of a significant number of reports of associated fetal abnormalities arising in such pregnancies is incompatible with the allegations of teratogenic effects.
Golden and Perinan (52)	Case report of a pregnant woman exposed to multiple medications, including amitriptyline, and hospitalized for possible viral encephalitis.	Amitriptyline	Premature infant (32 wk) with bilateral clinical anophthalmia	No conclusions can be drawn.
Wertelecki (1980)	Case report of a mother who had overdosed on amitriptyline and perphenazine during a suicide attempt.	Amitriptyline (725 mg); perphenazine (58 mg)	Infant born with severe birth defects, including microcephaly, "cotton-like" hair, cleft palate, micrognathia, ambiguous genitalia, foot deformities.	

Table 5 Continued

Authors	Design	Drugs	Results	Comment
Bracken and Holford (1981)	Case control study of 1370 infants with malformations and 2968 healthy infants	Antidepressants	Of all mothers, 44.5% used at least one prescribed drug during pregnancy. Case mothers were more likely than control mothers to use antidepressants, narcotics, analgesics, and tranquilizers during the first trimester.	
Abramovici et al. (54)	Case report of a mother who had suffered a severe depression during the first and second month of pregnancy and was treated with progressively larger doses of chlorimipramine	Chlorimipramine (250-925 mg day/IV)	Pregnancy was interrupted for nonmedical reasons and the embryo had ventricular inversion, dextroversion, hypoplastic aorta arising from a right ventricle, interventricular septal defect, ocular lens vacuolization, lack of fusion of frontonasal process.	Definite cause-effect relationship cannot be established in this case.

study of 17 children exposed to imipramine and 31 children exposed to amitriptyline in utero reported one child exposed to imipramine born with defective abdominal muscles and gut. Of the group exposed to amitriptyline, one abortion occurred and one child was born with hypospadias. Idanpaan-Heikkila and Saxen (62) reviewed records of mothers of children with birth defects. Five malformed infants had been born to mothers who had been taking tricyclics during pregnancy. Four had central nervous system anomalies, and one had multiple bone anomalies. These retrospective studies suggest a casual relationship between tricyclic ingestion during pregnancy and congenital anomalies. However, the small number of cases and the concomitant use of other medications in the study population prevents the drawing of any definitive conclusions.

Many women of childbearing age are prescribed antidepressants, and as limb bud development starts around the 35th day, it is probable that many fetuses have been exposed to these drugs at a critical time, even before the mother may be aware that she is pregnant. The fact that there has not been an increase in limb deformities or other major physical anomalies in the past few decades, during which time there has been widespread use of tricyclics, supports the relative safety of these drugs.

There are no studies or reports on monoamine oxidase inhibitors during pregnancy. Female patients who were pregnant or who intended to become pregnant were excluded from therapeutic trials of all new antidepressants (43). In view of this, tricyclics should be used in preference to other antidepressants in treating depression during pregnancy.

Human teratogenicity studies are reviewed in Table 5.

LACTATION

Antidepressants and Breast Feeding: Clinical Reports

Major depressive episodes occur in approximately 10% of women in the postpartum period, and antidepressants are essential for treatment. Their transfer into breast milk and thereby to the infant through lactation has been difficult to determine because of the limited sensitivity of the analytic methods available.

Past reports of tricyclic antidepressants in breast milk have been negative or inconclusive owing to insensitivity of the assay procedure (63-67). Tranylcypromine was also reported not to be excreted in appreciable quantities in breast milk (64,68), and Knowles (63) reported on 103 nursing mothers who received dextroamphetamine for postpartum depression, and observed no instances in which a baby showed evidence of stimulation or insomnia.

In recent years, more sensitive assays of plasma and milk have been able to detect levels of antidepressants that previously had been missed (Table 6).

Table 6 Antidepressants and Breast Milk

Author (Ref.)	Study	Medication	Maternal plasma level	Milk level	Infant plasma level
Vorherr (76)		Amitriptyline	0.2-1.3 mg/100 mL	0.1 mg/100 mL	Not assayed
Erickson et al. (69)	Assayed milk and serum of nursing mother and her 2-mo-old nursing infant. Mother was taking amitriptyline 150 mg/day for 3 wk.	Amitriptyline	90 ng/mL	Not assayed	0
		Nortriptyline	146 ng/mL	Not assayed	0
Sovner and Orsulak (71)	32-yr-old woman with history of depression who had been treated with imipramine before becoming pregnant, when it was discontinued. It was resumed 1 mo after delivery at 200 mg hs.	Imipramine	21 ng/mL	16.5 ng/mL (average value)	Not assayed
		Desipramine	41 ng/mL	26 ng/mL (average value)	Not assayed
					No behavioral changes in the infant were detected by mother or pediatrician.
Bader and Newman (70)	36-yr-old woman with a history of depression treated with 100 mg amitriptyline during the postpartum period.	Amitriptyline	83 ng/mL	135 ng/mL	0
		Nortriptyline	59 ng/mL	52 ng/mL	0
Kemp et al. (73)	26-yr-old nursing mother treated with 150 mg doxepin starting at 30 days post-	Doxepin	57 $\mu g/L^{-1}$	74.2 $\mu g/L^{-1}$	0
		N-Desmethyldoxepin	98 $\mu g/L^{-1}$	129.3 $\mu g/L^{-1}$	15 $\mu g/L$

	serum and milk were assayed 7-99 days after treatment was begun.				were noted in the infant.
Matheson et al. (74)	36-yr-old nursing mother treated for depression with doxepin at 2 wk postpartum. Dosage was 10 mg/day; increased to 25 mg t.i.d. 4 days before the child became ill.	Doxepin *N*-Desmethyldoxepin	15 μg/L 57 μg/L	18 μg/L 9 μg/L	4 μg/L 58 μg/L 8-wk-old wholly breastfed infant was found one morning very pale, limp, and almost not breathing. Breastfeeding was stopped and the infant returned to normal in 24 hr.
Stancer et al. (72)	35-yr-old nursing mother treated with desipramine, 300 mg hs for depression.	Desipramine	257 ng/mL (on day 7) 271 ng/mL (on day 14)	316 ng/mL (on day 7) 328 ng/mL (on day 14)	Levels insufficient to result in a measurable concentration of desipramine or its metabolite, on both days that the levels were measured.
		2-Hydroxydesipramine	234 ng/mL (on day 7) 253 ng/mL (on day 14)	381 ng/mL (on day 7) 327 ng/mL (on day 14)	
Verbeeck et al. (75)	Six lactating women 3- to 8-mo postpartum were given a single 50-mg dose of trazodone after which plasma and milk were assayed.	Trazodone	1000 ng/mL^{-1}	100 ng/mL^{-1}	

Most of these recent studies show the parent compound as well as metabolites in breast milk. Amitriptyline and its metabolite nortriptyline were found in breast milk (69,70), but none was detected in the infant's serum. In assays for imipramine and desipramine (71) and for desipramine and 2-hydroxy-desipramine (72), concentrations of these drugs in the breast milk have reached levels similar to those in plasma. In Sovner's case report (71), maternal serum levels were below therapeutic, and it is possible that higher concentrations may be found in the serum of women who achieve higher levels and subsequently could affect the child. Doxepin and its metabolite were both found in breast milk and were also the only compounds found in the infant's serum (72,74). In one study (74), the level of *n*-desmethyldoxepin was as high in the infant's serum as in the mother's. The authors attribute this accumulation to the infant's limited hepatic hydroxylation and conjugation with glucuronic acid. Trazodone (75) has also been detected in breast milk, and although its milk/plasma ratio after a single dose was small, it is not known to what extent its metabolite, 1-*m*-chlorophenylpiperazine distributes into the milk and is transferred to the infant.

With the exception of doxepin and its metabolite, other antidepressants have not been detected in infants' serum. Possibly, these medications have a larger volume distribution in the child as compared with that of an adult. Also, an increased first-pass effect in the mother could lower plasma levels to a greater degree than expected.

Biochemistry of Antidepressants and Their Transfer into Milk

One of the primary determinants of a drug's ability to enter breast milk is its pKa. Because the pH of breast milk (6.6-7.0) is more acidic than that of plasma (7.4), basic compounds are often trapped and attain higher levels in milk (76). Most of the tricyclics and trazodone are weak bases and, therefore, are transferred into the milk. The protein-binding characteristics of a drug also influences its distribution into the breast milk, as well as its persistence in the milk. Generally, drug binding to milk protein is less than to that of plasma proteins (76). Imipramine and the other tricyclics have high lipid-solubility and, therefore, a greater likelihood of being transferred into the milk. Molecular size is another factor, in that diffusion of small un-ionized molecules across various lipid membranes will be faster than that of large molecules (76). Both the tricyclics and trazodone exist predominantly in the un-ionized form, another factor that enhances their being found in the milk. Specific transport mechanisms for facilitating drug entry for the antidepressants into human breast milk have not being investigated.

Other factors to be considered include the amount of milk a child consumes, the dose of medication administered to the mother, the proximity in time of drug administration and infant nursing, as well as the metabolism and drug clearance by the mother. The composition of milk also goes through phases, and the ability of a drug to cross from plasma to milk changes. Initially, during postpartum days 1-4, colostrum is secreted, which is alkaline and has a lower fat content than whole milk. The alveolar epithelium represents a lipid barrier with water-filled protein pores (76), which is most permeable for drugs during the colostral phase of milk secretion. This is replaced by transitional milk, which gradually assumes the characteristics of whole milk. The fat content of milk is generally higher in the morning (65) and also with feeding. There is an increased concentration of drug compounds in the milk during the infant feeding (73). This may be related to the high lipid solubility of these compounds and the marked four- to fivefold increase in lipid content of milk that occurs during feeding.

Even small drug doses may have significant effects on infants (77). The infant's enhanced gastrointestinal permeability, as compared with adults, and the immaturity of their drug-metabolizing enzymes, such as the limited hydroxylation and conjugation with glucuronic acid, may enhance drug accumulation.

Nonpuerperal Galactorrhea

Two antidepressants have also caused galactorrhea in nonpuerperal females. There are two case reports (78,79) of clomipramine and one case report of imipramine. Clomipramine is thought to cause galactorrhea and amenorrhea by increasing prolactin levels. The symptoms resolved when the medication was stopped in one case (78) and when it was decreased and bromocriptine added in the other (79). In a third case report (80), galactorrhea was noted in a patient who received imipramine for 6 months. The medication was stopped and lactation subsided, only to recur when it was started again 2 weeks later. The authors hypothesize that imipramine possibly causes the galactorrhea by removing the hypothalimic inhibition of prolactin secretion.

PSYCHIATRIC DISORDERS IN THE POSTPARTUM PERIOD

Historical Background

Since the fourth century B.C., there are recorded episodes of women developing illnesses during the postpartum period. In the third book of the *Epidemics* (81), Hippocrates reports that a woman who gave birth to twins, experienced severe insomnia and restlessness on the sixth day postpartum, became delirious on the 11th day, and then comatose, and died on the 17th day. Esquirol in 1838 (82) discussed 92 cases of postpartum psychiatric illness, noting that postpartum illness could occur in a variety of syndromes, and he suggested several causal factors such as heredity, previous attacks, and traumatic events. Webster, in 1848 (83), studied 131 cases of puerperal mental illness, comprising 12% of the female patients admitted to Bethlem Hospital. Of these, 62% were well within 1 year, compared with the cure rate of 54% for the entire hospital population. Marcé published the only comprehensive book in the world on the subject in 1858 (1). He reported on 310 cases of mental illness associated with childbearing: 9% began during pregnancy, 58% developed during the puerperal period, and 33% developed 6 weeks after delivery. There were no important features that distinguished the psychoses of pregnancy from those occurring in the nonpregnant, nonpuerperal state. Conversely, the postpartum cases had many characteristics that distinguished them from other varieties of mental illness. In the 19th century, some authors denied that pregnancy was a true etiological factor, whereas others concluded that the puerperium was a precipitating, but not the fundamental, cause (84). Strecker and Ebaugh in 1926 (85) surveyed 50 consecutive cases who constituted 3% of all female admissions to three psychiatric facilities: 26% had a diagnosis of dementia praecox, 36% had manic-depressive illness, and 34% had delirium. They concluded that because the postpartum cases could be fitted into standard categories of psychiatric illness, the designation of postpartum psychoses should be discarded from psychiatric terminology. This category was eliminated from the standard nomenclature of diseases. Even today, the event of childbirth is disregarded in classification. Consequently, it is impossible to separate a sample of postpartum cases from psychiatric hospital files without reading every female case history. The three types of disorders occurring during the postpartum period that will be discussed include (1) Adjustment disorder with depressed mood—"maternity blues," (2) major depressive disorder, (3) Psychotic disorder not otherwise specified—atypical psychosis.

Adjustment Disorder with Depressed Mood: Maternity Blues

In a 1952 paper, Haas (86) reported "It is known to every clinician that at about the fifth or sixth day of the lying in period many women get nervous, irritable, depressed and demanding. This mood is somewhat similar to premenstrual tension. What the psychological implications of these manifestations are is unknown. Usually this mood subsides within a few days." According to Yalom (87), the term "milk fever" was first used by Savage in 1875 to describe the dysphoria that appeared to coincide with the onset of lactation. "Maternity blues" is another term used to describe this clinically well-delineated phenomena which occurs in about 50% of women in the postpartum period and seems to be independent of culture, socioeconomic (6, 88), and marital status (6). The symptoms, which are transient, self-limiting, lasting only a few days, and are limited to the first 2 weeks after childbirth, include tearfulness, mild depression and anxiety, lability of mood, fatigue, irritability, and insomnia. The most characteristic symptom is crying, which is sporadic, brief, and without precipitating factors. Often, it is not even congruent with the patient's mood. Mothers are also often easily distractible and have difficulty concentrating. However, psychological tests have produced no evidence of cognitive impairment (87). These symptoms usually resolve spontaneously without any long-term complications. Although they do not present serious problems in clinical practice, they may be important in our further understanding of affective disorders.

There seem to be consistant high rates of this self-limited disorder in most of the studies. High scores in a depression scale in late pregnancy were associated with more severe blues (6), and a sense of pessimism in late pregnancy was a predictor for postpartum blues by Condon (90). High ratings in severity of the blues were correlated with depression by several investigators (3, 91,92).

Most of the endocrine studies during the puerperium have been performed in women suffering from the blues, rather than from major depression or psychoses. Kennerly (93) reports that the high frequency and regular timing of the blues suggest an association with changes in the maternal hormones at childbirth: maternal levels of estrogen and progesterone increase during late pregnancy and fall precipitously after childbirth. Pitt (6) hypothesized that this precipitous drop may be the causative factor in the mood changes he observed in the postpartum period. Large changes also occur in the blood levels of adrenal steroids, and serum prolacin levels fall immediately following birth.

In conclusion, attempts to correlate postpartum blues with depression occurring at other times during a woman's life have yielded conflicting results. Some authors report an association (88,94), whereas others find no correlation (6,87,93,95,96).

Some of the studies correlate postpartum blues with antenatal depressive symptoms that occur during the latter part of gestation (89,90,95,96).

Blues and Subsequent Affective Disorders

Handley (95) found depressed mood in the first 5 postpartum days associated with an increased risk of depressed mood at 6 months. Kendell (3) showed that high ratings for depression and lability were correlated with occurrence of clinical depression at 3 weeks postpartum. Once delivery occurs, it is necessary to distinguish the mothers for whom the blues are transitory, from those who are at risk of developing postnatal depression or psychoses. Mothers with severe blues, with a history of psychiatric problems or a family history of psychiatric illness should be monitored closely.

Major Depression

When the symptoms of the maternity "blues" persist beyond the second postnatal week, a diagnosis of major depression is made. Approximately 10% of postpartum women develop a major depression.

Tod (5) reported an increased rate of depression that he associated with a previous inadequate personality, previous psychiatric history, and abnormal obstetrical history. Nilsson (7) found a 19% rate of disturbance in the puerperium, and Kendell (3) cites a dramatic increase in psychiatric admissions during the first 3 months postpartum. A depressive illness was the most common illness identified. First pregnancy, unmarried status, cesarian section, all were associated with the increased risk.

Cox (97), in a prospective study, interviewed 103 women at their first antenatal visit and followed them until their third to fifth postpartum month; 13% had a marked and disabling illness at this time. These mothers had been depressed continuously since delivery; 16% had milder depression that lasted for 6 weeks before resolving.

Pugh (2) calculated an increased rate in admissions during the first 6 weeks of the puerperium and found this to be significant only for bipolar illness. In an 8- to 9-year follow-up of 82 women with bipolar disorder, Bratfos (98) found almost a 40% postpartum disturbance. Reich (99) compared postpartum illness in 20 bipolar women and compared them with family members. He found the rate (40%) of postpartum relapses to be significantly higher than the frequency of nonpuerperal episodes.

Welner (100) suggests that, in most studies, the patient and childbirth-related illness have not been studied as a homogeneous group. He believes that there is a difference between a non-childbirth-related illness that occurs in the postpartum period and a postpartum illness that occurs in a patient with a positive history of psychiatric illness.

With more accurate classifications of psychiatric disorders and more prospective studies, a better understanding of these disorders will be obtained.

Puerperal Psychosis

Unlike depression, which may go unrecognized, puerperal psychosis is quickly identified. The rate can be 2:1000 live births (97) and usually occurs within the first 6 weeks of the postpartum period, with the highest prevalence between days 3 and 14 (101). The psychotic symptoms can be manifestations of a brief reactive psychosis, a major depression or mania, or schizophrenia. If delirium is present, infection, central nervous system trauma, and other medical causes must be investigated.

Prodromal symptoms include sleep disturbances, restlessness, fatigue, depression, irritability, headache, and emotional lability (102). If the psychotic symptoms are components of a major depression, the patient is often tearful, preoccupied with guilt and feelings of worthlessness, and has psychomotor retardation and sleep disturbances. In a postpartum mania, the patient may be euphoric, noisy, needing very little sleep, and is often loud, critical, and labile. Delusions and hallucinations, which can be components of a major depression or mania, can also be characteristic symptoms of schizophrenia.

Unusual behavior that is out of keeping with the mother's usual personality should alert the clinician. Suspiciousness, inappropriate interaction with the baby or with staff, responses to internal stimuli, delusions, or hallucinations are signs indicating a psychosis. Suicidal risk can be high if thoughts of suicide are present and if the mother expresses beliefs that she deserves to be punished or that others, including the baby, would be happier without her. Infant suicidal thoughts may also be present and close supervision of the mother and child is essential.

Further puerperal psychotic illness following a subsequent pregnancy can be as high as one in five (97), and the risk is particularly great if there is a family history of a psychiatric disorder and previous puerperal psychoses.

In bipolar patients the frequency of postpartum relapses was reported to be significantly greater than the frequency of nonpuerperal episodes during the childbearing years (99), although there were no recurrences of mania outside the postpartum period in a group of 21 patients who had been admitted for mania during the postpartum period (103). However, one patient in the postpartum group was readmitted for an affective illness during the 3-year follow-up that occurred during a subsequent postpartum period.

CONCLUSIONS

The studies reviewed indicate that women are more susceptible to minor psychiatric symptoms during pregnancy and in the puerperium than at other times. Major disorders appear to peak right after delivery and all patients should be informed about the possibility of dysphoria after delivery. It is important to distinguish those mothers for whom the blues are transitory from those at risk for developing a depression or psychosis. Those with severe blues and a history of psychiatric problems or a family history of psychiatric illness should be monitored closely.

If a major depression occurs, antidepressants should be used, but if a mother is breastfeeding, remember that tricyclics and trazodone are weak bases, with high lipid solubility, and they exist predominantly in the unionized form, factors that are all responsible for their transfer into breast milk. Doxepin and its metabolite were the only tricyclics found in the infant's serum in high concentrations, suggesting that the infant's metabolizing capabilities are immature, and this drug should be avoided.

Trazodone has been found in breast milk, but little is known about its metabolite; therefore, it also should not be used. Nortriptyline should not be used in slow metabolizers, for it will accumulate in the infant's system. Tricyclics such as imipramine and its metabolite have also been found in breast milk, but have not been reported to cause behavioral changes in the few studies cited. These agents should be used in preference to monoamine oxidase inhibitors and other classes of antidepressants because of the lack of any data on these other drugs.

Animal studies of prenatal exposure to antidepressants show definite teratogenic risks. There are several case reports of human teratogenicity that have not been validated by controlled studies. Nonetheless, women of childbearing age for whom antidepressants are indicated should be advised to avoid becoming pregnant. However, if a major psychiatric disorder does occur during pregnancy, medication needs to be considered, and the potential teratogenic risk must be weighed against the consequences of withholding treatment.

With increased attention paid to behavioral teratogenicity and receptor studies, more sensitive indicators will be available. Human behavioral studies are needed, as well as increased research on the mechanism of drug action and computerized registers to help in clarifying the safety of these drugs during pregnancy and in the postpartum period.

REFERENCES

1. Marcé, L. V. (1958). Traité de la folie des femmes enceintes, des nouvelles accouchées et des nourrices. Paris, J.B. Bailliére et fils. Quoted in Hamilton, J. A. (1982). *Postpartum Psychiatric Problems.* St. Louis, C.V. Mosby, pp. 13-27.
2. Pugh, T. F., Jerath, B. K., Schmidt, W. M., and Reed, R. B. (1963). Rates of mental diseases related to childbearing. *N. Engl. J. Med. 268*:1224-1228.
3. Kendell, R. E., Wainwright, S., Hailey, A., and Shannon, B. (1976). The influence of childbirth on psychiatric morbidity. *Psychol. Med. 6*:297-302.
4. Paffenbarger, R. S. and McCabe, L. J. (1966). The effect of obstetric and perinatal events on risk of mental illness in women of childbearing age. *Am. J. Public Health 56*:400-407.
5. Tod, E. D. M. (1964). Puerperal depression: A prospective epidemiological study. *Lancet 2*:1264-1266.
6. Pitt, B. (1973). Maternity blues. *Br. J. Psychiatry 122*:431-435.
7. Nilsson, A. and Almgren, P. E. (1970). Parinatal emotional adjustment: A prospective investigation of 165 women. *Acta Psychiatr. Scand. Suppl. 220*:62-141.
8. Dalton, K. (1971). Prospective study into puerperal depression. *Br. J. Psychiatry 118*:689-692.
9. Kumar, R. and Robson, K. (1978). Neurotic disturbance during pregnancy and the puerperium: Preliminary report of a prospective survey of 119 primiparae. In *Mental Illness in Pregnancy and the Puerperium.* Edited by M. Sandler. New York, Oxford University Press, pp. 40-51.

10. Cox, J. L. (1979). Psychiatric morbidity and pregnancy: A controlled study of 263 semi-rural Ugandan women. *Br. J. Psychiatry 134*:401-405.
11. Gupta, M. A., Gupta, A. K., and Ellis, C. N. (198x). Antidepressant drugs in dermatology. *Arch. Dermatol. 123*:647-652.
12. Krauer, B., Krauer, F., and Hytten, F. E. (1980). Drug disposition and pharmacokinetics in the maternal-placental-fetal-unit. *Pharmacol. Ther. 10*:301-328. 328.
13. Reboud, P., Groulade, J., and Groslambert, P. (1963). The influence of normal pregnancy and the postpartum state on plasma proteins and lipids. *Am. J. Obstet. Gynecol. 86*:820-828.
14. Rowland, M. and Tozer, T. N. (1980). *Clinical Pharmacokinetics: Concepts and Applications.* Philadelphia, Lea & Febiger.
15. Crawford, J. S. and Rudolfsky, S. (1966). Some alterations in the pattern of drug metabolism associated with pregnancy, oral contraceptives and the newlyborn. *Br. J. Anaesthesiol. 38*:446-454.
16. Davison, J. M. (1980). The urinary system. In *Clinical Physiology in Obstetrics.* Edited by F. Hytten and G. Chamberlain. Oxford, Blackwell Scientific Publications, pp. 289-327.
17. Davison, J. S., Davison, M. C., and Hay, D. M. (1970). Gastric emptying time in late pregnancy and labour. *J. Obstet. Gynaecol. 77*:37-41.
18. Kerns, L. L. (1986). Treatment of mental disorders in pregnancy. A review of psychotropic drug risks and benefits. *J. Nerv. Ment. Dis. 174*:652-659.
19. Wood, S. M. and Hytten, F. E. (1981). The fate of drugs in pregnancy. *Clin. Obstet. Gynecol. 8*:255-259.
20. Rayburn, W. F. and Andresen, B. D. (1982). Principles of perinatal pharmacology. In *Drug Therapy in Obstetrics and Gynecology.* Edited by W. F. Rayburn and F. Zuspan. Norwalk, Conn., Appleton-Century-Crofts.
21. Douglas, B. H. and Hume, A. S. (1967). Placental transfer of imipramine, a basic, lipid-soluble drug. *Am. J. Obstet. Gynecol. 99*:573-575.
22. Hume, A. and Douglas, B. H. (1968). Placental transfer of desmethylimipramine. *Am. J. Obstet. Gynecol. 101*:915-917.
23. Van Petten, G. R. (1975). Fetal cardiovascular effects of maternally administered tricyclic antidepressants. In *Basic and Therapeutic Aspects of Perinatal Pharmacology.* Edited by P. L. Morselli, S. Garattini, and F. Sereni. New York, Raven Press, pp. 83-88.
24. Shearer, W. T., Schreiner, R. L., and Marshall, R. E. (1972). Urinary retention in a neonate secondary to maternal ingestion of nortriptyline. *J. Pediatr. 81*: 570-572.
25. Webster, P. A. C. (1973). Withdrawal symptoms in neonates associated with maternal antidepressant therapy. *Lancet 2*:318-319.
26. Eggermont, E., Raveschot, J., Deneve, V., and Casteels-Van Daele, M. (1972). The adverse influence of imipramine on the adaptation of the newborn infant to extrauterine life. *Acta Paediatr. Belg. 26*:197-204.
27. Sjöqvist, F., Bergfors, P. G., Borgå, O., Lind, M., and Ygge, H. (1971). Plasma disappearance of nortriptyline in a newborn infant following placental transfer from an intoxicated mother: Evidence for drug metabolism. *J. Pediatr. 80*:496-500.

28. Pelkonen, O., Korhonen, P., Jouppila, P., Kärki, N. Placental transfer and fetal metabolism of drugs. In: *Basic and therapeutic aspects of perinatal pharmacology*. (Eds). P. L. Marselli, S. Garattini, F. Sereni, Raven Press, New York, 1975. 65-74.
29. Yaffe, S. J., Rane, A., Sjöqvist, F., Boréus, L.-O., and Orrenius, S. (1970). The presence of a monooxygenase system in human fetal liver microsomes. *Life Sci. 9*:1189-1200.
30. *Physician's Desk Reference* (1988). Oradell, N. J., Medical Economics.
31. Larsen, V. (1963). The teratogenic effects of thalidomide, imipramine HCl and imipramine-*N*-oxide HCl on white Danish rabbits. *Acta Pharmacol. Toxicol. 20*:186-200.
32. Delahunt, C. S., and Lassen, L. J. (1964). Thalidomide syndrome in monkeys. *Science 146*:1300-1305.
33. Guram, M. S., Gill, T. S., and Geber, W. F. (1980). Teratogenicity of imipramine and amitriptyline in fetal hamsters. *Res. Commun. Psychol. Psychiatry Behav. 5*:275-282.
34. Robson, J. M., and Sullivan, F. M. (1963). The production of foetal abnormalities in rabbits by imipramine. *Lancet 1*:638-639.
35. Harper, K. H., Palmer, A. K., and Davies, R. E. (1965). Effect of imipramine upon pregnancy of laboratory animals. *Arzneimittelforsch 15*:1218. [Quoted in Tuchmann-Duplessis, H. (1984) Drugs and other xenobiotics as teratogens. *Pharmacol. Ther. 26*:273-344.]
36. Aeppli, L. (1969). Teratologische Studien mit Imipramin auf Ratte und Kaninchen. Ein Beitrag sur Planung und Interpretation teratologischer unter Suchungen unter Berucksichtigung von Biochemie and Toxikologie der Prufsubstanz. *Arzneimittelforsch 19*:1617-1640. [Quoted in Fiori, M. (1977). Tricyclic antidepressants: A review of their toxicology. In: *Current Developments in Psychopharmacology,* Vol. 4. Edited by B. E. Walter and L. Valzelli. New York, Spectrum Publications.]
37. Simpkins, J. W., Field, F. P., Torosian, G., and Soltis, E. E. (1985). Effects of prenatal exposure to tricyclic antidepressants on adrenergic responses in progeny. *Dev. Pharmacol. Ther. 8*:17-33.
38. Ali, S. F., Buelke-Sam, J., Newport, G., Slikker, W., Jr., and Harmon, J. R. (1985). Neurochemical alterations in rats prenatally exposed to imipramine. *Teratology 31*:11B.
39. Gilani, S. H. (1975). The effect of imipramine on the development of the chick embryo. *Teratology 11*:8A.
40. Jelinek, V., Zikmund, E., and Reichlova, R. (1967). L'influence de quelques medicaments psychotropes sur le développement du foetus chez le rat. *Thérapie 22*:1429-1433. [Quoted in Tuchmann-Duplessis, H. (1984). Drugs and other xenobiotics as teratogens. *Pharmacol. Ther. 26*:273-344.]
41. Oberholzer, R. J. H. (1964). Contribution a' l'étude d'une action tératogene éventuelle de l'imipramine. *Med. Hyg. 22*:557. [Quoted in Tuchmann-Duplessis, H. (1984). Drugs and other xenobiotics as teratogens. *Pharmacol Ther. 26*:273-344.]

42. Hendrickx, A. G. (1975). Teratologic evaluation of imipramine hydrochloride in bonnet (*Macaca radiata*), and rhesus monkeys (*Macaca mulatta*). *Teratology 11*:219-222.
43. Preskorn, S. H., and Othmer, S. C. (1984). Evaluation of bupropion hydrochloride. The first of a new class of atypical antidepressants. *Pharmacotherapy 4*:20-34.
44. Poulson, E., and Robson, J. M. (1964). Effect of phenelzine and some related compounds on pregnancy and on sexual development. *J. Endocrinol. 30*:205-215.
45. Coyle, I. R., and Singer, G. (1975). Changes in developing behavior following prenatal administration of imipramine. *Pharmacol. Biochem. Behav. 3*:799-807.
46. Coyle, I. R., Wayner, M. J., and Singer, G. (1976). Behavioral teratogenesis: A critical evaluation. *Pharmacol. Biochem. Behav. 4*:191-200.
47. Echandia, E., and Broitman, S. (1983). Effect of prenatal and post-natal exposure to therapeutic doses of chlorimipramine on emotionality in the rat. *Psychopharmacology 79*:236-241.
48. Dorner, G. (1975). Further evidence of permanent behavioral changes in rats treated neonatally with neurodrugs. Endokrinologie 68:345-348.
49. Jason, K. M., Cooper, T. B., and Friedman, E. (1981). Prenatal exposure to imipramine alters early behavioral development and beta adrenergic receptors in rats. *J. Pharmacol. Exp. Ther. 217*:461-466.
50. DeCeballos, M. L., Benedi, A., DeFelippe, C., and Del Rio, J. (1985). Prenatal exposure of rats to antidepressants enhances agonist affinity of brain dopamine receptors and dopamine-mediated behavior. *Eur. J. Pharmacol. 116*:257-262.
51. DeCeballos, M. L., Benedi, A., Urdin, C., and Del Rio, J. (1985). Prenatal exposure of rats to antidepressant drugs down regulates beta-adrenoceptors and 5HT2 receptors in cerebral cortex. *Neuropharmacology 24*:947-952.
52. Golden, S., and Perman, K. (1980). Bilateral clinical anophthalmia: Drugs as potential factors. *South. Med. J. 73*:1404-1407.
53. Freeman, R. (1972). Limb deformities: Possible association with drugs [Letter]. *Med. J. Aust. 1*:606-607.
54. Abramovici, A., Abramovici, I., Kalman, G., and Liban, E. (1981). Teratogenic effect of chlorimipramine in a young human embryo. *Teratology 24*:42A.
55. McBride, W. G. (1972). Limb deformities associated with iminodibenzyl hydrochloride [Letter]. *Med. J. Aust. 1*:492.
56. Wilson, J. G. (1972). Present status of drugs as teratogens in man. *Teratology 7*:3-16.
57. Rachelefsky, G. S., Flynt, J. W., Ebbin, A. J., and Wilson, M. G. (1972). Possible teratogenicity of tricyclic antidepressants [Letter]. *Lancet 1*:838-839.
58. Crombie, D. L., Pinsent, R. J., and Fleming, D. (1972). Imipramine in pregnancy [Letter]. *Br. Med. J. 1*:745.
59. Australian Drug Evaluation Committee (1973). Tricyclic antidepressants and limb reduction deformities. *Med. J. Aust. 1*:768-769.
60. Banister, P., Dafoe, C., Smith, E., and Miller, J. (1972). Possible teratogenicity of tricyclic antidepressants [Letter]. *Lancet 1*:838-839.

61. Kuenssberg, E. V., and Knox, J. D. (1972). Imipramine in pregnancy [Letter]. *Br. Med. J. 2*:292.
62. Idanpaan-Heikkila, J., and Saxen, L. (1973). Possible teratogenicity of imipramine/chloropyramine. *Lancet 2*:282-284.
63. Knowles, J. A. (1965). Excretion of drugs in milk—a review. *J. Pediatr. 66*:1068-1082.
64. Takyi, B. E. (1970). Excretion of drugs in human milk. *Am. J. Hosp. Pharm. 28*:317-326.
65. O'Brien, T. (1974). Excretion of drugs in human milk. *Am. J. Hosp. Pharm. 31*:844-854.
66. Ayd, F. J., Jr. (1973). Excretion of psychotropic drugs in human breast milk. *Int. Drug Ther. Newslett. 8*:33-40.
67. Eschenoff, E., and Reider, J. Quoted as Bader, T. E. and Newman, K. (1980). Amitriptyline in human breast milk and the nursing infant's serum. *Am. J. Psychiatry 137*:855-856.
68. Matrangan, A. Quoted in O'Brien T. E. (1974). Excretion of drugs in human milk. *Am. J. Hosp. Pharm. 31*:844-854.
69. Erickson, S. H., Smith, G. H., and Heidrich, F. (1979). Tricyclics and breast feeding. *Am. J. Psychiatry 136*:1483.
70. Bader, T. F., and Newman, K. (1980). Amitriptyline in human breast milk and the nursing infant's serum. *Am. J. Psychiatry 137*:855-856.
71. Sovner, R., and Orsulak, P. (1979). Excretion of imipramine and desipramine in human breast milk. *Am. J. Psychiatry 136*:451-452.
72. Stancer, H. C., and Reed, K. L. (1986). Desipramine and 2-hydroxydesipramine in human breast milk and the nursing infant's serum. *Am. J. Psychiatry 143*: 1597-1600.
73. Kemp, J. Ilett, K. F., Booth, J., and Hackett, L. P. (1985). Excretion of doxepin and *N*-desmethyldoxepin in human milk. *Br. J. Clin. Pharmacol. 20*:497-499.
74. Matheson, I., Pande, H., and Alertsen, A. R. (1985). Respiratory depression caused by *N*-desmethyldoxepin in breast milk. *Lancet 2*:1124.
75. Verbeeck, R. R., Ross, S. G., and McKenna, E. A. (1986). Excretion of trazodone in breast milk. *Br. J. Clin. Pharmacol. 22*:367-370.
76. Vorherr, H. (1974). Drug excretion in breast milk. *Postgrad. Med. 56*(4):97-104.
77. Rivera-Calimlim, L. (1977). Drugs in breast milk. *Drug. Ther. Hosp. 2*:20-22.
78. Fowlie, S., and Burton, J. (1987). Hyperprolactinaemia and nonpuerperal lactation associated with clomipramine. *Scot. Med. J. 32*:52.
79. Anand, V. S. (1985). Clomipramine induced galactorrhoea and amenorrhoea. *Br. J. Psychiatry 147*:87-88.
80. Klein, J. J., Segal, R. L., and Warner, R. P. (1964). Galactorrhoea due to imipramine *N. Engl. J. Med. 271*:510-512.
81. Jones, W. H. (1923). Hippocrates with an English translation, Vol. 1. London, William Heinemann Vol. 1. [Quoted in Hamilton, J. A. (1962). *Postpartum Psychiatric Problems.* St. Louis, C. V. Mosby, p. 126]
82. Esquirol, J. E. D. (1838). Des maladies mentales considérées sous les rapports medical, hygiénique et médico-légal. Paris, J. B. Bailliére. [Quoted in Hamilton, J. A. (1962). *Postpartum Psychiatric Problems.* St. Louis, C. V. Mosby, p. 126.]

83. Webster, J. (1848). Remarks on statistics, pathology and treatment of puerperal insanity. *Lancet 2*:611-612.
84. Tetlow, C. (1955). Psychoses of childbearing. *J. Ment. Sci. 101*:629-639.
85. Strecker, E. A., and Ebaugh, F. G. (1926). Psychoses occurring during the puerperium. *Arch. Neurol. Psychiatry 15*:239-252.
86. Haas, S. (1952). Psychiatric implications in gynecology and obstetrics. In *Psychology of Physical Illness*. Edited by L. Bellack. London, Churchill.
87. Yalom, I. D., Lunde, D. T., Moos, R. H., and Hamburg, D. A. (1968). Postpartum blues syndrome. *Arch. Gen. Psychiatry 18*:16-27.
88. Stein, G. S. (1980). The pattern of mental and body weight change in the first post-partum week. *J. Psychosom. Res. 24*:165-171.
89. Davidson, J. R. T. (1972). Postpartum mood changes in Jamaican women: A description and discussion on its significance. *Br. J. Psychiatry 121*:659-663.
90. Condon, J. T., and Watson, T. L. (1987). The maternity blues: Exploration of a psychological hypothesis. *Acta Psychiatr. Scand. 76*:164-171.
91. Melges, F. T. (1968). Postpartum psychiatric syndromes. *Psychosom. Med. 30*:95-108.
92. Cox., J. L., Connor, Y., and Kendell, R. E. (1982). Prospective study of the psychiatric disorders of childbirth. *Br. J. Psychiatry 140*:111-117.
93. Kennerley, H., and Gath, D. (1968). Maternity blues reassessed. *Psychiatr. Dev. 1*:1-17.
94. Ballinger, C. B., Buckley, D. E., Naylor, G. J., and Stansfield, D. A. (1979). Emotional disturbances following childbirth: Clinical findings and urinary excretion of cyclic AMP. *Psychol. Med. 9*:293-300.
95. Handley, S. L., Dunn, T. L., Waldron, G., and Baker, J. M. (1980). Tryptophan, cortisol and puerperal mood. *Br. J. Psychiatry 136*:498-508.
96. Harris, B. (1980). Prospecitve trial of L-tryptophan in maternity blues. *Br. J. Psychiatry 137*:223-235.
97. Cox, J. L. (1986). *Postnatal Depression, A Guide for Health Professionals.* Edinburgh, Churchill Livingstone.
98. Bratfos, O., and Haug, J. O. (1966). Puerperal mental disorders in manic-depressive females. *Acta Psychiatr. Scand. 42*:285-294.
99. Reich, T. and Winokur, G. (1970). Postpartum psychoses in patients with manic depressive disease. *J. Nerv. Ment. Dis. 151*:60-69.
100. Welner, A. (1982). Childbirth-related psychiatric illness. *Compr. Psychiatry 23*:143-154.
101. Inwood, D. G., ed. (1985). *Postpartum Psychiatric Disorders.* Washington, D. C., American Psychiatric Press.
102. Robinson, G. E., and Stewart, D. E. (1985). Postpartum psychiatric disorders. *Can. Med. Assoc. J. 134*:31-37.
103. Kadrmras, A., Winokur, G., and Crowe, R. (1979). Postpartum mania. *Br. J. Psychiatry 135*:551-554.

20

Systematic Approaches to Treatment-Resistant Depressions

ROBERT H. GERNER

University of California, Los Angeles, West Los Angeles VA Medical Center, and Center for Mood Disorders, Los Angeles, California

NICHOLAS ROSENLICHT

University of California, Davis, VA Medical Center, Martinez, and Center for Mood Disorders, Los Angeles, California

It has been universally accepted that depression is one of the "treatable" psychiatric disorders. This expectation postdates the dominance of psychopharmacologic intervention, before which time depressions typically were expected to endure for many months or years. Thus, our present definition of "treatment resistance" has become modified by the profound impact of antidepressant medications. Furthermore, although we now have the tool of a very specific diagnostic nosology, we must acknowledge that some syndromes are not well described by the DSM-III-R (1) and have not been the topic of extensive clinical studies. In other words, we do not have in-depth knowledge of depressions that do not correspond to the criteria of major depression (unipolar and bipolar) as described by DSM-III-R. Minor depressions, dysthymia, atypical depressions, and secondary depressions also have not been well characterized. Yet, such patients do exist and require consideration and treatment. Although their depression is called "minor," many of these patients suffer marked dysfunction and develop a chronic depressive course that may be as devastating as that of major depression (2).

Most published studies of antidepressant efficacy show a consistent rate of response between 60 and 70%. Although these studies are generally very

---

The views in this chapter do not necessarily reflect the official view of the Veterans Administration.

well designed, there are several aspects of their methodology that limit the extrapolation of their findings to the general population of patients in need of treatment. For example, such patients usually have unipolar depression, and often have no major medical problems, nor require additional psychotropic medication. Furthermore, the doses of antidepressant medication are well-defined and improvement is determined by rating scales, which may not be adequate to characterize a lack of subjective improvement in many patients (i.e., the physical symptoms improve but the patient continues to express dysphoria to a mild degree). Finally, in research patients, the depression must be moderate to severe and have endured for at least 4 weeks before entrance into the study, whereas the duration of treatment outcome assessment usually ranges from only 4 to 6 weeks in most studies. Therefore, these studies often give us limited guidance for treating patients with atypical depressions, those who may have a medical disorder requiring altered doses of antidepressants, or patients that require prolonged treatment for chronic affective illness.

The concept of treatment resistance for a psychiatric illness is speculative. Such a hypothesis implies that we can make a specific diagnosis and have specific knowledge of a standard treatment and outcome.

FACTORS ASSOCIATED WITH TREATMENT RESISTANCE

Before we conclude that any pharmacologic or psychotherapeutic treatment is not effective we must assess whether or not progress is being impeded by other factors: most commonly iatrogenic (medication) or concomitant medical disorders. Table 1 shows the most common factors associated with resistant

Table 1 Common Depressogenic Factors

Disorders
Hypothyroidism
Hypercalcemia (secondary to hyperparathyroidism)
Premenstrual syndrome (late luteal phase disorder)
Chronic fatigue syndrome
Medications
Reserpine
Clonidine
Methyldopa (Aldomet)
All nonsteroidal anti-inflammatory drugs (NSAIDs)
Birth control pills
β-blockers (with the probable exception of atenolol)
Danazole (Danocrine)
Some antibiotics

depression. This is not an exhaustive list, however, and other factors associated with treatment-resistance can be found in chapters 9, 11, and 13.

Endocrine

When considering treatment-resistant depressions, it is requisite to obtain a full battery of thyroid function tests including thyroxine (T_4), triiodothyronine (T_3)-uptake, and thyrotropin (TSH) (3). Thyrotropin is elevated when the brain perceives a deficiency in circulating thyroid hormone. Normally, individuals have very low TSH levels in the range 0-7 μU/mL, depending upon the type of assay used. However, in depressed patients we believe that TSH levels should be optimal (i.e., less than 2 μU/mL). There is considerable evidence that mild, subclinical thyroid dysfunction may be associated with depression or reduced responsiveness to antidepressant medications, especially in women. Recently, Reus (4) observed that some patients have a low rate of conversion of T_4 to T_3 (which is the most active form of thyroid hormone) and produce increased reverse T_3 (rT_3) which is an inactive hormone, "hidden" in the usual T_3 assay. Thus, rT_3 measurements may be indicated for some patients in whom subtle thyroid dysfunction is suspected.

We treat patients in whom we suspect a subclinical hypothyroid state with levothyroxine (Synthyroid) (although T_3 can be used for more rapid effect, as described later) and measure TSH levels at 4 to 6-week intervals until it is less than 2 μU/mL. Thereafter, we monitor T_4 and T_3 at regular intervals to ensure they do not become abnormally elevated. This is a separate intervention from the use of thyroid hormone to augment the response of other antidepressants.

In a similar fashion, all patients with "high-normal" serum calcium concentrations should be evaluated for subclinical hyperparathyroidism by obtaining a serum parathormone level. The incidence of psychiatric symptoms associated with hypercalcemia is high and ranges from 30% at "borderline" elevations to virtually every patient at levels exceeding 16 mEq% (5). Consultation with an endocrinologist would also be indicated.

Premenstrual syndrome (late luteal dysphoria) may start as early as midphase of the menstrual cycle, although it is more commonly reported in the week before menses. It can best be identified by the marked normalization of affect following the onset of menses. However, many females report an exacerbation of a more chronic depression premenstrually and this should be approached in the context of treating a more chronic endogenous depression that is worsened by the presence of premenstrual syndrome.

Infection

The chronic fatigue syndrome (6) is likely to be a sequela of a prior viral infection (e.g., Epstein-Barr virus) and may present with symptoms similar to endogenous depression. Although the diagnosis and treatment of this syndrome is complicated and controversial, it is important to include in the differential diagnosis of major depression.

Iatrogenic

Nonsteroidal anti-inflammatory drugs may also cause or exacerbate a depressive syndrome in a dose-dependent manner. Reducing the dose or substituting aspirin or acetominophen may be of benefit.

Danocrine is an antiestrogen commonly used to treat endometriosis. The antiestrogen effect can produce marked mood changes, in addition to somatic masculinization.

We have also observed that some antibiotics may produce or exacerbate depression; however, because they are usually given for a relatively brief period, this is a relatively unimportant factor when considering changing treatment. We suggest waiting until the course of antibiotics is completed before changing the antidepressant medication in a treatment-resistant depressed patient.

Antihypertensive agents, such as clonidine, α-methyldopa, reserpine, and β-blockers, all functionally reduce norepinephrine turnover and should be substituted with other antihypertensive agent(s). We have rarely seen an instance for which hypertension could not be adequately controlled with other agents.

Treatment Adequacy

Once these factors have been considered as a potential cause of treatment resistance, the next area of concern is the adequacy of treatment. It has been accepted practice to initiate treatment with a heterocyclic antidepressant or related compound. Lack of adequate treatment at the onset of depression is linked with the risk of persistent illness (7). Yet several studies have confirmed the troubling fact that many depressed patients are undertreated (8,9). For example, Keller et al. (10) evaluated the treatment of 217 depressed outpatients and found that only 34% had received at least 4 weeks of consecutive antidepressants. Only 12% were treated with 150-mg equivalents of imipramine, and only 14% of those with protracted depression had ever received at least 150-mg equivalents of imipramine. Kocsis (11) reported that 59% of an outpatient sample responded to "high" doses (300 mg daily) of imipramine, compared with 13% of those taking placebo, despite many patients having chronic depression.

Many psychodynamically oriented clinicians may be reluctant to aggressively pursue pharmacologic intervention for depressive illness and, in essence, collude with the patient's symptom of hopelessness. Ayd (8) reported that 66% of a "treatment-resistant" patient group had complete recovery after appropriate treatment with antidepressants or electroconvulsive therapy (ECT), and only 10% remained treatment-refractory.

The use of oral dosage as the criterion for adequate drug therapy has now been complemented by the use of antidepressant blood level monitoring. This has intrinsic appeal for clinical and research purposes because oral dosage is only partly correlated with blood levels, whereas blood levels are highly related to brain tissue drug levels (12). Furthermore, some of the antidepressants are metabolized into "active metabolites" that may affect different neurotransmitters than the parent compound and possess a different side effect profile. For example, amitriptyline is demethylated into nortriptyline, imipramine into desipramine, and doxepin into desmethyldoxepin. Blood levels of both compounds are usually reported, and the sum of both used for clinical monitoring. By convention, blood levels are usually obtained 10-14 hr after the last dose and after the patient has achieved a steady-state blood level (i.e., after a constant daily dose has been maintained for approximately 1 week). Systematic studies of blood levels are available for amitriptyline, imipramine, nortriptyline, and desipramine, although plasma level ranges for other agents are less reliable. Even for the four tricyclic drugs, data on correlation between drug level and clinical response are controversial (12,13).

Although the range of "therapeutic levels" may differ among laboratories, two clinically relevant issues are always present. Because drug toxicity is often related to blood level and not to dosage, the clinician may increase the medication dosage for patients with "low levels." Furthermore, if blood levels are used to monitor treatment outcome, then one may also appropriately increase the dosage if serum drug levels are in the low range. In general, patients with blood levels above 400 ng% may be nearing the cardiotoxic range and may benefit from a reduction in dosage. This bracketing or "window" of blood levels may be especially important for medically ill or older patients who can experience increased drug toxicity. The metabolism of antidepressants in these patients is often prolonged and can result in elevation of steady-state blood levels at relatively low doses (14). Patients who fail to respond at higher therapeutic drug levels are, in our opinion, unlikely to benefit from a further increase in dosage or blood level.

It is also important to consider the quality of the drug being used, and several investigators have reported depressive relapse when the patient was switched from a proprietary brand to a generic preparation (15). We have also observed numerous cases of this phenomenon. Currently, the Food and Drug Administration (FDA) requires only 20% bioavailability of generic compounds, compared with standard drugs, and generic preparations do not go through the extensive clinical trials that are required for proprietary brands (16).

Once appropriate blood levels and doses have been achieved, treatment should be continued for at least 2 weeks, without any symptomatic sign of improvement, before concluding that the treatment may be ineffective (17). The patient is not usually a reliable rater of initial improvement, because change in depressive cognition often lags behind improvement in somatic symptoms by several weeks.

Side Effects

Both clinicians and patients may be reluctant to achieve doses that would be likely to be therapeutic because of concern for side effects. Indeed, a substantial minority of carefully selected patients in antidepressant studies drop out of treatment because of side effects. Although those receiving placebo also complain of "side effects," in a clinical setting this factor becomes academic because the treatment emergent symptoms must be addressed regardless of the etiology. We, and others, have developed several strategies for dealing with the major side effects that might interfere with compliance (18, 19). Those outlined in Table 2 do not include true "toxic" reactions, which can occur with excessive dosage and/or blood levels.

Many patients become acclimated to these side effects and may require dosage adjustment only initially to improve compliance. Informing patients that dosage adjustment or counteractive medications are available will assuage their concerns enough for them to tolerate continued treatment. For example, sympathomimetic side effects can be quite troubling, and symptoms such as tremors, tachycardia, and palpitations may respond to adjunctive β-blockers. We have given atenolol (25-50 mg b.i.d. or t.i.d.) because this drug has a

Table 2 Common Treatable Antidepressant Side Effects

Anticholinergic
Dry mouth
Blurred vision
Constipation
Urinary hesitancy or retention
Sympathomimeticlike
Tremors
Palpitations or tachycardia
Diaphoresis
Insomnia
Myoclonus
Cardiovascular
Orthostatic hypotension

long effective action (about 8-12 hr), with less penetration of the blood-brain barrier and less concern about exacerbating the depressive symptoms. Some patients feel that propranolol may be more effective at doses of 20 mg every 4-6 hr (or sustained-release propranolol at 80 mg b.i.d.). Very few patients manifest substantial lowering of blood pressure as a complication of these drugs. Unfortunately, the side effect of diaphoresis, often occurring at night, is less responsive to adjunctive β-blockers.

Nocturnal myoclonus, which occurs in a dose-dependent fashion with the monoamine oxidase inhibitors (MAOI) may be ameliorated by adding lorazepam 1-2 mg every 4 hr or by clonazepam 0.5-2.0 mg every 6-8 hr.

Drug-induced anticholinergic side effects appear to occur within clinical practice in a fashion similar to that observed in in vitro studies by Richelson (20), with the most anticholinergic being amitriptyline, then protriptyline, trimipramine, doxepin, imipramine, nortriptyline, desipramine, and maprotiline, whereas trazodone, fluoxetine, buproprion, and MAOIs appear to cause fewer anticholinergic side effects. Because some patients can develop a central anticholinergic syndrome (21), the more potent anticholinergic antidepressants should generally be avoided in older or medically ill patients. The peripheral anticholinergic side effects can be treated with urocholine, a cholinomimetic agent, in the following fashion. We start with 25 mg t.i.d., because of its relatively short half-life, and may increase dosage over a few days as necessary to 50-100 mg t.i.d. We have found this moderately effective in counteracting blurred vision, dry mouth, and urinary hesitancy.

Orthostatic hypotension is probably caused by α-receptor blockade (20), with descending frequency in doxepin, trimipramine, amitriptyline, trazodone, nortriptyline, imipramine, maprotiline, desipramine, and protriptyline. In our experience pretreatment orthostasis does not predict the presence of orthostasis from antidepressants. The MAOIs were originally utilized as antihypertensive agents and may produce profound hypotension. In our experience, heterocyclic-induced hypotension is very difficult to treat and dosage reduction is rarely beneficial. Four interventions have been found useful in some patients, although there has been no systematic comparison: metoclopromide; fludrocortisone; stimulants such as methylphenidate or dextroamphetamine; and sodium chloride. Both salt and fludrocortisone (which increase sodium retention) are relatively contraindicated in patients who have congestive heart failure or renal disease. Sodium chloride tablets can be given at 600-1800 mg twice a day, and fludrocortisone at 0.1 mg/day up to 0.6 mg/day in two divided doses, increasing by 0.1 mg/day increments every 3-7 days. Metoclopromide, at 5 mg two to three times a day, may be better tolerated, although it has a mild neuroleptic effect with potential extrapyramidal side effects. Response for these three agents may occur within several days of initiation. Methylphenidate or dextroamphetamine will reduce orthostatic hypotension (22) and, in our experience, with no hypertensive effects when combined in modest doses with the MAOIs, phenelzine or isocarboxazide. We have observed only one instance of dextroamphetamine-induced hypertension when added to tranylcypromine. We usually start with adding 2.5 mg of either stimulant in the morning and then increasing dosage by 2.5-5 mg in two to three divided doses, with a final dose in the 5-20 mg/day range. Response occurs within 1-2 days at any given dosage. Orthostatic blood pressure change and subjective improvement in "dizziness" mark the maintenance dose for any of these treatments. Finally, some patients may require extended treatment for hypotension for the duration of antidepressant therapy.

The MAOI-induced hypertension is rapid in onset after ingesting tyramine-containing food or indirect acting stimulants (23), and the episode typically remits within 1 hr if a catastrophic intracerebral bleed does not occur. We have found two effective counteractive treatments for this syndrome. Two or three nifedapine capsules (10 mg each) are punctured with a pin or teeth and the capsule and contents are swished in the mouth and swallowed. Blood pressure starts to subside within 1-2 min. This regimen may be repeated at 20-min intervals.

An alternative treatment is the use of chlorpromazine, which reduces blood pressure by its α-blocking action. Although chlorpromazine may act more slowly than nifedapine, 25-50 mg orally or intramuscularly should rapidly reverse the hypertensive episode. Phentolamine is a potent α-receptor blocker and hypotensive agent, but is now available only in intravenous formulation, making it less suitable for outpatients.

PATIENT CHARACTERISTICS

Some patients appear to be more likely to respond than others, even though they have the same DSM-III-R diagnosis. Goldberg et al. (24) conducted a survey of 133 experts in psychopharmacology who indicated that patients most likely to respond to heterocyclic antidepressants were those with endogenous depression, early-morning awakening, motor retardation, anorexia and weight loss, loss of interest in work and hobbies, diminished libido, diurnal mood swing—better in the evening, and a past response to pharmacotherapy. Regrettably, there is, as yet, little specific data to support these predictors, although findings of diurnal improvement (25) are consistent with this survey. Individuals without these features are less likely to meet DSM-III criteria for a primary major depression. This leaves the clinician with the dilemma of how to intervene in these cases of "atypical" depression. Akiskal (26) observed several factors associated with nonremitting depression: strong genetic loading, multiple object deaths, disabled spouse, medical disease, use of alcohol and sedatives, and agoraphobic symptoms.

Biological Variables

The diagnosis of depressive subtypes by biological variables is, at best, problematic. This is especially true for cerebrospinal fluid (CSF), urine, and blood measurements of biogenic amines or their metabolites [e.g., 3-methoxy-4-hydroxyphenolglycol (MHPG), 5-hydroxyindoleacetic acid (5-HIAA), homovanillic acid (HVA)] and platelet [H^3]imipramine binding sites. Furthermore, these variables have not predicted response to treatment, although they may be correlated with some behavioral factors such as suicidality (27). The dexamethasone suppression test (DST) and the thyrotropin-releasing hormone (TRH) stimulation test are often abnormal in depression and may eventually be helpful as diagnostic or prognostic tools, but they cannot now discriminate treatment responders from nonresponders (28).

Because various antidepressants have different effects on the reuptake of norepinephrine (NE), serotonin (5-HT), and dopamine (DA), researchers have examined whether or not different types of depression may respond preferentially to a specific neurotransmitter-reuptake inhibitor. Early studies used amitriptyline as a 5-HT-active agent and nortriptyline or imipramine as a NE-reuptake inhibitor. Initial results appeared promising; however, more recent data have shown that amitriptyline is metabolized to nortriptyline, an NE inhibitor, and both nortriptyline and imipramine also produce alterations in 5-HT, as well as norepinephrine. The current relatively specific polycyclic antidepressants are shown in Table 3.

Psychological Variables

One clinical dichotomy for selecting a specific antidepressant has been between agitated and anergic types of depression. Robinson et al. (29) compared 73 depressed outpatients treated with trazodone with 76 treated with maprotiline and found no difference in response rates between those with and without agitation. Similar results were reported by Asberg et al. (30) who compared the efficacy of zimelidine (a serotonergic antidepressant) to desipramine (which is active at noradrenergic sites). These and other studies support the contention that antidepressants are equally effective regardless of the patient's presenting symptoms or their predominant site of action.

Table 3 Neurotransmitter-Specific Antidepressants

Norepinephrine	Serotonin	Dopamine
Desipramine	Trazodone	Buproprion
Maprotyline	Fluoxetine	Nomifensine[a]

[a]No longer available.

Another key symptom that is frequently used to judge antidepressant choice is insomnia. Because insomnia normalizes as the depression remits, this factor is of only temporary importance. There is much clinical anecdotal material for which antidepressants are most sedating and more likely to be beneficial to the agitated insomniac depressive. Unfortunately, there has been a paucity of rigorous data on this subject. Contrary to some speculation, the sedative action of many antidepressants is not solely related to their degree of serotonin activity, it is also dependent upon other receptor-blocking activity (20).

TREATMENT APPROACH

Table 4 represents a typical treatment paradigm that can be considered as an "adequate" antidepressant trial. A lack of benefit, or only partial improvement to this regimen, can be considered treatment-resistance for practical clinical purposes.

Although many clinicians use other treatment paradigms successfully, it is most important to develop a systematic approach to antidepressant therapy so that the clinician can gain information from treatment nonresponse, rather than become demoralized by it. Thus, there is almost no indication for switching from one tricyclic to another, until that group has been exhausted, because there appear to be no specific differences in their clinical efficacy. Furthermore, the following approaches to resistant depression may be incorporated at an early stage into a treatment plan, rather than follow the three stages shown in Table 4. The order of adding these therapeutic maneuvers depends upon the clinical situation and the physician's judgment because no comparative studies have been performed to validate this treatment

Table 4 Standard Antidepressant Treatment

1. 4-6 wk of a heterocyclic antidepressant
   Blood levels (if available)
   Maximum tolerated dosage for at least 2 wk
2. Change to an alternate heterocyclic antidepressant with different neurotransmitter action
   Blood levels (if available)
   Maximum tolerated dosage for at least 2 wk
3. MAOI for 4-6 wk
   - Phenelzine (Nardil) (> 1 mg/kg)
   - Isocarboxazid (Marplan) (> 0.5 mg/kg)
   - Tranylcypromine (Parnate) (> 0.5 mg/kg)

algorithm. We try to achieve a balance between the severity of the illness and the length of time for each potential treatment in arriving at a choice. We usually continue heterocyclic treatment and add additional medication, because in our experience, patients' conditions are likely to deteriorate substantially before a new treatment can become effective.

Table 5 outlines several approaches to treatment-resistant depression.

Lithium as Adjunctive Therapy

Although lithium alone has not generally been found to have a robust antidepressant effect, the addition of lithium to heterocyclic antidepressants and MAOIs has enhanced response. For example, Price et al. (31) treated 84 patients who were refractory to at least 4 weeks of antidepressant therapy by adding lithium carbonate, 900 mg/day, and adjusting serum levels to range between 0.5 and 1.3 mEq/L. Thirty-one percent of the patients demonstrated a marked improvement, and 25% had a partial response. Unipolar patients seemed to respond in greater proportion (59%) when compared with bipolar patients (36%), confirming similar observations from earlier studies (32,33). Blood levels may be correlated with response because Zusky et al. (34) found no benefit with the addition of relatively low doses of lithium (up to 900 mg/day) in 16 heterocyclic nonresponders. Therefore, it seems reasonable to achieve lithium levels in the 0.8-1.2 mEq/L range. Furthermore, the response to lithium augmentation may require at least 4 weeks.

Lithium also has a place in augmenting MAOI therapy. Fein et al. (35) demonstrated alleviation of depression with the combination of lithium and phenylzine in seven treatment-resistant patients. Similarly, Price et al. (36) reported that 11 of 12 antidepressant nonresponders improved with the combination of tranylcypromine (40-60 mg/day) and lithium (600-1200 mg/day).

Table 5 Approaches to Treatment-Resistant Depression

Lithium augmentation
Thyroid supplementation
Alprazolam
Combination MAOI-heterocyclic antidepressant
L-Tryptophan
Stimulants
Carbamazepine (Tegretol)
ECT
Other

Thyroid Hormones as Adjunctive Therapy

The use of thyroid supplementation in resistant depressed patients has been practiced for more than a decade (37,38). The essential hypothesis of this strategy was that increased thyroid levels in the central nervous system (CNS) would increase β-adrenergic receptor sensitivity and enhance the antidepressant effect of tricyclic antidepressants (39). Both T_3 and T_4 hormone preparations have been used for this purpose (40-43). However, toxicity from T_3 may result at doses in excess of 50 μg/day, and some individuals may require 5-10 μg/day. Triiodothyronine has a more rapid onset of action than T_4. Furthermore, use of T_3 can reduce T_4 levels by its potent feedback inhibition, and thyroid function must then be monitored by obtaining TSH and T_3 levels (preferably by T_3 radioimmunoassay). We prefer to use T_4 (0.025-0.05 mg/day) and monitor serum T_4 levels. However, thyroid augmentation has not been consistently beneficial, and the results from several recent double-blind studies have not shown a treatment effect of T_3 (44,45) in tricyclic antidepressant nonresponders. Although Joffe et al. (46) found that T_3 was significantly more effective than T_4 in 38 imipramine and desipramine nonresponders, at the present time, the data are still equivocal. For a more detailed discussion on thyroid augmentation, see Chapter 13.

Monoamine Oxidase Inhibitors as Adjunctive Therapy

The combination of MAOIs with heterocyclic antidepressants is becoming more widely accepted for the treatment of refractory depression. Fears concerning catastrophic adverse reactions seem unfounded, for the most part, if reasonable caution is exercised. In a landmark study, White and Simpson (47) concluded that adverse effects from this drug combination, in many cases, probably resulted from a rapid dosage increase. Since then, others have demonstrated the relative safety of combining these agents. Oefele et al. (48) examined the frequency of adverse drug reactions in patients treated with several tricyclic and MAOI combinations and found that the combination most likely to result in adverse reactions was clomipramine and tranylcypromine. There is no systematic data on combining MAOIs with other antidepressants. However, the combination of MAOIs with fluoxetine or clomipramine would appear to be contraindicated. Schmauss et al. (49) reviewed the charts of 94 patients who had been unsuccessfully treated with at least two different antidepressants and then treated with tranylcypromine and trifluoperazine (Stelazine) plus a tricyclic agent. The results showed 31% with a "very good" response and 27% with a "good" improvement. Similar results have been reported by Feighner et al. (22).

When using an MAOI-heterocyclic antidepressant combination, it is generally recommended that either the two medications be started simultaneously, or that the MAOI be added to the tricyclic to minimize the potential risk of a hypertensive episode. Nevertheless, we have seen several cases for whom tricyclics were added to phenylzine or isocarboxyzide without adverse effects. Dosage of the MAOI should be slowly increased (every 3-4 days) to a standard dosage, and then the heterocyclic antidepressant monitored as described previously.

Stimulants as Adjunctive Therapy

There has been a resurgence of interest in the use of stimulants, such as dextroamphetamine, methylphenidate, and pemoline, as possible treatments for resistant depression, both alone and in combination with other medications. Chiarello and Cole (50) recently reviewed the literature on analeptic drugs in depression and concluded that certain depressed individuals respond quite well. For example, depressed patients with medical illness often respond to stimulant drugs. Woods et al. (51) reviewed the charts from 68 depressed patients with a medical illness who were treated with stimulants and found that 73% showed improvement. Furthermore, response was rapid, and 93% showed improvement within 2 days, with minimal side effects. In addition, Kaufmann et al. (52,53) reported a rapid response in mood in medically ill depressed patients given methylphenidate (10-20 mg b.i.d.) or dextroamphetamine (2.5-10 mg daily). In addition to depressed patients with medical illnesses, other patients may also benefit from this regimen, in particular geriatric depressives. It is our usual practice to use a stimulant concurrently with a tricyclic antidepressant in low to moderate doses. Although a range of doses for methylphenidate and dextroamphetamine appears effective, less systematic data are available on pemoline. Pemoline may be useful at doses between 17.5 and 70 mg/day, but because of its prominent dopaminergic action, it has been less well tolerated owing to agitation.

The combination of stimulants with tricyclic antidepressants or MAOIs appears to be a safe and effective method of treating refractory depression (50). Feighner et al. (22) described treatment of 16 patients with depression for at least a 2-year duration who failed to respond to tricyclic antidepressants, MAOIs, or both. Three were treated with a tricyclic and MAOI, five with an MAOI and a stimulant, and eight with all three drugs simultaneously. Doses of dextroamphetamine (10-20 mg/day) and methylphenidate (10-15 mg/day) were used. Overall, 16 patients improved and two declined, although no serious side effects were encountered. Orthostatic hypotension, irritability, and insomnia were the most commonly reported side effects. We have not experienced an abuse potential in depressed patients taking stimulants, nor has any tolerance to antidepressant effect been observed.

Other Agents as Adjunctive Therapy

L-Tryptophan has also been shown to be a possible adjunctive agent for augmenting antidepressant therapy (32,54-56). Because it is a precursor to serotonin, it has primarily been used to augment serotonergically active tricyclic and MAOI antidepressants. Its dosage range can vary widely between 2 and 20 g/day, with the average dose being 2-4 g/day. Pyridoxine (vitamin B_6) (100 mg b.i.d.), a cofactor in the conversion of tryptophan to serotonin, may enhance the augmentation of tryptophan. Combining L-tryptophan with either a tricyclic or the MAOIs phenelzine or isocarboxyzide has not produced excessive serotonergic activity in our experience. However, when tryptophan is used to augment tranylcypromine or a serotonergic antidepressant, such as fluoxetine, it may precipitate a life-threatening "serotonergic syndrome" characterized by myoclonus, chills, delerium, and other neurotoxic signs (57). [Recent association of blood dyscrasias to L-tryptophan remains controversial.]

Carbamazepine is a tricyclic anticonvulsant that has been used to treat mania that is unresponsive to lithium, as well as an adjunct to lithium for prophylaxis against mood swings. More recently, it has been reported to possess antidepressant qualities that may be correlated with serum drug levels (58). In one study, Ballenger reported that 35% of depressed patients resistant to standard treatment showed a marked response to carbamazepine, and 57% showed a mild to moderate response (59,60). Bipolar patients and those with severe depression had the best response rate at doses of approximately 1 g/day. Of the patients who did not respond to carabamazepine alone, many showed improvement when lithium was added. (A more detailed discussion of the use of carbamazepine can be found in Chap. 8.)

Alprazolam, a triazolobenzodiazepine tranquilizer, also has antidepressant effects when compared with several tricyclic antidepressants (61). Effective antidepressant doses vary widely among individuals, but average about 3.0 mg/day. It may be added to any other antidepressant regimen with little risk of drug interaction, but it should be carefully tapered at the end of treatment to avoid withdrawal symptoms. We recommend tapering it by 0.125-0.25 mg every 4-7 days.

Reserpine, yohimbine, and estrogen have also been used to potentiate the antidepressant response of other drugs, but most results with these treatments have been tentative, with inconclusive guidelines for subject selection and risk/benefit ratio (42,62-64). There is one report of verapamil (240-400 mg/day) being effective for depression (65).

Electroconvulsive Therapy

All patients with chronic or treatment-resistant depression should be considered for electroconvulsive therapy (ECT). Severely depressed patients, particularly those who are acutely suicidal or have psychotic symptoms, may respond particularly well to ECT in contrast with pharmacotherapy (32,66, 67). When one considers the morbidity and potential mortality from suicide, as well as the debilitating effects of a chronic illness treated unsuccessfully for years, it may be unfair to withhold a treatment with ECT in patients with refractory depressions (68). Therefore, it is appropriate to discuss this treatment early on if initial antidepressant treatment has failed. A more detailed discussion on when to refer patients for ECT is provided in Chapter 11.

CONCLUSIONS

Bearing in mind issues relating to the duration of each treatment trial, potential side effects, and patient compliance, we initially use the treatment algorhithm displayed in Table 6. Clinical variables will often result in deviation from this scheme, but a systematic approach is important in avoiding erratic treatment attempts. We suggest that each clinician develop such a plan to enhance the systematic treatment for their patients with refractory depression.

If response occurs, it is our suggestion that the particular combination of medications be continued for several months to prevent relapse. Although

Table 6 Sample Plan for Treatment-Refractory Depression

First:	Drug A (heterocyclic) for 4-6 wk
	Blood level (if applicable)
Second:	Discontinue drug A while adding drug B (heterocyclic with different neurotransmitter specificity) for 4-6 wk
	Blood level (if applicable)
Third:	Discuss alternative treatments in a hopeful manner and systematically
	Add thyroid supplement for 1- to 2-wk trial
	or add stimulant for 1-wk trial
	or add lithium for 4-wk trial
	or add MAOI for 4-wk trial
	or add alprazolam for 4-wk trial
Fourth:	Discuss ECT
	Systematically develop a combination treatment
	1. Enhance 5-HT systems by use of trazodone, L-tryptophan, and phenylzine or isocarboxyzide
	2. Enhance NE/DA system with stimulant, noradrenergic antidepressant, and MAOI
	3. Add carbamazepine (Tegretol)

5-HT, serotonin; NE, morepinephrine; DA, dopamine.

there are no firm guidelines for discontinuing treatment, we often start by tapering one agent completely and then another. It is not unusual for some patients to relapse and require the reintroduction of treatment for several additional months, and occasional patients may require their drug combination for an indefinite period.

The utilization of combined antidepressant drug therapy has engendered apprehension in some clinicians because of the implication that polypharmacy is inherently dangerous. However, once a physician becomes conversant with the pharmacology of these agents, their possible side effects, and indications for therapeutic intervention, there is no logical reason to withhold such potentially effective treatments from refractory patients. The risks from such treatment may be minimal when compared with the known morbidity and mortality of refractory depression.

REFERENCES

1. American Psychiatric Association (1987). *Diagnostic and Statistical Manual of Mental Disorders*, 3rd ed., revised. Washington, D.C., American Psychiatric Association.
2. Akiskal, H. S. and Lemmi, H. (1983). Clinical, neuroendocrine, and sleep diagnosis of "unusual" affective presentations: A practical review. *Psychiatr. Clin. North Am. 6*:69-84.
3. Gold, M. S., Pottash, A. L. C., and Extein, I. (1981). Hypothyroidism and depression. *JAMA 245*:1919-1922.
4. Reus, V. (1989). Behavioral aspects of thyroid disease in women. *Psychiatr. Clin. North Am. 12*:153-165.
5. Martin, J. B. and Reichlin, S., eds. (1987). *Clinical Neuroendocrinology*. Philadelphia, F.A. Davis, pp. 659-660.
6. Holmes, G. P., Kaplan, J. E., Gantz, N. M., et al. (1988). Chronic fatigue syndrome: A working case definition. *Ann. Intern. Med. 108*:387-389.
7. Ceroni, G. B., Neri, C., and Pezzoli, A. (1984). Chronicity in major depression. *J. Affect. Disord. 7*:123-132.
8. Ayd, F. (1983). Treatment-resistant depression. *Int. Drug Ther. Newslett. 18*:25-27.
9. Quitkin, F. M. (1985). The importance of dosage in prescribing antidepressants. *Br. J. Psychiatry 147*:593-597.
10. Keller, M. B., Klerman, G. L., Lavori, P. W., Fawcett, J. A., Coryell, W., and Endicott, J. (1982). Treatment received by depressed patients. *JAMA 248*:1848-1855.
11. Kocsis, J. H., Frances, A. J., Voss, C., et al. (1988). Imipramine treatment for chronic depression. *Arch. Gen. Psychiatry 45*:253-257.
12. Hanin, I., Koslow, S. H., Kocsis, J. H., et al. (1985). Cerebrospinal fluid levels of amitriptyline, nortriptyline, imipramine and desmethylimipramine—relationship to plasma levels and treatment outcome. *J. Affect. Disord. 9*:69-78.

13. Coccaro, E. F., Adan, F., Allen, D., and Cooper, T. B. (1987). Plasma-serum differences in the assessment of tricyclic antidepressant blood levels. *Int. Clin. Psychopharmacol.* *2*:217-224.
14. Kitani, K. (1986). Hepatic drug metabolism in the elderly. *Hepatology* *6*:316-319.
15. Colaizzi, J. L. and Lowenthal, D. T. (1986). Critical therapeutic categories: A contradiction to generic substitution? *Clin. Ther.* *8*:370-379.
16. Greenblatt, D. J. and Shader, R. I. (1987). Bioequivalence of generic drugs in clinical psychopharmacology. *J. Clin. Psychopharmacol.* *7*:A21-A23.
17. Jarvik, L., Mintz, J., Steuer, J., and Gerner, R. H. (1982). Treating geriatric depression. *J. Am. Geriatr. Soc.* *30*:713-717.
18. Gerner, R. H. (1983). Systematic treatment approach to depression and treatment resistant depression. *Psychiatr. Ann.* *13*:37-49.
19. Pollack, M. H. and Rosenbaum, J. F. (1987). Management of antidepressant induced side effects: A practical guide for the clinician. *J. Clin. Psychiatry* *48*: 3-8.
20. Richelson, E. (1983). Are receptor studies useful for clinical practice? *J. Clin. Psychiatry* *44*:9:4-9.
21. Curran, H. V., Sakulsri, M., and Lader, M. (1988). Antidepressants and human memory—an investigation of 4 drugs with different sedative and anticholinergic profiles. *Psychopharmacology* *95*:516-519.
22. Feighner, J. P., Herbstein, J., and Damlouji, N. (1985). Combined MAOI, TCA, and direct stimulant therapy of treatment-resistant depression. *J. Clin. Psychiatry* *46*:206-209.
23. Lippmann, S. (1987). Practical MAOI food and drug avoidances. *Psychosomatics* *28*:591.
24. Goldberg, S. C., Tilley, D. H., Friedel, R. O., et al. (1988). Who benefits from tricyclic antidepressants: A survey. *J. Clin. Psychiatry* *49*:224-228.
25. Carpenter, L. L., Kupfer, D. J., and Frank, E. (1986). Is diurnal variation a meaningful symptom in unipolar depression? *J. Affect. Disord.* *11*:255-264.
26. Akiskal, H. S. (1982). Factors associated with incomplete recovery in primary depressive illness. *J. Clin. Psychiatry* *43*:266-271.
27. Asberg, M., Eriksson, B., Martensson, B., Traskman-Bendz, L., and Wagner, A. (1986). Therapeutic effects of serotonin uptake inhibitors in depression. *J. Clin. Psychiatry* *46*(suppl. 4):23-35.
28. Myers, E. D. (1988). Predicting the response of depressed patients to biological treatment: The dexamethasone suppression test versus clinical judgment. *Br. J. Psychiatry* *152*:657-659.
29. Robinson, D. S., Corcella, J., Feighner, J. P., et al. (1984). A comparison of trazodone, amoxapine and maprotiline in the treatment of endogenous depression: Results of a multicenter study. *Curr. Ther. Res.* *35*:549-560.
30. Asberg, A. (1981). Controlled cross-over study of a 5-HT uptake inhibiting and NA-uptake inhibiting antidepressant. *Acta Psychiatr. Scand. Suppl.* *290*:244-255.
31. Price, L. H., Charney, D. S., and Heninger, G. R. (1986). Variability of response to lithium augmentation in refractory depression. *Am. J. Psychiatry* *143*:1387-1392.

32. Paykel, E. S. and van Woerkom, A. E. (1987). Pharmacologic treatment of refractory depression. *Psychiatr. Ann. 17*:327-331.
33. Garbutt, J. C., Mayo, J. P., Jr., Gillette, G. M., et al. (1986). Lithium potentiation of tricyclic antidepressants following lack of T_3 potentiation. *Am. J. Psychiatry 143*:1038-1039.
34. Zusky, P. M., Biederman, J., Rosenbaum, J. F., Manschreck, T. C., Gross, C. C., Weilberg, J. B., and Gastfriend, D. R. (1988). Adjunct low dose lithium carbonate in treatment resistant depression: A placebo controlled study. *J. Clin. Psychopharmacol. 8*:120-124.
35. Fein, S., Paz, V., Rao, N., and LaGrassa, J. (1988). The combination of lithium carbonate and an MAOI in refractory depressions. *Am. J. Psychiatry 145*:249-253.
36. Price, L. H., Charney, D. S., and Heninger, G. R. (1986). Variability of response to lithium augmentation in refractory depression. *Am. J. Psychiatry 143*:1387-1392.
37. Stein, D. and Avni, J. (1988). Thyroid hormone in the treatment of affective disorders. *Acta Psychiatr. Scand. 77*:623-636.
38. Joffe, R. T., Roy-Byrne, P. P., and Uhde, T. W. (1984). Thyroid function and affective illness: A reappraisal. *Biol. Psychiatry 19*:1685-1690.
39. Whybrow, P. C. and Prange, A. J. (1981). A hypothesis of thyroid-catecholamine-receptor interaction. *Arch. Gen. Psychiatry 38*:106-113.
40. Fischer, J. M. and Schwinghammer, T. L. (1983). Enhancement of tricyclic antidepressants by thyroid. *Drug Intell. Clin. Pharmacy 17*:718-719.
41. Garbutt, J., Malekpour, B., Brunswick, D., et al. (1980). Dr. Garbutt and associates reply. *Am. J. Psychiatry 137*:384.
42. Prange, A. J. and Loosen, P. T. (1982). Hormone therapy in depressive diseases. In *Typical and Atypical Antidepressants in Practice*. Edited by E. Costa and G. Racagni. New York, Raven Press, pp. 289-296.
43. Swartz, C. M. (1982). Dependency of tricyclic antidepressant efficacy on thyroid hormone potentiation: Case studies. *J. Nerv. Ment. Dis. 170*:50-52.
44. Thase, M. E., Kupfer, D. J., and Jarrett, D. B. (1985). Active L-triiodothyronine (T_3) in imipramine-resistant recurrent unipolar depression. Presented at Fourth World Congress of Biological Psychiatry, Philadelphia, Sept. 8, 1985.
45. Gitlin, M. J., Weiner, H., Fairbanks, L., Hershman, J., and Friedfeld, N. (1987). Failure of T_3 to potentiate tricyclic antidepressant response. *J. Affect. Disord. 13*:267-272.
46. Joffe, R. T. and Singer, W. (1988). Thyroid hormone potentiation of antidepressants. Presented at 141st American Psychiatric Association Meeting. Montreal, May 10, 1988.
47. White, K. and Simpson, G. (1983). Combined MAOI-tricyclic antidepressant treatment: A reevaluation. *J. Clin. Psychopharmacol. 3*:221-226.
48. Oefele, K. V., Grohmann, R., and Ruther, E. (1986). Adverse drug reactions in combined tricyclic and MAOI therapy. *Pharmacopsychiatry 19*:243-244.
49. Schmauss, M., Kapfhammer, H. P., Meyr, P., and Hoff, P. (1986). Combined MAO-inhibitor and tri-(tetra)cyclic antidepressant in therapy resistant depression: A retrospective study. *Pharmacopsychiatry 19*:251-252.

50. Chiarello, R. J. and Cole, J. O. (1987). The use of psychostimulants in general psychiatry. *Arch. Gen. Psychiatry 44*:286-295.
51. Woods, S. W., Tesar, G. E., Murray, G. B., and Cassem, N. H. (1986). Psychostimulant treatment of depressive disorders secondary to medical illness. *J. Clin. Psychiatry 47*:12-15.
52. Kaufmann, M. W. and Murray, G. B. (1982). The use of d-amphetamine in medically ill depressed patients. *J. Clin. Psychiatry 43*:463-464.
53. Kaufmann, M. W., Cassem, N., Murray, G., and MacDonald, D. (1984). The use of methylphenidate in depressed patients after cardiac surgery. *J. Clin. Psychiatry 45*:82-84.
54. Cooper, A. J. and Magnus, R. V. (1984). Strategies for the treatment of depression. *Can. Med. Assoc. J. 130*:383-390.
55. Kielholz, P. (1986). Treatment for therapy-resistant depression. *Psychopathology 19*(suppl. 2):194-200.
56. Hale, A. S., Procter, A. W., and Bridges, P. K. (1987). Clomipramine, tryptophan and lithium in combination for resistant endogenous depression: Seven case studies. *Br. J. Psychiatry 151*:213-217.
57. Price, W. A., Zimmer, B., and Kucas, P. (1986). Serotonin syndrome: A case report. *J. Clin. Pharmacol. 26*:77-78.
58. Trimble, M. R. (1988). Carbamazepine and mood: Evidence from patients with seizure disorders. *J. Clin. Psychiatry 49* (supp.):7-11.
59. Ballenger, J. C. and Post, R. M. (1985). Anticonvulsants in psychiatric disease. *Hosp. Ther.* Nov.:73-89.
60. Ballenger, J. C. (1988). The clinical use of carbamazepine in affective disorders. *J. Clin. Psychiatry 49* (suppl.):13-19.
61. Warner, M. D., Peabody, C. A., Whiteford, H. A., and Hollister, L. E. (1988). Alprazolam as an antidepressant. *J. Clin. Psychiatry 49*:148-150.
62. Amsterdam, J. D. and Berwish, N. (1987). Treatment of refractory depression with combination reserpine and tricyclic antidepressant therapy. *J. Clin. Psychopharmacol. 7*:238-242.
63. Schmauss, M., Laakmann, G., and Dieterle, D. (1986). Effects of α_2-receptor blockade in addition to tricyclic antidepressants in therapy-resistant depression: A retrospective study. *Pharmacopsychiatry 19*:251-252.
64. Zohar, J., Shapira, B., Oppenheim, G., et al. (1985). Addition of estrogen to imipramine in female resistant-depressives. *Psychopharmacol. Bull. 21*:705-706.
65. Pollack, M. H., Rosenbaum, J. F., and Hyman, S. E. (1987). Calcium channel blockers in psychiatry. *Psychosomatics 28*:356-360.
66. Simpson, G. M., Pi, E. H., Gross, L. G., et al. (1988). Plasma levels and therapeutic response with trimipramine treatment of endogenous depression. *J. Clin. Psychiatry 49*:113-116.
67. Rifkin, A. (1988). ECT versus tricyclic antidepressants in depression: A review of the evidence. *J. Clin. Psychiatry 49*:3-7.
68. Kramer, B. (1987). Electroconvulsive therapy use in geriatric depression. *J. Nerv. Ment. Dis. 175*:233-235.

21

Causes and Treatments of Rapid-Cycling Affective Disorder

THOMAS A. WEHR

Clinical Psychobiology Branch, National Institute of Mental Health, Bethesda, Maryland

INTRODUCTION

Patients with *rapid-cycling mood disorders* have been arbitrarily defined as having four or more affective episodes per year (1,2). To this criterion, we have added a circular course, in which episodes of normal or elevated mood regularly alternate with episodes of depression at some time during the history of the illness (3).

In his description of circular insanity (*la folie circulaire*) in 1854, Falret noted that these patients are very often women, and that the cycles of illness are often unremitting and resistant to treatment (Table 1; 4). These observations are still relevant today.

We have found the following features to be characteristic of a group of 51 patients with rapid-cycling affective disorder referred to the Intramural Research Program of the National Institute of Mental Health (NIMH) (3):

1. Nearly all (92%) of the patients were women (in contrast with 44% of a control group of non-rapid-cycling patients with bipolar illness).
2. All of the patients were classified as having bipolar affective disorder according to the Research Diagnostic Criteria (RDC), and all met RDC criteria for endogenous depression.
3. Nearly half (47%) had thyroid disease, mostly hypothyroidism secondary to lithium treatment.

Table 1 A Description of Rapid-Cycling Affective Disorder by Falret in 1854

La Folie Circulaire (Circular Insanity)
J. P. Falret (1854)

Definition: "A perpetual circle of depression and manic excitement interrupted by a period of lucidity, which is typically brief but occasionally long lasting."

Severity and duration of cycles: "Circular insanity . . . varies in intensity and in duration . . . At times the circle is complete in 3 weeks or a month; sometimes it takes many months or years."

Prevalence: "It does not appear especially common; but there are many causes that interfere with an accurate appreciation of the actual frequency . . . the evolution of mental illness is not carefully enough appreciated . . . such patients often remain in society."

Heredity: "We were . . . able to detect, despite the euphemisms employed by the family members, that oftentimes the ancestors did have a similar type of mental condition . . . circular insanity is very hereditary."

Sex ratio: "Circular insanity, with short or with long phases, is infinitely more frequent in females than in males."

Prognosis: "Remarkably, mania and melancholia when they occur in isolation are more treatable than when they occur together in circular insanity . . . So far, we have never observed a complete cure, nor even a lasting improvement."

4. Although women were especially susceptible to rapid cycling, it did not appear to be caused by the menstrual cycle.
5. In about half (51%) of the patients, antidepressant medications appeared to induce the rapid cycling in a reversible manner (see Tables 2, 3, 4, 6).

CLINICAL PICTURE OF MANIA AND DEPRESSION IN RAPID-CYCLING AFFECTIVE DISORDER

We found the clinical picture of depression and mania in rapid-cycling patients to be similar in character to the mood states in non-rapid-cycling patients (3). About half the patients had bipolar I affective disorder and half had bipolar II (Table 2). Half had been hospitalized for mania or depression, and half had been psychotic at some time during the course of their illness. Half had been treated with electroconvulsive therapy (ECT), and one-fourth had previously attempted suicide. Most had had extensive treatment with various psychotropic drugs and were referred to NIMH because they were considered to be refractory to treatment. Therefore, this appeared to be an especially treatment-resistant group of patients.

Table 2 Patient Characteristics in Rapid-Cycling Affective Disorder

		Sex (%)		Diagnosis (%)			
Author (Ref.)	N	M	F	BP	BPI	BPII	UP
Stancer et al. (42)	7	43	57				
Dunner et al. (2)	<40	30	70	100	55	45	0
Kukopulos et al. (21)	118	30	70	92	15	77	8
Squillace et al. (43)	20	20	80				
Alarcon (9)	15	7	93				
Wehr et al. (3)	51	8	92	100	53	47	0

COURSE OF ILLNESS IN PATIENTS WITH RAPID-CYCLING AFFECTIVE DISORDER

The age of onset of affective illness in the rapid-cycling patients was similar to the more conventional forms of bipolar illness, with most patients having their first episode in their teens and 20s. In fact, the pattern of age of onsets for this group is almost identical with the pattern for bipolar patients in general (Fig. 1 and Table 3) (5).

In rapid-cycling patients, the illness nearly always (98%) began with a depressive episode, in contrast with the non-rapid-cycling control group, whose illness can begin with mania or hypomania in 25%. Because later episodes of mania and rapid cycling often occur in the context of antidepressant drug treatments, it is possible that a substantial number of these patients might not have exhibited a bipolar course in the prepharmacologic era.

In most cases (63%), the illness began with a non-rapid-cycling course (see Table 3). Patients usually experienced one or more irregular, intermittent episodes for several years before the onset of rapid cycling (see Fig. 1). This is one of several findings that suggests that patients with rapid cycles are not fundamentally different from those with non-rapid-cycling forms of illness.

Rapid cycling typically is characterized by two kinds of processes: (1) a slow process ("the cycling process"), corresponding to the circular cycle of the alternating episodes; and (2) a rapid process ("the switch process"), corresponding to the sudden transitions, or switches, that often occur as patients move from depression to mania, or vice versa. Various biological correlates of each type of process have been described. For example, levels of urinary 3-methoxy-4-hydroxyphenylglycol (MHPG), the norepinephrine metabolite, gradually increase and decrease in synchrony with the cycling process in some

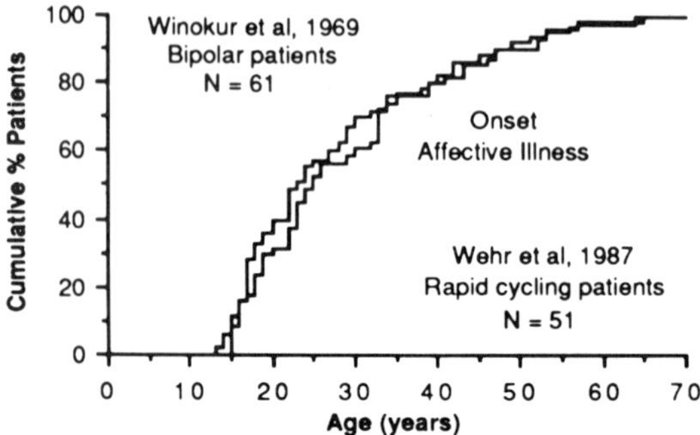

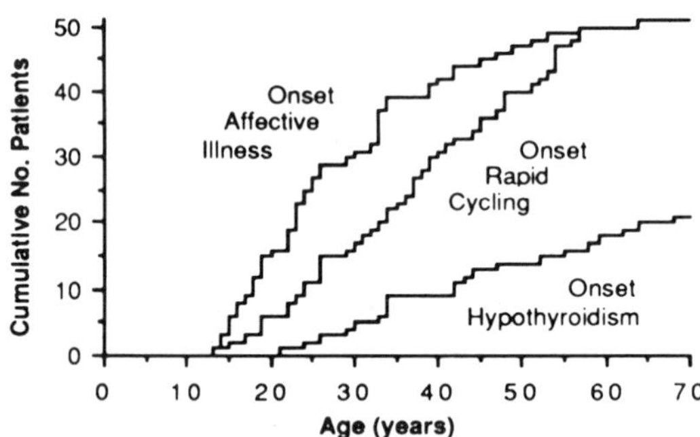

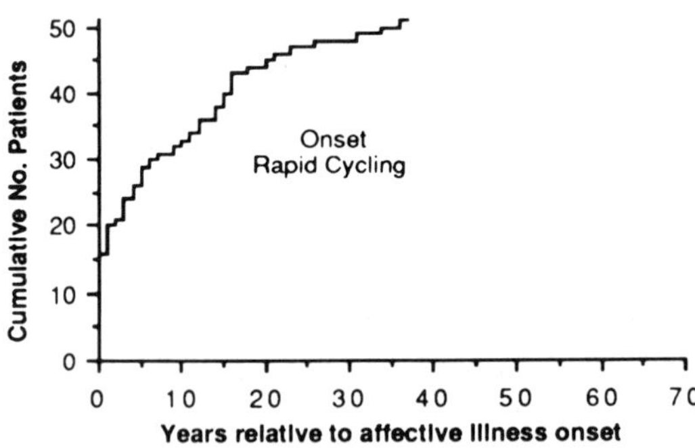

Figure 1 (a) Superimposed cumulative sums of onsets of affective illness in 61 bipolar patients reported by Winokur et al. (5) and in 51 rapid-cycling bipolar patients reported by Wehr et al. (3). (b) Cumulative sums of onsets of affective illness, rapid cycling, and thyroid disease in 51 patients with rapid-cycling bipolar illness (3). (c) Cumulative sums of onsets of rapid cycling relative to onset of affective illness in 51 patients with rapid-cycling bipolar illness (3).

Table 3 Course of Illness in Rapid-Cycling Affective Disorder

Author (Ref.)	N	Age of onset of: Affective illness mean	Affective illness median	Rapid cycling mean	Rapid cycling median	Onset with rapid cycling (%)	Episodes per year
Stancer et al. (42)	7	31.7	33				12.9
Dunner et al. (2)	33	30.3					>4.0
Kukopulos et al. (21)	118	33.2		40.7		27	7.8
Squillace et al. (43)	20	23.8					7.3
Alarcon (9)	15	30.1	28	32.4	28	67	36.0
Wehr et al. (3)	51	30.0	26	37.9	37	37	15.1

patients, whereas body temperature and motor activity change abruptly with the switch from depression into mania (6).

Cycling and switching appear to be somewhat independent processes. Sometimes, the severity of either depression or mania can wax and wane without the patient switching into the opposite state. We refer to this phenomenon as cycling above or below the line (cycling without switching; Fig. 2; 7). Sometimes patients repeatedly switched back and forth between mania and depression every 24-48 hr at certain phases in their long-term mood cycles (switching without cycling; see Fig. 2; 7).

In our patients, the duration of mood cycles ranged from several days to many weeks (Fig. 3). Although the frequency of cycling appeared to be somewhat irregular, long records of the course of illness often revealed surprisingly regular, although complex, patterns of recurrence. For example, one patient's recurrences, which were monitored for more than 4 years, were actually found to result from a coupling of two biological cycles with stable periods of 35.5 days and 43 days (Figs. 4 and 5) (8). The regularity of this complex pattern would never have been suspected from casual observations, or from records of only a few cycles of the illness.

REPRODUCTIVE CYCLES AND MOOD CYCLES

Over three-fourths of the 47 rapid-cycling women had histories of pregnancy (3). Most first pregnancies had occurred before the onset of affective illness (68%) and rapid cycling (90%). Of the women who had been pregnant (N=41), 40% had had postpartum affective episodes.

In the rapid-cycling women, no convincing relationship could be established between manic-depressive cycles and menstrual cycles. In 49% of the patients, rapid cycling either began (N=9) or persisted (N=14) after menopause.

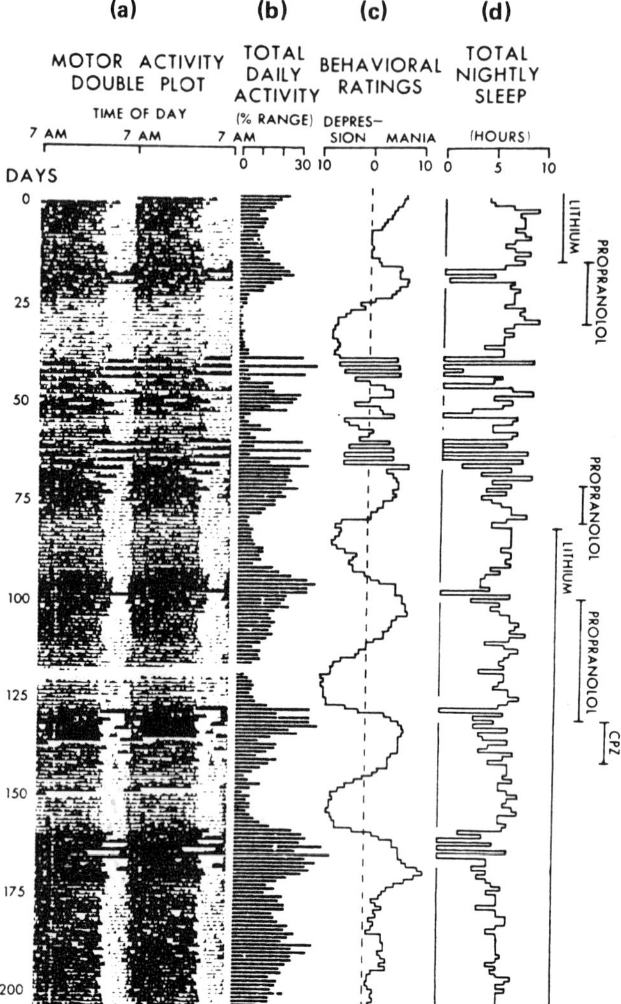

Figure 2 (a) Wrist motor activity recording raster plot; (b) total 24-hr activity levels; (c) nurses' behavioral ratings of mania and depression; (d) duration of nightly sleep (based on nurses' half-hourly sleep checks), and psychotropic drug treatments in a rapid-cycling manic-depressive woman. The raster plot was constructed by graphing 15-min bins of motor activity data in 24-hr segments that are plotted successively beneath one another and double-plotted to the right. Vertical dark bands reflect daily recurring waking activity; vertical light bands reflect nightly recurring sleep. Daytime activity is increased (darker) during mania and decreased (lighter) during depression. At the time of switches from depression to mania the patient usually experienced one or more nights of total insomnia (reflected in the continuation of the dark horizontal bands of daytime activity across the light vertical bands produced by nighttime sleep). (Reprinted from Ref. 7.)

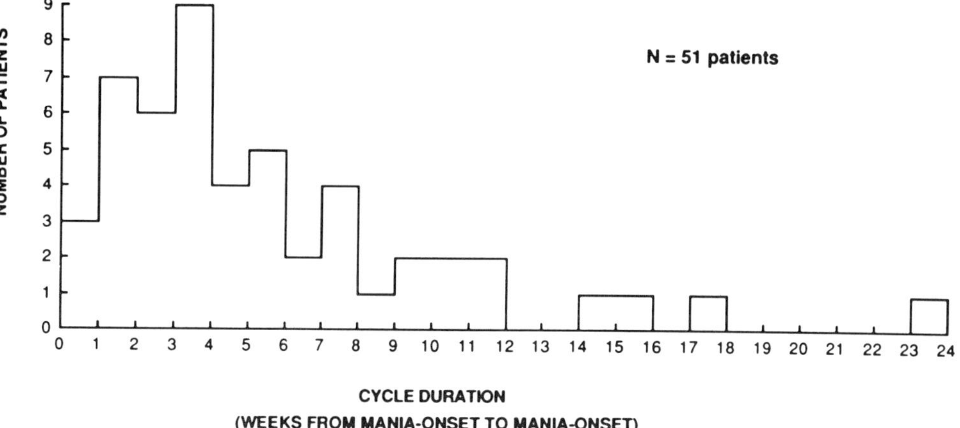

Figure 3 Frequency distribution of average lengths of manic-depressive cycles (onset of mania to onset of mania) in 51 rapid-cycling patients reported by Wehr et al. (3).

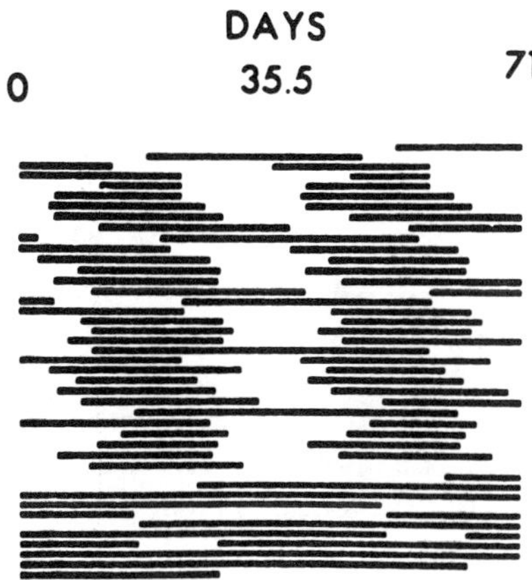

Figure 4 Raster plot of manic-depressive cycles in a rapid-cycling woman. Data from daily mood self-ratings are plotted in 35.5-day segments successively beneath one another. Mania is shown as dark horizontal line segments, depression as open spaces between line segments. The graph is double-plotted to the right to facilitate visual inspection of the courses of the mood cycles. The vertical alignment of manic and depressive phases of the cycles reflects a 35.5-day periodicity in their pattern of recurrence. Every four or five cycles, the cycle lengthens and passes through 360°, or "wraps around," relative to the 35.5-day pattern. Because of the periodic lengthenings of the cycle, its average period is approximately 43 days. This complex pattern persisted for 4 years, and it suggests that a 43-day mood cycle is interacting with another, unidentified 35.5-day biological rhythm. The 35.5-day rhythm was not the menstrual cycle (the patient was postmenopausal).

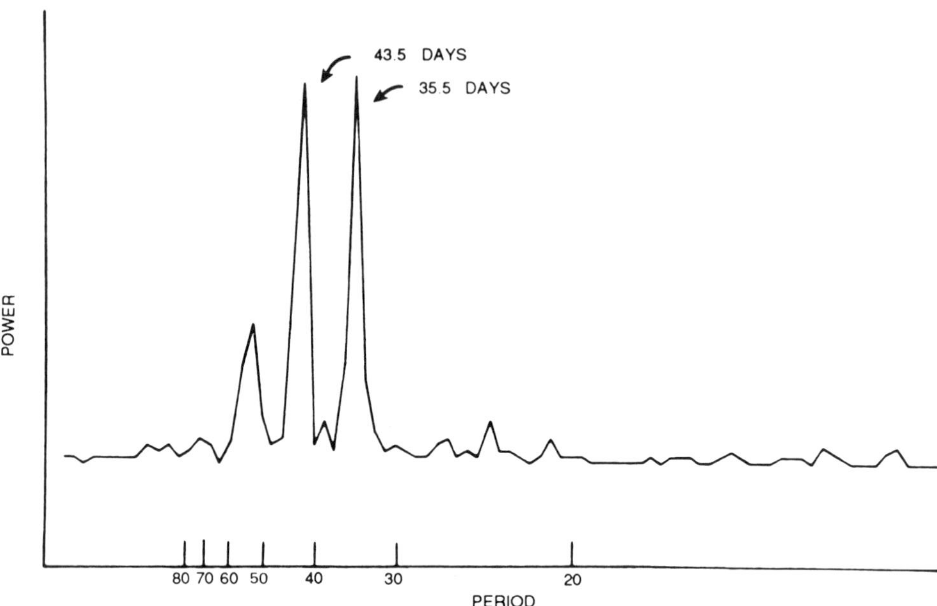

Figure 5 Spectral (frequency) analysis of the mood data depicted in Figure 4, showing 35.5-day and 43-day periodicities in the data.

In a further 40% of the patients (N = 19), the mood cycle length was shorter than 3 weeks or longer than 5 weeks and did not appear to be related to the menstrual cycle. In most of the five remaining patients (11%), mood cycles were similar in duration to the menstrual cycle. In two patients, for whom extensive longitudinal observations were available, the two cycles could be seen to go gradually in and out of phase with one another (i.e., to exhibit different cycle durations). In a third patient, rapid cycling persisted during a pregnancy. For the remaining two, insufficient data were available to assess the relationship between the two types of cycles. Thus, although women appear especially vulnerable to rapid cycling, the reason for their vulnerability is still unknown.

Alarcon made the interesting observation that the extremely rare patients with 48-hr mood cycles (1 day up, 1 day down) are an exception to the general rule about women and rapid cycling, and almost all of these rapid cyclers are men (9).

SLEEP-WAKE CYCLES AND MOOD CYCLES

Many patients experience dramatic changes in the timing and duration of sleep during the course of their rapid manic-depressive cycles. The results of experiments, in which the timing and duration of patients' sleep has been manipulated, suggest that sleep changes are not merely symptoms of the illness, but may play an intimate role in the biological mechanisms that are responsible for the mood cycles. Patients often experience profound insomnia when they switch from the depressed to the manic phase of the cycle. Sometimes, the insomnia takes the form of alternate nights of total sleep loss (i.e., 48-hr sleep-wake cycles; see Fig. 2) (7). These same patients can be made to switch from depression into mania when they are deprived of sleep for one night during the depressive phase (Fig. 6) (7). Thus, the reduction of sleep that occurs at the onset of mania may actually help to cause the switch from depression to mania, or to exacerbate it (10).

The results of sleep deprivation experiments have implications for treatment and prevention of affective states in patients with cyclic mood disorders. First, the severity of mania might be attenuated by sleep-enhancing treatments (10), and second, the depressive episodes might be terminated by therapeutic sleep deprivation.

The biological mechanisms of the antidepressant and mania-inducing effects of sleep deprivation are not yet known. One possibility currently being investigated is that sleep deprivation elevates mood by stimulating nocturnal thyrotropin (TSH) secretion. In healthy individuals, TSH secretion remains

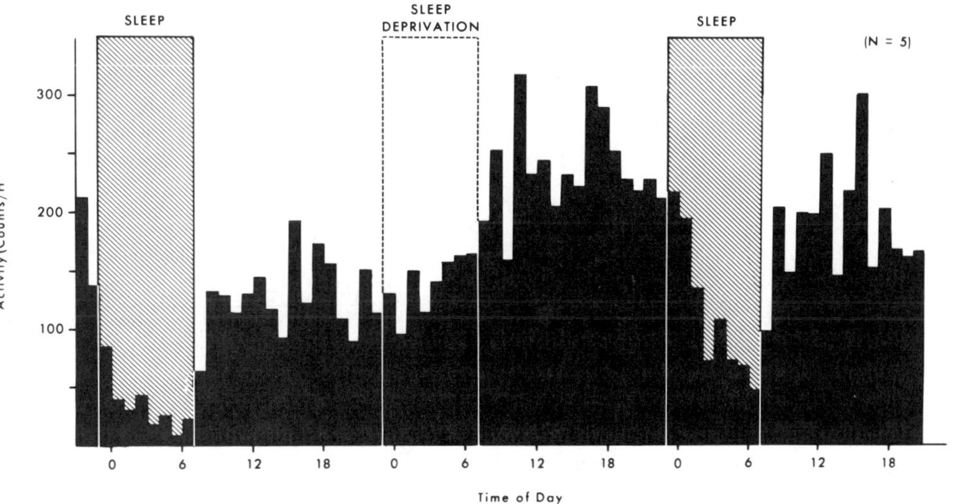

Figure 6 Marked increase in wrist motor activity levels in five rapid-cycling patients who switched from depression to mania during one night's total sleep deprivation. (Reprinted from Ref. 10.)

at low, basal levels during the daytime, but exhibits a secretory surge at night, which is thought to be necessary for the tropic support of the thyroid gland (Fig. 7) (11). Patients with rapid-cycling affective disorder (like other types of depressed patients) lack this nocturnal surge in TSH secretion (see Fig. 7) (12), and their TSH levels remain low during the night. Sleep deprivation stimulates TSH secretion, tends to restore its deficient nocturnal surge, and elevates mood (12). Whether the effects of sleep deprivation on mood are mediated by its effects on the hypothalamic-pituitary-thyroid axis has not yet been determined.

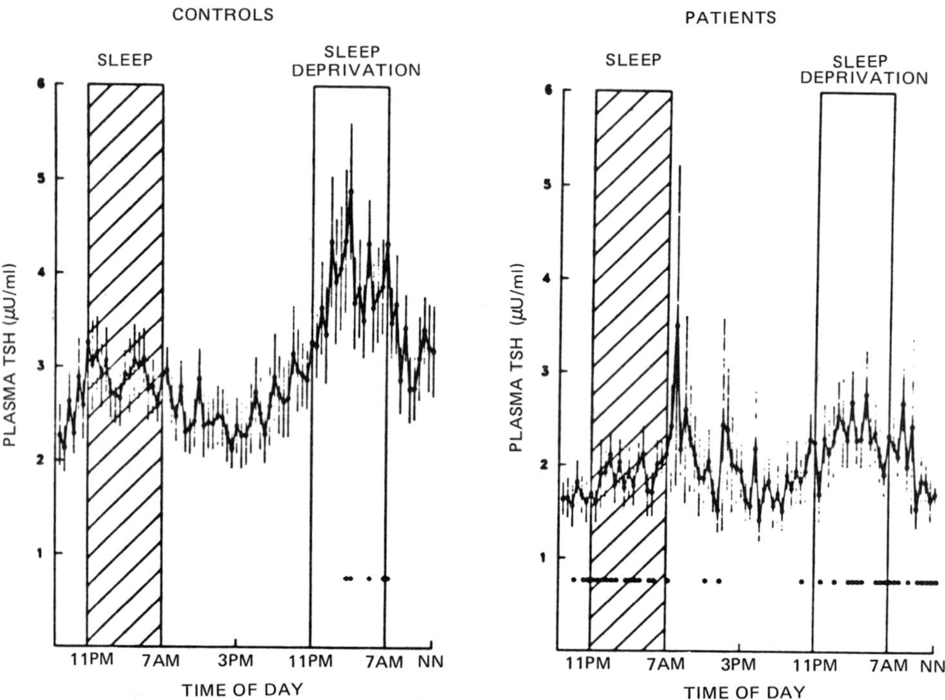

Figure 7 Around-the-clock profiles of plasma thyrotropin (TSH) levels in normal individuals (*left*) and depressed rapid cycling patients (*right*) studied during a night of normal sleep and a subsequent night of total sleep deprivation. TSH levels are lower in the patient group, especially at night. Sleep deprivation increases TSH levels and, in patients, improves mood. (Reprinted from Ref. 12).

THYROID DISEASE AND RAPID CYCLING

Early in the 20th century, the Norwegian psychiatrist, Gjessing, observed that rapid mood cycles were associated with cycles in nitrogen retention and excretion (13). He used thyroid treatments to drive the organism to a fixed and extreme state of negative nitrogen balance and found that the rapid mood cycles ceased. Since Gjessing, there have been reports that thyroid function might be abnormal in rapid-cycling affective disorder and that thyroid hormones might be used to treat it.

We found that the nocturnal surge in TSH secretion is lacking in depressed rapid-cycling patients (although this feature does not distinguish them from non-rapid-cycling depressed patients). Cho et al. (14) and our group (15) also reported a relatively high prevalence of lithium-induced hypothyroidism in rapid-cycling patients. However, our recent study in which we controlled for gender, age, and exposure to lithium, casts some doubt on this finding (3). We found that 47% of rapid cycling women and 39% of non-rapid-cycling women with bipolar illness had thyroid disease, usually hypothyroidism. Patients were considered to have thyroid disease only if thyroid hormone levels were repeatedly abnormal and thyroid treatments were prescribed. In these patients, the thyroid disease was diagnosed sometime after the onset of affective illness in 90% of each group, in rapid-cycling patients, sometime after the onset of rapid-cycling in 80%, and, during lithium treatment, in 60-70% of cases. More than 20% of the patients in each group had first-degree relatives with thyroid disease. The high prevalence of thyroid disease during lithium treatment in both rapid-cycling and non-rapid-cycling women was consistent with Transbol et al.'s report of a high prevalence of hypothyroidism in women over 40 years of age who were treated with lithium (16). The high prevalence of thyroid disease in rapid-cycling patients may simply reflect that most of these patients are women, that thyroid disease is much more common in women than in men, and that most of the patients had been treated with lithium, a known thyrotoxin. These findings do not necessarily argue against the possibility that thyroid disease is connected in some way to the susceptibility for rapid cycling. Women are much more susceptible to rapid cycling than men. Women's susceptibility to rapid cycling could be related to their much greater susceptibility to thyroid disease.

Since Gjessing, there have been other reports that thyroid hormones might be used to treat rapid-cycling affective disorder. Stancer and Persad found that treatment-resistant patients, especially women, appeared to respond to hypermetabolic doses of thyroxine (17). In subsequent controlled studies, Whybrow et al. (personal communication) and our group (unpublished data) have found that some rapid cycling patients became euthymic during treatment with hypermetabolic doses of thyroxine. However, patients ultimately appeared to develop tolerance to this effect and resumed cycling within a year. Therefore, the usefulness of thyroid treatments in rapid-cycling affective disorder has still not been convincingly demonstrated.

ANTIDEPRESSANT DRUGS AND RAPID CYCLING

In about one-third of our bipolar patients, the onset of their first manic or hypomanic episode occurred during treatment with antidepressant drugs (3). In 73%, the onset of rapid cycling occurred with various thymoleptic drugs, especially tricyclic antidepressant (94%; Table 4). These findings raise the possibility that mania and rapid cycling might be induced by antidepressant drugs. In fact, we found that rapid cycling appeared to depend on the continuing administration of antidepressant drugs in 51% of the rapid-cycling patients. In these patients, cycling occurred rapidly during periods of drug administration and dramatically slowed or stopped when the drugs were withdrawn (Fig. 8). In 17 of these patients (33% of the entire rapid-cycling group), longitudinal observations carried out after drugs were discontinued and replaced with placebo confirmed that rapid cycling did not occur when antidepressants were not administered. For 10 of these 17 patients (20% of the entire rapid-cycling group), longitudinal observations carried out both during periods of antidepressant treatment and periods of no treatment confirmed that rapid cycling depended on antidepressant treatment (Table 5).

There have been several reports that antidepressant medications may increase the frequency of recurrences after the acute treatment of a depressive episode. In the German literature, several investigators have claimed that antidepressants sometimes transform the illness from an episodic course with

Table 4 Effects of Treatments in Rapid-Cycling Affective Disorder

Author (Ref.)	N	Onset during antidepressant treatment (%)	Remission (%)
Stancer et al. (42)	7		0
Dunner et al. (2)[a]	17		24
Kukopulos et al. (21)	118	>50	
Alarcon (9)	15	55	
Wehr et al. (3)	51	73	32

[a]Nearly 100% taking antidepressants.

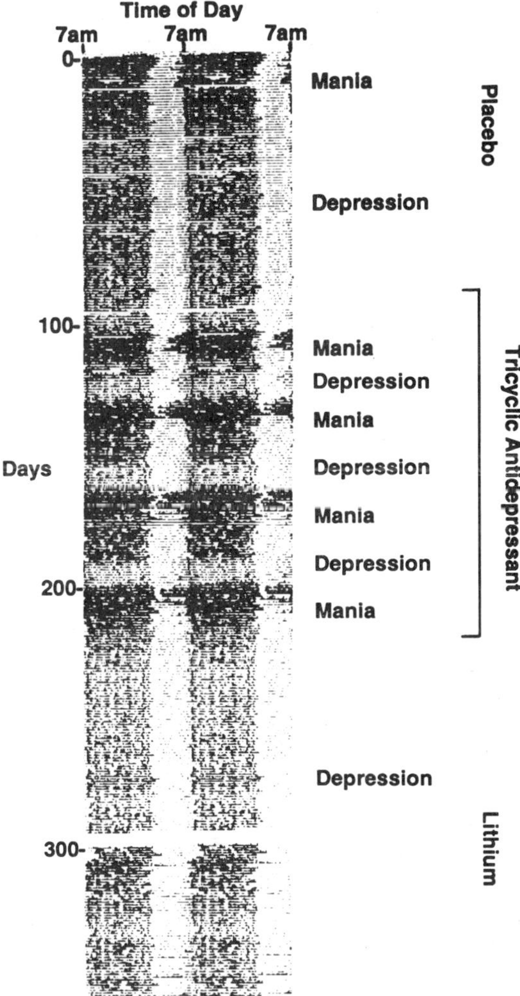

Figure 8 Record of motor activity in a manic-depressive patient showing reversible induction of rapid cycling by a tricyclic antidepressant. Level of activity was recorded every 15 min by an electronic device worn on the wrist. Twenty-four-hour segments of activity data beginning at 7:00 AM are plotted successively beneath one another, and the entire display is double-plotted to the right as a visual aid. Dark vertical elements correspond to activity during wakefulness; light vertical elements correspond to rest during sleep. Depression is characterized by low activity (lighter sections, as indicated), mania by high activity and reduced sleep (darker sections, as indicated).

Table 5 Mean Cycle Duration (Days) and Number of Cycles Observed On and Off Tricyclic Antidepressants in 10 Rapid-Cycling Patients

Patient	Off	On	Off	On	Off
	X ± SD (N)	X ± SD (N)	X ± SD (N)	X ± SD (N)	X ± SD (N)
1.	90 ± 8 (14)	65 ± 12 (13)			
2.	127 (1+)	42 ± 11 (25)	128 ± 30 (3)		
3.	63 (1+)	23 ± 9 (4)	52 (1+)		
4.	98 (1+)	22 ± 13 (26)	85 ± 16 (2+)	6 ± 0 (2)	
5.		59 ± 9 (15)	269 ± 98 (4)		
6.		42 (1)	188 (1)		
7.		23 ± 1 (5)	105 (1+)		
8.		39 ± 13 (29)	221 (1)	53 ± 6 (6)	
9.		47 ± 9 (7)	151 (1)	41 ± 10 (3)	104 (1+)
10.		52 ± 16 (8)	213 (1)	46 ± 6 (4)	42 ± 5 (3)

The plus symbol (+) indicates that the patient did not complete a full cycle during the observation period (some patients may have stopped cycling).
Source: Data from patients 2, 3, 4, 7, and 10 from Ref. 8.

free intervals to a chronic course with continuous cycles (*Chronifizierung*) (18-21). In some cases, the drugs produce a destabilization (*Labilizierung*) characterized by the occurrence, for the first time, of hypomania followed by continual cycling between hypomania and depression. This type of antidepressant-induced rapid cycling was first described in 1956 in a tuberculosis patient treated with iproniazid (Fig. 9; 22), and since that time, numerous reports of similar cases have appeared (Table 6) (18-31). In most instances, these reports were based on uncontrolled studies that were partly or wholly retrospective.

In contrast, we have conducted placebo-controlled, prospective, double-blind studies. However, in interpreting our results it is noteworthy that the patients studied were those who required referral to a specialized research center. Furthermore, it is difficult to determine what percentage of bipolar patients in other settings might develop drug-induced rapid cycling when treated with antidepressants because rapid cycling has seldom been looked for, and patients who exhibit the response have either been excluded from studies or their antidepressants have been stopped and observations discontinued before they began to cycle (32).

The mechanism by which antidepressants induce rapid cycling is unknown. However, there is a similarity between the rapid-cycling response and the more conventional antidepressant response. The rapid-cycling response usually

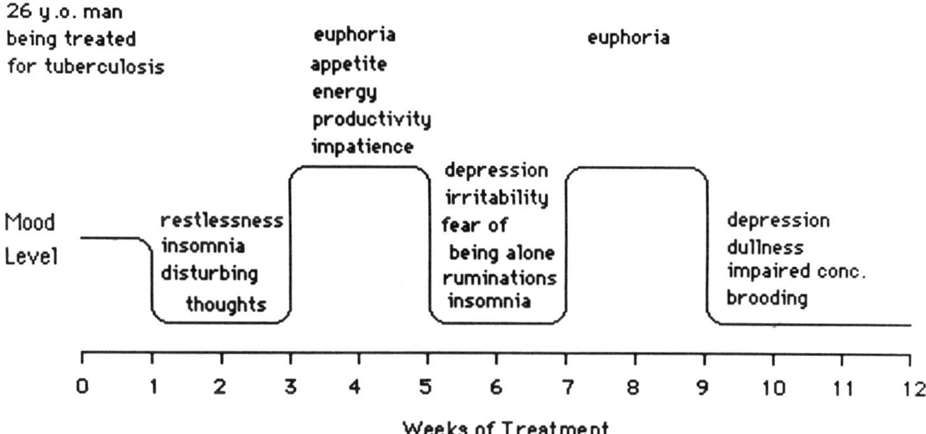

Figure 9 Schematic diagram of clinical notes describing MAOI-induced rapid cycling in a patient who was treated for tuberculosis with the drug. This description by Crane in 1956 (22) antedates the use of these drugs as antidepressants and may be the first report of antidepressant-induced rapid cycling.

Table 6 Induction of Rapid Cycling by Antidepressants

Authors (Ref.)	No. patients (%)	Drug
Crane (22)	1	MAOI
Arnold and Kryspin-Exner (18)	1	Tricyclic
Till and Vuckovic (19)	7 (27)	Tricyclic
Coppen et al. (23)	2 (67)	Tricyclic
Van Scheyen (24)	2 (2)	Tricyclic
Wehr and Goodwin (25)	6	Tricyclic, MAOI
Siris et al. (26)	1	Tricyclic
Kukopulos et al. (20)	59 (51)	Tricyclic, MAOI
Lerer et al. (27)	1	Tricyclic
Ko et al. (28)	1	L-Dopa
Mattson and Seltzer (29)	1	MAOI
Extein et al. (30)	1	Tricyclic
Oppenheim (31)	1	Tricyclic
Oppenheim (1984)	1	Estrogen
Wehr et al. (10)	26[a] (51)	Tricyclic
Total	105	

[a]Cumulative total

begins when a patient who has been depressed is treated with an antidepressant. After 3 weeks or so, the patient switches out of depression and into mania or hypomania. So far, the response resembles that of other bipolar patients. However, after another 3 weeks or so, the patient switches back into depression, and then back into mania or hypomania. The rapid cycling has begun. During the drug-induced rapid cycles, however, the intervals between the beginning and the end of each depressive episode are similar in duration to the interval between the onset of treatment and the conventional antidepressant response (i.e., about 3 weeks). It is as though the patient cycles through the antidepressant response over and over again. Perhaps the process that drives the cycle is the same process that drives most depressed patients toward their remission about 3 weeks after they begin treatment (Fig. 10).

The fact that antidepressants can induce rapid cycling has seldom been considered in descriptions of the clinical course of affective patients or in interpretations of their response to treatment. For example, novel drugs or procedures reported to be effective in the maintenance treatment of recurrent affective disorder have often been instituted after extended or repeated periods of treatment with antidepressants drugs. In these cases, investiga-

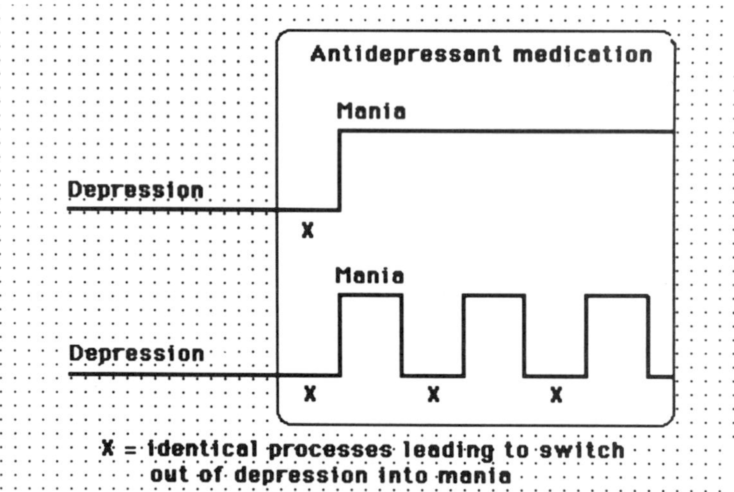

Figure 10 Schematic diagram showing possible relationship between the more common case of antidepressant-induced switch out of depression into mania (*top*), and the less common case of antidepressant-induced rapid cycling between depression and mania (*bottom*). The diagram highlights the similarity in durations (indicated by x) of depressive phases of the rapid cycles and the usual latency of onset of action after initiation of treatment.

tors have usually attributed cessation of mood swings to the new treatment regimens, but have neglected the possibility that withdrawal of previous antidepressants may be partly responsible for the change. Studies of the natural course of affective disorder may have been contaminated by the effect of antidepressants, and increases in the frequency of affective episodes, thought to be associated with increasing age and with duration of illness, could have resulted, in part, from the cycle-accelerating effects of antidepressant medications (33).

THE MECHANISM OF RAPID CYCLING

The mechanism of rapid cycling is unknown, but there have been several hypotheses put forth. Halberg proposed that cycles of several weeks duration could arise (1) if depression and mania were caused by abnormal phase relationships between circadian rhythms and sleep, and (2) if the circadian rhythms were not entrained to the 24-hr day-night cycle (as they usually are), but were to free-run according to their own intrinsic rhythm (usually about 25 hr), generating beat frequencies of one cycle every few weeks (34). Kripke et al. studied circadian rhythms in rapid-cycling patients and interpreted their results as supporting Halberg's hypothesis (35). However, there are methodological shortcomings in their study, and there is little additional evidence to support the theory. According to another hypothesis, rapid cycles might be generated by oscillations in neuroendocrine feedback systems caused by loss of glandular tissue, or delayed responses or insensitivity to hormonal negative-feedback (25,36).

We have proposed the hypothesis that rapid cycling might be a derivative of seasonal affective disorder. The inspiration for this hypothesis comes from an animal model. The edible dormouse (*Glis glis*) is a nocturnal, arboreal rodent that lives in northern Europe. In the wild, it hibernates once a year. If this animal is kept indoors in a laboratory, it no longer exhibits annual hibernation cycles, but shifts to a pattern of rapid cycles in behavior and physiology that appear to be abortive hibernation cycles (37). These cycles include characteristics that are reminiscent of manic-depressive illness, such as changes in appetite, weight, the duration and timing of sleep, levels of activity, degree of interaction with the environment, libido, and in hypothalamic-pituitary-thyroid and hypothalamic-pituitary-adrenal axes (Fig. 11). The rapidity of cycling appears to depend on ambient temperature; the warmer the room the more rapid the cycles.

Affective illness is also sensitive to seasonal changes in the physical environment. Episodes of depression and mania are more likely to begin in the spring and fall than at other times of year (reviewed in reference 38). These tendencies are most fully expressed in individuals whose episodes recur on

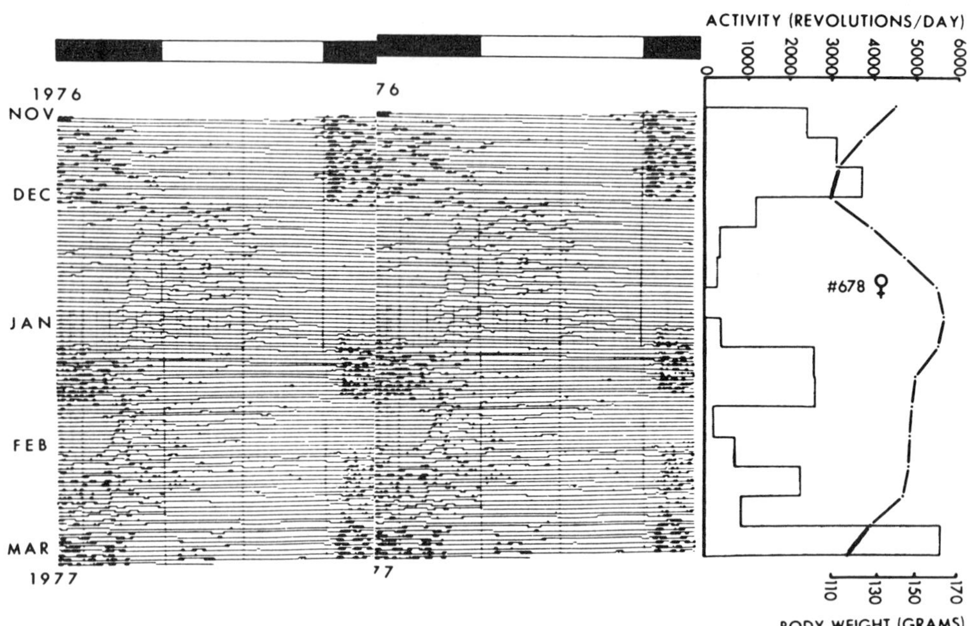

Figure 11 Raster plot of continuously recorded wheel-running activity, total wheel revolutions per day, and daily weight, in a wild rodent (*Glis glis*), which normally hibernates out-of-doors, but was studied while living in a climate-controlled laboratory (see legend Fig. 8 for explanation of raster plot). Removed from its natural environment, this animal appears to have shifted from its usual pattern of seasonal cycles in activity and weight to rapid cycles spanning several weeks. (Reprinted from Ref. 37.) Compare with Figure 8.

an annual basis and produce regular patterns of winter depression, summer depression, or combined summer and winter depression (reviewed in reference 38). Some types of seasonal affective disorder appear to be driven by seasonal changes in environmental light. According to our hypothesis, rapid-cycling affective disorder might arise from seasonal rhythms that have escaped from control by annual cycles in nature because humans live in an artificial environment (similar to the edible dormouse in the laboratory setting). A corollary is that antidepressants might induce rapid cycling through their capacity to alter sensitivity to environmental temperature (as the environmental temperature modulates the frequency of rapid cycling by the edible dormouse) (Fig. 12).

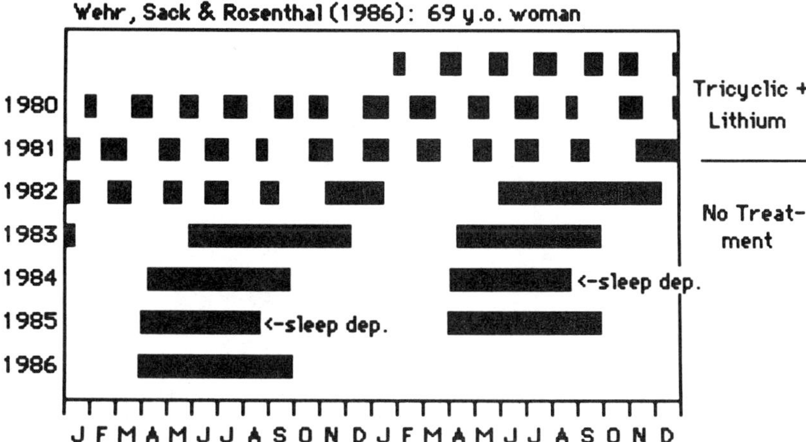

Figure 12 Raster plot showing manic-depressive cycles in a patient who exhibited rapid cycling during treatment with a tricyclic antidepressant and lithium and seasonal cycling when she was not treated with drugs. (See legend Fig. 4 for explanation of raster plot). This raster plot was constructed by plotting *1-year* segments of data successively beneath one another, and depicting *depressive* phases as dark horizontal line segments and *manic* phases as open spaces between the line segments. (Wehr et al., unpublished data).

RELATIONSHIP OF RAPID-CYCLING TO NON-RAPID-CYCLING AFFECTIVE DISORDERS

Although rapid cyclers are uncommon and comprise 15% or fewer of patients in lithium or affective disorder clinics (3), there are more reasons than not to consider them to be related to more typical bipolar patients (1).

1. Rapid cycling appears to represent an extreme development of the intrinsic features of bipolar illness. Similar to rapid cycling, bipolar illness, in general, is distinguished by (a) a tendency to remit and recur spontaneously and with increasing frequency (33); (b) a tendency for manic episodes to be immediately preceded or followed by depressive episodes, with no intervening normal period (5); and (c) for mania to alternate with depression (39).
2. Many patients with rapid-cycling affective disorder begin their illness as non-rapid-cycling patients (3).
3. The pattern of age of onset in rapid-cycling patients is identical with that of non-rapid-cycling patients (see Fig. 1) (3,5).

Table 7 Family History In Rapid-Cycling Affective Disorder

		% Affective illness in first degree relatives			
Author (Ref.)	N	Total	BP	UP	RCAD
Stancer et al. (42)	7	71	29	57	
Dunner et al. (2)	29		38	34	
Alarcon (9)	15	55	27	27	9
Wehr et al. (3)	51	59	27	41	12

BP, bipolar disorder; UP, unipolar disorder; RCAD, rapid-cycling affective disorder.

4. The clinical pictures of manic and depressive episodes are the same in rapid-cycling and non-rapid-cycling forms of bipolar illness.
5. More than 50% of rapid-cycling patients have first-degree relatives with affective illness, and most of these do not have rapid cycling (Table 7) (3). In other words, rapid-cycling affective disorder is genetically related to non-rapid-cycling affective disorder.

TREATMENT OF RAPID-CYCLING AFFECTIVE DISORDER

In a follow-up study of the 51 rapid-cycling patients treated in our program, we found that 41% continued to cycle rapidly; 16% had stopped rapid cycling, but continued to have very slow cycles of mania and depression or protracted periods of depression; 6% had nearly complete remission, with only brief and infrequent episodes of mania or depression; and 32% had complete remissions (3) (Fig. 13; see Table 4).

Treatments most often associated with remission were lithium and, less frequently, low doses of monoamine oxidase inhibitors (MAOIs), alone or in combination (Tables 8 and 9) (3). Two patients had remissions when they discontinued all drugs. Four had temporary remissions lasting 9 months to 5 years during treatment with lithium, hydroxyzine, hypermetabolic doses of thyroxine, or during pregnancy. Twenty-seven patients who failed to respond to lithium were subsequently treated with carbamazepine, sometimes in combination with lithium or other drugs. Two patients responded to the combination of carbamazepine and tranylcypromine or thioridazine. The remainder of the carbamazepine-treated group (N=25; 93%) continued to experience rapid cycling. Two patients who were treated with verapamil responded. Almost without exception, treatments involving tricyclic antidepressants, neuroleptics, or ECT were unsuccessful in stopping the rapid cycling. In those patients who continued to experience rapid cycling, in spite of treatment with lithium and/or carbamazepine, these drugs appeared to be beneficial insofar as they abbreviated and attenuated the manic phase of the cycles.

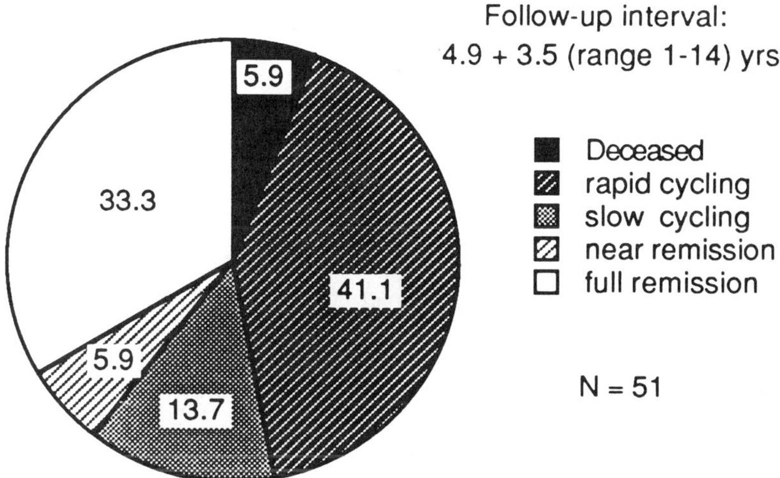

Figure 13 Outcome in 51 rapid-cycling patients. (From data in Ref. 3.)

Other factors that coincided with cessation of rapid cycling, and may have contributed to patients' remissions, included discontinuation of tricyclic antidepressants or neuroleptics (N = 12), temporary treatment with the MAOI, clorgyline (N = 2), and transient thyroxine toxicity (N = 1). Except for prior suicide attempts, no clinical features distinguished the nonresponders from the responders to treatment.

As described earlier, 47% of the rapid-cycling patients developed hypothyroidism, usually during lithium treatment (3). Consequently, it is important to monitor thyroid function in these patients and to institute replacement treatment when appropriate. Whether or not treatment of hypothyroidism improves their clinical state or the response to antidepressant medication is unknown, but this possibility needs to be considered.

In considering the treatment of treatment-resistant rapid-cycling-patients, withdrawal of antidepressant medication is the first intervention that should be considered. Seven (14%) of our 51 patients eventually became euthymic after withdrawal of antidepressants (N = 6) or neuroleptics (N = 1) while they continued to be treated with lithium alone (3). In some patients who ultimately responded to treatment with lithium alone, lithium had been ineffective in treating antidepressant-induced rapid cycling. Thus, patients should not be considered to be lithium nonresponders until they have been treated unsuccessfully with lithium alone. In those patients whose cycling persists during lithium treatment, carbamazepine is occasionally effective; however, it is usually only the severity of the manic phase that is attenuated by carbamazepine alone or in combination with lithium. Sometimes, patients

Table 8 Interventions That by Themselves or in Combination with Other Interventions Were Associated with Complete or Nearly Complete Remissions in 19 (37%) of 51 Patients Treated for Rapid-Cycling Affective Disorder

Intervention	Patients treated N (%)[a]	Patients in remission N (%)[b]
Discontinuation		
TCA and/or NL	42 (82)	12 (29)
Maintenance treatment		
Lithium	51 (100)	12 (24)
MAOI	37 (73)	4 (11)
Carbamazepine	27 (53)	2 (7)
Verapamil	2 (4)	2 (100)
TCA	49 (96)	2 (4)
NL	32 (63)	1 (3)
ECT	24 (47)	0
High-dose T_4	6 (12)	0
No drug	30 (59)	2 (7)

[a]Percentage of total sample.
[b]Percentage of treated patients.

whose cycling stops when antidepressants are discontinued, remain depressed for long periods, in spite of treatment with lithium carbonate. In our experience it was difficult to treat these depressions without including rapid cycling once again. In some cases, we have attempted to bring patients out of depression gradually without inducing mania by using low doses of MAOIs, especially clorgyline (40). This strategy has been successful in four cases. Treatments that are associated with lasting remission are summarized in Table 9.

The percentage of patients who respond with rapid cycling to antidepressant treatment is unknown, but it is probably quite low in primary care settings. The practical point is that whenever rapid cycling occurs in a patient receiving an antidepressant, the possibility that the drug has caused the rapid cycling should be considered. In these patients, discontinuation of the antidepressant and administration of lithium or other mood stabilizers may lead to sustained remissions. The good outcome in nearly 40% of our treatment-resistant rapid-cycling patients attests to this strategy and contrasts with the negative findings with conventional treatment approaches reported by Prien et al. in 18 rapid-cycling patients (41).

Table 9 Maintenance Treatments Associated with Sustained Remissions in Rapid-Cycling Affective Disorder (N = 51)

Treatment	No. of patients
Lithium	7
Lithium + MAOI	2
Lithium + verapamil	1
Verapamil + TCA	1
Carbamazepine + neuroleptic	1
Carbamazepine + MAOI	1
MAOI	1
TCA	1
Neuroleptic	0
ECT	0
No drug	2
Total	17 (33%)

With drug-induced rapid cycling, it is important to remember that its discovery and treatment were dependent upon the discontinuation of medications for extended periods. This practice is often routine in research environments, but is uncommon in clinical settings. We have found that the application of research methods, such as drug-free periods of clinical observation and controlled interventions in which only one treatment variable is changed at a time, are particularly useful in the management of rapid-cycling patients. In this fashion, a significant number of these patients can ultimately attain substantial improvement in their cycling mood disorder.

REFERENCES

1. Dunner, D. L. and Fieve, R. R. (1974). Clinical factors in lithium carbonate prophylaxis failure. *Arch. Gen. Psychiatry 30*:229-233.
2. Dunner, D. L., Patrick, V., and Fieve, R. R. (1977). Rapid cycling manic-depressive patients. *Compr. Psychiatry 18*:561-566.
3. Wehr, T. A., Sack, D. A., Rosenthal, N. E., and Cowdry, R. W. (1988). Rapid cycling affective disorder: Contributing factors and treatment responses in 51 patients. *Am. J. Psychiatry 145*:179-184.
4. Sedler, M. J. and Dessain, E. C. (1983). Falret's discovery: The origin of the concept of bipolar affective illness. *Am. J. Psychiatry 140*:1127-1133.
5. Winokur, G., Clayton, P., and Reich, T. (1977). *Manic Depressive Illness.* St. Louis, C.V. Mosby.
6. Wehr, T. A. (1977). Phase and biorhythm studies of manic-depressive illness. *Ann. Intern. Med. 87*:321-324.

7. Wehr, T. A., Wirz-Justice, A., Goodwin, F. K., Breitmeier, J., and Craig, C. (1982). 48-Hour sleep-wake cycles in manic-depressive illness: Naturalistic observations and sleep deprivation experiments. *Arch. Gen. Psychiatry 39*:559-565.
8. Wehr, T. A. and Goodwin, F. K. (1983). Biological rhythms and manic-depressive illness. In *Circadian Rhythms and Psychiatry*. Edited by T. A. Wehr and F. K. Goodwin. Pacific Grove, Calif., Boxwood Press, pp. 129-184.
9. Alarcon, R. D. (1985). Rapid cycling affective disorders: A clinical review. *Compr. Psychiatry 26*:522-540.
10. Wehr, T. A., Sack, D. A., and Rosenthal, N. E. (1987). Sleep reduction as a final common pathway in the genesis of mania. *Am. J. Psychiatry 144*:201-204.
11. Parker, D. C., Pekary, A. E., and Hershman, J. M. (1976). Effect of normal and reversed sleep-wake cycles upon nyctohemeral rhythmicity of plasma thyrotropin: Evidence suggestive of an inhibitory influence in sleep. *J. Clin. Endocrinol. 43*:318-329.
12. Sack, D. A., James, S. P., Rosenthal, N. E., and Wehr, T. A. (1988). Deficient nocturnal surge of TSH during sleep and sleep deprivation in rapid cycling bipolar illness. *Psychiatry Res. 23*:179-191.
13. Gjessing, R. R. (1976). *Contribution to the Somatology of Periodic Catatonia.* Edited by L. Gjessing and F. A. Jenner. Oxford, Pergamon Press.
14. Cho, J. T., Bone, S., Dunner, D. L., Colt, E., and Fieve, R. R. (1979). The effect of lithium treatment on thyroid function in patients with primary affective disorder. *Am. J. Psychiatry 136*:115-116.
15. Cowdry, R. W., Wehr, T. A., Zis, A. P., and Goodwin, F. K. (1983). Thyroid abnormalities associated with rapid cycling bipolar illness. *Arch. Gen. Psychiatry 40*:414-420.
16. Transbol, I., Christiansen, C., and Baastrup, P. C. (1978). Endocrine effects of lithium. *Acta Endocrinol. 87*:759-767.
17. Stancer, H. C. and Persad, E. (1982). Treatment of intractable rapid cycling manic-depressive disorder with levothyroxine. *Arch. Gen. Psychiatry 39*:311-312.
18. Arnold, O. H. and Kryspin-Exner, K. (1965). Zur Frage der Beeinflussung des Verlaufes des manisch-depressiven Krankheitsgeschehens durch Antidepressiva. *Wien. Med. Wochenschr. 45/46*:929-934.
19. Till, E. and Vuckovic, S. (1970). Uber den Einfluss der thymoleptischen Behandlung auf den Verlauf endogener Depressionen. *Int. Pharmacopsychiatry 4*:210-219.
20. Kukopulos, A., Reginaldi, D., Laddomada, P., Floris, G., Serra, G., and Tondo, L. (1980). Course of the manic-depressive cycle and changes caused by treatments. *Pharmacopsychiatry 13*:156-167.
21. Kukopulos, A., Caliari, B., Tundo, A., Minnai, G., Floris, G., Reginaldi, D., and Tondo, L. (1983). Rapid cyclers, temperament, and antidepressants. *Compr. Psychiatry 24*:249-258.
22. Crane, G. E. (1956). The psychiatric side-effects of iproniazid. *Am. J. Psychiatry 112*:494-501.
23. Coppen, A., Whybrow, P. C., Noguera, R., Maggs, R., and Prange, A. J., Jr. (1972). The comparative antidepressant value of L-tryptophan and imipramine

with and without attempted potentiation by liothyronine. *Arch. Gen. Psychiatry 26*:234-241.

24. Van Scheyen, J. D. (1973). Recurrent vital depressions. *Psychiatr. Neurol. Neurochir. 76*:93-112.
25. Wehr, T. A. and Goodwin, F. K. (1979). Rapid cycling in manic-depressives induced by tricyclic antidepressants. *Arch. Gen. Psychiatry 36*:555-559.
26. Siris, S., Chertoff, H. R., and Perel, J. M. (1979). Rapid-cycling affective disorder during imipramine treatment: A case report. *Am. J. Psychiatry 136*:341-342.
27. Lerer, B., Birmacher, B., Ebstein, R. P., and Belmaker, R. H. (1980). Forty-eight-hour depressive cycling induced by antidepressant. *Br. J. Psychiatry 137*: 183-185.
28. Ko, G. N., Leckman, J. F., and Heninger, G. R. (1981). Induction of rapid mood cycling during L-dopa treatment in a bipolar patient. *Am. J. Psychiatry 138*: 1624-1675.
29. Mattson, A. and Seltzer, R. L. (1981). MAOI-induced rapid cycling bipolar affective disorder in an adolescent. *Am. J. Psychiatry 138*:677-679.
30. Extein, I., Pottash, A. L. C., and Gold, M. S. (1982). Does subclinical hypothyroidism predispose to tricyclic-induced rapid cycles? *J. Clin. Psychiatry 43*: 290-291.
31. Oppenheim, G. (1982). Drug-induced rapid cycling: Possible outcomes and management. *Am. J. Psychiatry 139*:939-941.
32. Wehr, T. A. and Goodwin, F. K. (1987). Do antidepressants cause mania and worsen the course of affective illness? *Am. J. Psychiatry 144*:1403-1411.
33. Grof, P., Angst, J., and Haines, T. (1974). The clinical course of depression: Practical issues. In *Symposia Medica Hoechst 8*: *Classification and Prediction of Outcome of Depression*. Edited by J. Angst. New York, Schattauer Verlag, pp. 141-148.
34. Halberg, F. (1967). Physiologic considerations underlying rhythmometry with special reference to emotional illness. Bel-Air Symposium, Geneva. In *Ajuriaguerra J de* (*Hrsg.*), *Cycles Biologiques et Psychiatric*. Paris, 1968.
35. Kripke, D. F., Delaney, D. J., Atkinson, M., and Wolf, S. (1978). Circadian rhythm disorders in manic-depressives. *Biol. Psychiatry 13*:335-350.
36. Morley, A. (1970). Periodic diseases, physiological rhythms and feedback control—a hypothesis. *Abstr. Ann. Med. 3*:244-249.
37. Mrosovsky, N., Melnyk, R. B., Lang, K., Hallonquist, J. D., Boshes, M., and Joy, J. E. (1980). Infradian cycles in dormice. *J. Comp. Physiol. 137*:315-339.
38. Wehr, T. A. and Rosenthal, N. E. (1989). The seasonality of affective illness. *Am. J. Psychiatry 146*:829-839.
39. Kukopulos, A. and Reginaldi, D. (1973). Does lithium prevent depressions by suppressing manias? *Int. Pharmacopsychiatry 8*:152-158.
40. Potter, W. Z., Murphy, D., Wehr, T. A., Linnoila, M., and Goodwin, F. K. (1982). Clorgyline: A new treatment for refractory rapid-cycling patients? *Arch. Gen. Psychiatry 39*:505-510.
41. Prien, R. F., Kupfer, D. J., Mansky, P. A., Small, J. G., Tuason, V. B., Voss, C. B., and Johnson, W. E. (1984). Drug therapy in the prevention of recurrences

in unipolar and bipolar affective disorders: Report of the NIMH Collaborative Study Group comparing lithium carbonate, imipramine, and a lithium carbonate-imipramine combination. *Arch. Gen. Psychiatry 41*:1096-1104.
42. Stancer, H. C., Furlong, F. W., and Godse, D. D. (1970). A longitudinal investigation of lithium as a prophylactic agent for recurrent depressions. *Can. Psychiatr. Assoc. J. 15*:29-40.
43. Squillace, K., Post, R. M., Savard, R., and Erwin-Gorman, M. (1984). Life charting of recurrent affective illness. In *Neurobiology of Mood Disorders*. Edited by R. M. Post and J. C. Ballenger. Baltimore, Williams & Wilkins.

22

Sleep and Affective Disorders

STEVEN P. JAMES and JAY D. AMSTERDAM

University of Pennsylvania School of Medicine, Philadelphia, Pennsylvania

Complaints of disrupted sleep frequently accompany episodes of depression. In most instances, insomnia occurs with mood changes, and early-morning awakening is a common symptom of depression. Evidence suggests that these symptoms are more than simply secondary phenomena, and they may indicate physiological disturbances in affective illness.

Sleep is evaluated in the laboratory setting by three measurements: the electroencephalogram (EEG), the electrooculogram (EOG), and the electromyogram (EMG). The relationship between these three measurements determines the stage of sleep and is referred to as stage 1, 2, 3, 4, and rapid eye movement (REM) sleep. The first four stages of sleep are called non-REM (NREM), and stage 3 and 4 are also subdivided into slow-wave sleep (SWS).

In normal individuals sleep occurs with a regular and cyclic pattern. When a healthy young adult falls asleep, approximately 120 min of NREM sleep occurs before the first REM period begins. After the first REM period is completed (approximately 10-15 min), another cycle of NREM sleep commences and continues until the next occurrence of REM sleep. Thus, every 90-120 min REM sleep recurs, and this cycle continues throughout the night until the individual awakens the next morning.

This well-organized periodic activity in sleep is often disrupted in depression. Approximately 90% of depressed patients have complaints of insomnia. Once asleep, their sleep is shallow, with a decrease in slow-wave sleep (1).

Continual awakening during sleep is a fairly common finding, and frequent sleep stage changes occur throughout the night.

In other instances, depressed patients may report hypersomnolence, rather than insomnia (2). Although hypersomnolent patients represent no more than 10% of the total number of depressed individuals, a high proportion of these individuals are in their teens and 20s. Detre et al. (3) reported that hypersomnolent depressives were frequently found to overeat and gain weight, and to have a marked diurnal variation in mood, with increased depression in the morning.

Alterations in REM sleep are frequently found in affective disorders. Although early studies suggested that a decrease in the total amount of REM sleep was involved in the expression of depression (4), subsequent studies found that the distribution of REM sleep, rather than its duration, was related to affective disorders.

The finding that the onset of REM sleep occurred closer to the initiation of sleep (shortened REM latency) has been widely reported (5-13). In addition, early studies reported that an increasing severity of the depressed mood resulted in the rapid onset of REM sleep (14,15). Giles has also reported that a persistence in short REM latencies during a depression remission may also predict future depressive relapse (16). Finally, Kupfer et al. (17) have reported that the amount of delay of REM onset after administration of amitriptyline predicted the ultimate response to treatment.

Despite the findings that a short REM latency is associated with depression, not all studies are in agreement. Shipley et al. (18) did not confirm any significant change in REM latency in his depressed patients, and noted that the night-to-night variability in all sleep parameters limited the clinical usefullness of any one sleep recording parameter.

One possible explanation for the differences in REM latency between studies could be an increased variability in REM sleep. Several groups have evaluated this possibility with differing results. For example, Kerhofs et al. performed sleep records on depressed patients for three consecutive nights and found a tendency for REM sleep to occur earlier on each successive night (19). Ansseau et al. (20) recorded the sleep of depressed patients for four consecutive nights and observed a unimodal peak in the occurrence of REM latency between 50 and 59 min. Other groups, however, have found a bimodal distribution of REM sleep in patients undergoing repetitive polysomnography, with peak occurrence between 10 and 19 min for some, and 40 and 60 min in others (18,21,22).

The specificity of the laboratory finding must also be considered. An alteration in mood may be the result of various factors, including various psychological and medical conditions, in addition to endogenous depression. Attempts to find an association between a short REM latency and endogenous depression have resulted in inconclusive findings, and Lund and Berger (23) reported that REM latency could not distinguish primary from secondary depression.

Other psychiatric conditions have also been associated with the rapid onset of REM sleep. Mendels and Hawkins (24) first reported short REM latencies in patients with mania or hypomania, whereas additional studies of obsessive-compulsive patients (25), depressed alcoholics (26), primary alcoholics (27), schizophrenic patients (28), anorexic patients (29), and divorcing women have also reported short REM latencies. Although the procedures and definitions of which sleep architectural and normative values differ among these studies, there is clearly a lack of diagnostic specificity for decreases in REM latency in psychiatric disorders.

A short REM latency is also found in many nonpsychiatric conditions. For example, the presence of a shortened REM latency during overnight sleep studies and during daytime naps is a common finding in narcolepsy. At other times, decreased REM latencies may be associated with sleep apnea syndromes and sleep deprivation in healthy individuals (31). Finally, although the physiological significance is unknown, volunteers living in temporal isolation chambers have demonstrated a strong correlation between sleep onset and the commencement of REM sleep (32).

Other aspects of REM sleep are altered in depression. Gresham et al. (33) first reported that the normal ultradian distribution of REM sleep is disturbed in depression. Healthy individuals usually show an increased amount of REM sleep in the last third of the night, compared with the first two-thirds. Depressed patients, however, frequently show a shift of REM sleep to the first third of the night, with a subsequent reduction in the REM periods during the final third of sleep (34).

The change in the distribution of REM sleep may also influence the duration of each REM period. In normal subjects there is a lengthening of each successive REM period. In depression, this progression in REM sleep duration is less obvious and may even show differences within subgroups of patients. For example, unipolar depressed patients have been reported to have no increase in the duration of REM sleep across the night. Furthermore, these patients also demonstrate little increase in the duration of the first REM sleep episode when compared with normal subjects. Interestingly, these changes in the ultradian distribution of REM sleep have not been found in bipolar depressed patients.

In addition to REM latency and the ultradian distribution of REM sleep, *REM density*, which is a measure of the number of eye movements over time during REM sleep, is also reported to be altered in depressed patients. Thus, an increase in the frequency of eye movements leads to the impression that the REM episode is more intense. Snyder (4) first noted this observation in depressed patients, and Kupfer et al. (35) confirmed this finding, especially during the first REM period. Unlike normal subjects in whom each successive REM period results in an increased REM density, depressed patients may demonstrate more intense REM sleep during the first episode, with a decrease in successive REM periods.

Some investigators have proposed that the increase in REM density may help in the diagnostic distinction between psychotic and neurotic depression (4,19). However, similar to the reports of shortened REM latency in depression, the specificity of the reports of increased REM density also remain unclear. Gillin et al. (36) reported an absence of changes in REM density during episodes of depression in some patients, whereas Sitaram et al. (37) found a persistently increased REM density between depressive episodes when patients were clinically euthymic.

SLEEP AS A CIRCADIAN RHYTHM DISTURBANCE IN DEPRESSION

The periodic rhythm of sleep and wake is frequently disrupted during affective illness. The finding of predictable mood cycles in some bipolar patients has suggested the possibility that the mechanisms regulating these affective states may also influence the sleep-wake cycle. Although predictable mood swings based upon 24-hr, 48-hr, monthly, and annual patterns have been described, most of the investigations have focused on the circadian regulation of sleep and other daily biological rhythms.

Chronobiological research in depression has focused on the "phase-advance hypothesis" to explain the many circadian changes found in the sleep of affectively ill patients. Weitzman (38) reported that sleep architecture was dramatically altered when normal subjects were required to abruptly change their time of sleep from 10:00 PM to 10:00 AM for 3 weeks. Snyder noted that sleep changes in this paradigm were similar to changes seen in the sleep of depressed patients. Specifically, the common findings included a short REM latency; a prolonged initial REM period; a redistribution of REM sleep such that a greater percentage occurred in the first third and a reduction in the final third of sleep; and an increased number of awakenings in the latter part of the sleep period, with an increase in cortisol secretion in the first half of sleep.

Papousek (39) hypothesized that these changes supported the concept that the circadian rhythm of REM sleep in depression was the result of a phase displacement of REM activity. This observation became known as the *phase-advance hypothesis* of depression, and stated that the circadian rhythm of REM sleep became advanced in relation to normal sleep onset.

Although the organization of the circadian (biological) clock remains controversial, work by Wever (40) studying humans in temporal isolation has suggested that two major oscillators may regulate circadian rhythms. According to this model, one oscillator regulates REM sleep, temperature, and cortisol, whereas a second oscillator influences the sleep-wake cycle. In this paradigm, the short REM latency and altered distribution of REM sleep during the first third of the night is the result of an advance in the circadian rhythm of REM sleep in relation to sleep onset.

Considerable chronobiological research has focused on the association of other circadian rhythms (e.g., temperature or cortisol) to REM sleep abnormalities in depression. Pflug et al. collected the oral temperature of a manic-depressive several times each day for 1 year and found an earlier occurrence of the acrophase of temperature during depression, and a delay during mania. This observation was consistent with the phase-advance hypothesis. Other studies have also supported the phase advance hypothesis. For example, Wehr et al. (41) reported an advance of the temperature nadir in the sleep of depressed patients, and Wehr et al. (41) and Kripke et al. (42) reported a phase advance in temperature and REM onset in hypomanic patients. Unlike Wehr et al. (41), Kripke et al. (42) found a progressive advance of the temperature rhythm in both depression and mania, whereas Wehr et al. (41) found a delay in temperature only during depression. In contrast, other investigators have not been able to find phase changes in REM sleep or temperature in depression (43).

The circadian rhythms of cortisol have been examined in depressed patients in an effort to determine the applicability of the phase-advance hypothesis. Several studies (44) have reported a cortisol secretory nadir several hours earlier in depressed patients compared with controls, whereas others have found similar changes in the acrophase of cortisol secretion. As with the temperature data, however, not all reports have confirmed these phase changes (45).

In addition to depressed patients, there is also some evidence that mood changes can occur when normal subjects are placed in situations resulting in chronobiological alterations. Siffre (46) reported increased periods of depression when placed in an underground isolation chamber for 6 months, and a study of shift-work and mood (47) identified one subject thought to be internally desychronized, who subsequently committed suicide. Delay of the normal time of sleep (thereby causing an advance of REM sleep) has also been reported to result in depressed mood within healthy subjects (48).

A second chronobiological model of the assocation between sleep and affective illness is the "internal desynchronization model." Halberg (49) suggested that the expression of mania and depression might be the result of a "beat-phenomenon." In his model the circadian oscillator that regulates

REM sleep (as well as temperature, cortisol, etc.) is not locked into the 24-hr day and thus "free-runs" in comparison with the sleep-wake cycle. Under these conditions, dependent upon how much faster than the 24-hr day the circadian oscillator for REM sleep runs, the biological rhythms of REM sleep temperature and sleep would beat in and out of phase. Studies of subjects in temporal isolation support this model of internal desynchronization. Under the constant conditions of temporal isolation, the sleep-wake cycle normally lengthens to 24.5 hr, whereas the rhythm for REM sleep appears to run faster with the appearance of a short REM latency, prolonged first REM period, and an increased percentage of REM sleep and REM density in the first third of sleep (32,50).

Rapid-cycling manic-depression is a type of affective disorder proposed as an example of the internal desynchronization model. Wehr et al. have suggested that the cycle length of REM sleep and temperature is different from the sleep-wake cycle, with the oscillators that control these biological rhythms gradually going out of phase (internal desynchronization) and then back into phase (internal synchronization). This drifting in and out of phase may account for the predictability of the cycle length in some patients with rapid-cycling manic depression.

A full understanding of these models and their applicability to sleep and depression awaits more systematic study. That many individuals undergo chronobiological, alterations without mood swings (jet lag, shift work) limits the utility of the chronobiological models. In addition, both the phase-advance and internal desynchronization hypotheses are heavily depended on the two-oscillator model, and the presence of two oscillators remains unproved.

CHRONOBIOLOGICAL MANIPULATION OF THE SLEEP-WAKE CYCLE

Despite the need for more controlled studies of the phase-advance and internal desynchronization models, manipulation of the sleep-wake cycle frequently results in mood changes. Total sleep deprivation, partial sleep deprivation, phase advance of sleep, and REM deprivation, all have been reported to relieve depressive symptoms.

Total sleep deprivation (TSD) was first suggested as a treatment of depression, and subsequent reports confirmed this observation (51-54).

In general, one to two-thirds of depressed patients demonstrate a response to TSD, with the response usually occurring the day after the deprivation night. Factors that predict a response to TSD include endogenous features of depression and diurnal mood swings. The effect of the antidepressant response is limited, however, and after a night of recovery sleep the patient awakens depressed. Infrequently, patients when sleep-deprived have "switches" into hypomania or mania (54,55).

Attempts to determine whether or not chronobiological mechanisms are involved in TSD have been inconclusive. Duncan et al. compared baseline EEG characteristics of nine patients that responded to TSD with those of seven nonresponders and could not identify any one sleep parameter that predicted response. An evaluation of temperature rhythms before and after sleep deprivation in responders showed no change, although nonresponders had an attenuation of the temperature curve after TSD (53).

Examination of neurotransmitter metabolites may be more predictive of response than measures of body temperature or EEG parameters. Matussek et al. (56) found that responders to TSD had higher concentrations of 3-methoxy-4-hydroxyphenylglycol (MHPG) in urine and spinal fluid before sleep deprivation, compared with nonresponders. After sleep deprivation MHPG dropped in response, but increased in the nonresponders. Baseline homovanillic acid levels (HVA) in cerebrospinal fluid has also been lower in responders, although the significance of these observations is unclear (53).

Allowing patients to sleep for only half of their regular time also has an antidepressant effect (57). Deprivation of the second half of the night (PSD-L) appears to be more effective than deprivation in the early part of sleep (PSD-E). In one study, 30 patients were sleep-deprived in the second part of the night (PSD-L), which a response noted in two-thirds of the subjects (58). Goets and Tolle (59) deprived patients during the early portion of their usual sleep cycle (PSD-E) and noted only a minimal response in 50%, and the amount of improvement, was judged to be less than that of the PSD-L patients. Overall, PSD-L is believed to be as effective as TSD (60), and to prolong the effects of TSD when it is used as follow-up treatment (61).

A third chronobiological technique that has been used to treat depression is the phase advance of the sleep-wake cycle. Because the phase-advance hypothesis of depression suggests that REM sleep is abnormally advanced in relation to sleep onset, advancing the time of sleep onset theoretically corrects this relationship and should resolve the mood disturbance. Wehr et al. (62) found that advancing bedtime from the usual time of 11:00 PM to earlier in the evening, resulted in an antidepressant response. Sack et al. (63) and Soutre et al. (64) employed a similar phase-advance technique in depressed patients and reported a resolution of symptoms in most.

Although a phase advance of the oscillator that controls REM sleep may account for the sleep EEG findings, a number of factors limit the interpretation of the data. By phase advancing the sleep period, patients frequently experience a reduction in total sleep time, and partial sleep deprivation in the latter part of the night may occur. As noted earlier, both mechanisms may result in relief of depression; phase-advance therapy thus may be an alternative method to create sleep deprivation. In addition, phase advance and PSD-L, which both result in a selective loss of REM sleep and the reduction in REM time—rather than the timing of REM sleep—may ultimately mediate the antidepressant effect of sleep manipulation.

In a series of studies, Vogel first deprived nine patients of REM sleep and observed an antidepressant response in six. In a second study, 34 endogenous and 18 reactive depressives were awakened during each REM period every night for six consecutive nights, or until they were awakened 30 times. To control for the effects of awakening, subjects were also awakened during non-REM sleep to counterbalance the awakenings in REM sleep. Although only 1 of the 18 reactive patients responded to the REM awakenings, 17 (50%) of the endogenous depressives improved.

Ultimately, REM sleep deprivation appears to be a major clinical and theoretical model. Although various chronobiological mechanisms may mediate the antidepressant response, REM deprivation appears to occur in all these manipulations of the sleep cycle. Before these chronobiological manipulations can be clearly understood, the effects of REM deprivation must be more fully evaluated. Although the distribution of REM sleep clearly exhibits a circadian variation, other factors, which can be equally critical in producing the antidepressant response, may influence REM sleep.

Antidepressant medications, such as tricyclic, monoamine oxidase inhibitor, and the newer antidepressants, all are known to cause reductions in total REM sleep. Kupfer et al. (65) noted that clinical response to antidepressants could be predicted on the basis of change in REM latency after drug administration. Although antidepressants may influence chronobiological mechanisms in relieving depression, other models (such as neurochemical) may account for the efficacy if these agents.

NEUROCHEMICAL INFLUENCES ON SLEEP IN DEPRESSION

Because depressed patients demonstrate various changes in REM sleep and because many pharmacologic agents that influence specific neurotransmitters also alter REM sleep, these drugs may serve as potential neurochemical probes into the pathogenesis of depression. For example, reserpine results in depression in selected patients and also depletes catecholamine and serotonin stores in the central nervous system (CNS), without altering cholinergic mechanisms (66,67). Polysomnographic evaluation of sleep in humans after reserpine administration has also demonstrated a decrease in REM latency and an increase in total amount of REM sleep (68,69).

α-Methyl-p-tyrosine (AMPT) is another drug known to reduce catecholamine sources in the CNS through the inhibition of tyrosine hydroxylase.

It has been administered to humans in several small trials, and the results are similar to those of reserpine. Studies of patients with medical, neurologic, or depressive disorders revealed an increase in total REM sleep after AMPT administration (70,71). When AMPT has been administered to normal volunteers, similar increases in REM time and reduction in REM latency occurred. These findings are interpreted as supporting the hypothesis that catecholamines are important in affective illness.

An alternate model involves the cholinergic system. The placement of acetylate crystals in the midbrain and forebrain of rats resulted in sleep and an induction of REM sleep. In human studies of cholinomimetic compounds Sitaram et al. evaluated the sleep EEG before and after administration of the cholinergic agonist, arecholine, and reported that it induced the onset of REM sleep. This effect was also noted when the anticholinesterase, physostigmine, was given to normal subjects. Thus, an increase of cholinergic stores by either inhibition of the enzymatic pathway responsible for inactivation of acetylcholine or by infusion of a cholinergic agonist resulted in the initiation of REM sleep.

Taken collectively, these studies, which illustrate REM sleep changes with cholinergic and adrenergic drugs, imply a complicated regulatory system that involves multiple neurotransmitter systems.

SLEEP SATIETY AND DEPRESSION

Chronobiological manipulation or pharmacologic challenges induce sleep changes in normal subjects that are similar to sleep in depression. Increasing the time permitted to sleep also results in alterations reminiscent of depression. Aserinsky first noted that when normal subjects were allowed to sleep 2 hr longer than usual, an increase in REM density and progressively shorter REM periods were found. He went on to propose that these changes in REM sleep were measures of sleep satiety.

Gillin et al. stated that these changes in REM sleep were found in subjects satiated with sleep and suggested that depressed patients may also have sleep satiety. This hypothesis was supported by the earlier report of Kupfer et al. (34), which demonstrated that depressed patients do not show excessive sleepiness on the multiple sleep latency test (MSLT) (a procedure that quantitates drowsiness during the day). Moreover, those patients who were most alert during the MSLT were also more likely to respond to antidepressant therapy.

CONCLUSIONS

Although various models have been proposed for understanding the association between sleep and affective disorder, a predominant theory has not yet emerged. To make the complete diagnosis of endogenous depression, disturbances in sleep patterns can invariably be found. Whether these changes are best understood in the framework of chronobiological models, neurotransmitter studies, or other hypotheses remains to be determined.

REFERENCES

1. Gillin, J. C., Duncan, W., Murphy, D. L., Post, R. M., Goodwin, F. K., Wyatt, R. J., and Bunney, W. E., Jr. (1981). Age-related changes in sleep in depressed and normal subjects. *Psychiatr. Res.* *4*:73-78.
2. Michaelis, R. and Hofmann, E. (1973). Sur Phanomenologie und Atiopathogeneses der Hypersomnie bei endogen phasischen Depression. *The Nature of Sleep*. Edited by U. J. Javonovic. Stuttgart, Gustav Fischer Verlag, pp. 190-193.
3. Detre, T., Himmelhock, J., Swartzburg, M., Anderson, D. M., Byck, R., and Kupfer, D. J. (1972). Hypersomnia and manic-depressive disease. *Am. J. Psychiatry* *128*:1303-1305.
4. Snyder, F. (1969). Dynamic aspects of sleep disturbance in relation to mental illness. *Biol. Psychiatry* *1*:119-130.
5. Green, W. J. and Stajduher, P. P. (1966). The effect of ECT on the sleep-dream cycle in a psychotic depression. *J. Nerv. Ment. Dis.* *143*:123-134.
6. Hartmann, E. L. (1968). Longitudinal studies of sleep and dreams in manic-depressive patients. *Arch. Gen. Psychiatry* *19*:312-329.
7. Snyder, F. (1969). Dynamic aspects of sleep disturbance in relation to mental illness. *Biol. Psychiatry* *1*:119-130.
8. Hawkins, D. R., Mendels, J., Scott, J., Bensch, G., and Teachey, W. (1967). The psychophysiology of sleep in psychotic depression: A longitudinal study. *Psychosom. Med.* *29*:329-344.
9. Kupfer, D. J. and Foster, F. G. (1972). Interval between onset of sleep and rapid eye movement sleep as an indicator of depression. *Lancet* *2*:684-686.
10. Vogel, G. W., Vogel, F., McAbee, R. S., and Thurmond, A. J. (1980). Improvement of depression by REM sleep deprivation. *Arch. Gen. Psychiatry* *37*:247-253.
11. Svendsen, J. and Christensen, P. G. (1981). Duration of REM sleep latency as predictor of effect of antidepressant therapy. *Acta Psychiatr. Scand.* *64*:238-243.
12. Mendlewicz, J., Kerkohfs, M., Hoffmann, G., and Linkowski, P. (1984). Dexamethasone suppression test and REM sleep in patients with major depressive disorder. *Br. J. Psychiatry* *145*:383-388.
13. Kupfer, D. J. and Foster, F. G. &1972). Interval between onset of sleep and rapid eye movement sleep as an indicator of depression. *Lancet* *2*:684-686.
14. Spiker, D. G., Coble, P., Cofsky, J., Foster, F. G., and Dupfer, D. J. (1978). EEG sleep and severity of depression. *Biol. Psychiatry* *13*:485-488.
15. Giles, D. G., Roffwarg, H. P., Schlesser, M. A., and Rush, A. J. (1986). Which endogenous depressive symptoms relate to REM latency reduction? *Biol. Psychiatry* *21*:473-482.

16. Giles, D. E., Jarrett, R. B., Roffwarg, H. P., Rush, A. J. (1987). Reduced rapid eye movement latency: A prediction of recurrence in depression. *Neuropsychopharmacology 1*:33-39.
17. Kupfer, D. J., et al. (1972). Hypersomnia in manic-depressive disease. *Dis. Nerv. Sys. 33*:720-724.
18. Shipley, J. E., Kumar, A., Eiser, A., Feinberg, M., Flegel, P., and Greden, J. F. (1986). Clinical, EEG sleep, and DST correlates of sleep onset REM periods. *Sleep Res. 15*:97.
19. Kerkohfs, M., Hoffmann, G., De Martelaere, V., Linkowski, P., and Mendlewicz, J. (1985). Sleep EEG recordings in depressive disorders. *J. Affect. Disord. 9*:47-53.
20. Ansseau, M., Scheyvaerts, M., Doumount, A., Poirrier, R., Legros, J., and Franck, G. (1984). Concurrent use of REM latency, dexamethasone suppression, clonidine, and apomorphine tests as biological markers of endogenous depression: A pilot study. *Psychiatry Res. 12*:261-272.
21. Coble, P. A., Kupfer, D. J., and Shaw, D. H. (1981). Distribution of REM latency in depression. *Biol. Psychiatry 16*:453-466.
22. Schultz, H. and Trojan, B. (1979). A comparison of eye movement density in normal subjects and in depressed patients before and after remission. *Sleep Res. 8*:49.
23. Lund, R. and Berger, M. (1981). REM latency and duration in subgroups of depressive disorders. Presented at Annual Meeting, Association for the Psychophysiological Study of Sleep, June 1981, Hyannis Port, Mass.
24. Mendels, J. and Hawkins, D. R. (1971). Sleep and depression. IV Longitudinal studies. *J. Nerv. Ment. Dis. 153*:251-272.
25. Insel, T. R., Gillin, J. C., Moore, A., Mendelson, W. B., Loewenstein, R. S., and Murphy, D. C. (1982). The sleep of obsessive-compulsive patients. *Arch. Gen. Psychiatry 39*:1372-1377.
26. Spiker, D. G., Foster, F. G., Coble, P., Love, D., and Kupfer, D. J. (1977). The sleep disorder in depressed alcoholics. *Sleep Res. 6*:161.
27. Gillin, J. C., Kripke, D. F., Butters, N., Grant, I., Irwin, M., Naimie, M. D., and Schuckit, M. (1986). A longitudinal study of sleep in primary alcoholism. *Sleep Res. 15*:92.
28. Jus, K., Bouchard, M., Jus, A. K., Villeneuve, A., and Lachance, R. (1973). Sleep EEG studies in untreated, long term schizophrenic patients. *Arch. Gen. Psychiatry 29*:386-390.
29. Neil, J. F., Merikanges, J. R., Foster, F. G., Merikanges, K. R., Spiker, D. G., and Kupfer, D. J. (1980). Walking and all-night sleep EEG's in anorexia nervosa. *Clin. Electroencephalogr. 11*:9-15.
30. Cartwright et al. (1980). Source unknown.
31. Dement, W. C. (1960). The effect of dream deprivation. *Science 131*:1705-1707.
32. Czeisler, C. A., Zimmerman, J. C., Ronda, J. M., Moore-Ede, M. C., and Weitzman, E. D. (1980). Timing of REM sleep is coupled to the circadian rhythm of body temperature in man. *Sleep 2*:329-346.
33. Gresham, S. C., Agnew, W. F., Jr., and Williams, R. L. (1965). The sleep of depressed patients. *Arch. Gen. Psychiatry 13*:503-507.

34. Kupfer, D. J., Gillin, J. C., Coble, P. A., Spiker, D. G., Shaw, D., and Holtzer, B. (1980). REM sleep, naps, and depression. *J. Psychiatr. Res. 5*:17-25.
35. Kupfer, D. J., Foster, F. G., and Detre, T. P. (1973). Sleep continuity changes in depression. *Dis. Nerv. Syst. 34*:192-195.
36. Gillin, J. C., Duncan, W., Pettigrew, K. D., Frankel, B. L., and Snyder, F. (1979). Successful separation of depressed, normal, and insomniac subjects by EEG sleep data. *Arch. Gen. Psychiatry 36*:85-90.
37. Sitaram, N., Nurnberger, J. I., and Gershon, E. S. (1982). Faster cholinergic REM sleep induction in euthymic patients with primary effective illness. *Science 208*:200-201.
38. Weitzman, E. D., Kripke, D. F., Goldmacher, D., McGregor, P., and Nogeire, C. (1970). Acute reversal of the sleep-waking cycle in man. *Arch. Neurol. 22*:483-489.
39. Papousek, J. (1975). Chronobiologische aspekete der Zyklothyme. *Fortschr. Neurol. Psychiatr. 43*:381-440.
40. Wever, R. A. (1979). *The Circadian System of Man: Results of Experiments Under Temporal Isolation.* New York, Springer-Verlag, pp. 1-276.
41. Wehr, T. A., Gillin, J. C., and Goodwin, F. K. (1983). Sleep and circadian rhythms in depression. In *Perspectives in Sleep Research.* Edited by M. Chase. New York, Spectrum, pp. 195-225.
42. Kripke, D. F., Mullaney, D. F., Atkinson, M., and Wolf, S. (1978). Circadian rhythm disorders in manic-depressives. *Biol. Psychiatry 13*:335-344.
43. Avery, D. H., Wildschiodtz, G., and Rafaelsen, O. J. (1982). Nocturnal temperature in affective illness. *J. Affect. Disord. 4*:61-71.
44. Linkowski, P., Mendlewicz, J., Leclercq, R., et al. (1985). The 24-hour profile of adrenocorticotropin and cortisol in major depressive illness. *J. Clin. Endocrinol. Metab. 61*:429-438.
45. Sachar, E. L., Hellman, L., Rofwarg, H. P., Halpern, F. S., Fukushima, D. K., and Gallagher, T. F. (1973). Disrupted 24-hour patterns of cortisol secretion in psychotic depression. *Arch. Gen. Psychiatry 28*:19-24.
46. Siffre, M. (1975). Six months alone in a cave. *Natl. Geogr. 147*:426-435.
47. Rockwell, D. A., Winget, C. M., Rosenblatt, L. S., Higgins, E. A., and Hetherington, N. W. (1978). Biological aspects of suicide: Circadian disorganization. *J. Nerv. Ment. Dis. 166*:851-858.
48. Knowles, J. B. and MacLean, A. W. (1985). A critical evaluation of models of depression. Presentation at Fourth World Congress of Biological Psychiatry, Philadelphia, Sept. 8-13, 1985.
49. Halberg, F. (1968). Physiological considerations underlying rhythmometry, with special reference to emotional illness. In *Cycles Biologiques et Psychiatrie*, Symposium Bel-Air Ill. Edited by J. de Ajuriaguerra. Geneva, Masson et Cie, pp. 73-126.
50. Zimmerman, J. C., Czeisler, C. A., Laxminarzyan, S., Knauer, R. S., and Weitzman, E. D. (1980). REM density is dissociated from REM sleep timing during free running sleep episodes. *Sleep 2*:409-415.
51. Nasrallah, H. B. and Coryell, W. H. (1982). Dexamethasone nonsuppression predicts the antidepressant effects of sleep deprivation. *Psychiatry Res. 68*:61-64.

52. Fahndrich, E. (1981). Effects of sleep deprivation on depressed patients of different nosological groups. *Psychiatry Res.* *5*:277-285.
53. Gerner, R. H., Post, R. M., Gillin, J. C., and Bunney, W. E. (1979). Biological and behavioral effects of one night's sleep deprivation in depressed patients and normals. *J. Psychiatr. Res.* *15*:21-40.
54. Pflug, B. and Tolle, R. (1971). Disturbance of 24-hour rhythm, endogenous depression, and treatment of endogenous depression by sleep deprivation. *Int. Pharmacopsychiatry* *6*:187-196.
55. Post, R. M., Stoddard, F. G., Gillin, J. C., Buchsbaum, M., Runkle, D. C., Black, K., and Bunney, W. E. (1976). Slow and rapid alterations in motor activity, sleep and biochemistry in a cycling manic-depressive patient. *Arch. Gen. Psychiatry* *24*:470-477.
56. Matussek, N., Romisch, P., and Achenheil, M. (1977). MHPG excretion during sleep deprivation in endogenous depression. *Neuropsychobiology* *31*:23-29.
57. Gillin, J. C., Sitaram, N., Nurnberger, J. I., et al. (1983). The cholinergic REM induction test (CRIT). *Psychopharmacol. Bull.* *19*:668-670.
58. Schilgen, B. and Tolle, R. (1980). Partial sleep deprivation as therapy for depression. *Arch. Gen. Psychiatry* *37*:267-271.
59. Goetze, U. and Tolle, R. (1981). Antidepressant effect of partial sleep of partial sleep deprivation during the first half of the night. *Psychiatry Clin.* (*Basel*) *14*: 129-149.
60. Philip, M. and Werner, C. (1979). Prediction of lofepramine-response in depression based on response to partial sleep deprivation. *Pharmakopsychiatr. Neuropsychopharmakol.* *12*:346-348.
61. Van Bemmel, A. L. and Van den Hoofdakker, R. H. (1981). Maintenance of therapeutic effects of total sleep deprivation by limitation of subsequent sleep. *Acta Psychiatr. Scand.* *63*:453-462.
62. Wehr, T. A., Wirz-Justice, A., Goodwin, F. K., et al. (1979). Phase advance of the circadian sleep-wake cycle as an antidepressant. *Science* *20*:710-713.
63. Sack, D. A., Nurnberger, J., Rosenthal, N. E., Ashburn, E., and Wehr, T. A. (1985). Potentiation of antidepressant medications by phase advance of the sleep-wake cycle. *Am. J. Psychiatry* *142*:606-608.
64. Souetre, E., Salvati, E., Pringuey, D., and Darcourt, G. (1985). Sleep and mood of depressed patients are improved by a phase advance process. Presented to Fourth World Congress of Biological Psychiatry, Sept. 8-13, Philadelphia.
65. Kupfer, D. J. (1976). REM latency. A psychobiological marker for primary depressive disease. *Biol. Psychiatry* *11*:159-174.
66. Palfai, T., Wichlinski, L., Brown, H. A., and Brown, O. M. (1986). Effects of amnesic doses of reserpine or syrosingopine on mouse brain acetylcholine levels. *Pharmacol. Biochem. Behav.* *24*:1457-1459.
67. Weiner, N. (1980). Drugs that inhibit adrenergic nerves and block adrenergic receptors. In *The Pharmacological Basis of Therapeutics*. Edited by A. G. Gilman, L. S. Goodman, and A. Gilman. New York, Macmillan, pp. 176-210.
68. Hartmann, E. L. (1966). Reserpine: Its effect on the sleep-dream cycle in man. *Psychopharmacologia* *9*:242-247.

69. Coulter, J. D., Lester, B. K., and Williams, H. L. (1971). Reserpine and sleep. *Psychopharmacologia 19*:134-147.
70. Wyatt, R. J., Chase, T. N., Kupfer, D. J., Scott, J., Snyder, F., Sjoerdsma, A., and Engelman, K. (1971). Brain catecholamine and human sleep. *Nature 233*: 63-65.
71. Vaughan, T., Wyatt, R. J., and Green, R. (1972). Changes in REM sleep of chronically anxious depressed patients by alpha-methyl-paratyrosine (AMPT). *Psychophysiology 9*:96.

23

The Depressed Suicidal Patient

Assessment and Treatment Issues

DONALD W. BLACK

University of Iowa College of Medicine, Iowa City, Iowa

Suicide is a major health problem that accounts for about 1% of all deaths in the United States annually. It is a problem that affects not only surviving friends and family members, but also the victim's caregiver, because most suicides communicate their suicidal intentions to, and see physicians, in the period before they commit suicide. Because suicide is responsible for about 28,000 deaths annually and ranks eighth in frequency among causes of death in the United States, it is a problem with which physicians must familiarize themselves (1). Physicians must be prepared to educate patients and family members about risk of suicide, to assess risk for suicide, to act appropriately to intervene with suicide plans, and, one hopes, to prevent suicides as well.

Suicide is a complex human behavior that involves biological, social, and psychological factors. It is not a behavior that lends itself readily to simple analyses or formulations.

The following chapter reports on the epidemiology, clinical findings, biochemistry, assessment, and treatment of one group of suicides, namely, depressed suicides.

SUICIDE IN GENERAL AND CLINICAL POPULATIONS

Studies of suicides in the general population have often focused their attention on the person who has committed suicide. With use of a "psychological autopsy" method, survivors and other informants are contacted and interviewed to learn more about the psychological state of the deceased; hospital and clinic records may also be gathered. The result of this inquiry is to conduct, in essence, a proxy interview for the person who committed suicide to learn about this person's mental condition at the time of the act. Six studies of this nature have been reported in the past 30 years (2-7). Despite differences in methods, diagnostic criteria, location, and the year of study, all have yielded similar results (Table 1). They all found that over 90% of suicides suffer from a major psychiatric illness, and that half of the suicide victims were clinically depressed at the time. Approximately 33% of the suicides occurred in patients with chronic alcoholism, whereas schizophrenia, organic mental disorders, substance abuse, and anxiety disorders were less common contributors to suicide. The most recent study (6) departs from these conclusions by observing substance abuse in 45% and alcoholism in 54% of suicides. These disconcerting findings may reflect a growing problem with drug and alcohol abuse in the United States.

Typically, suicides are men (about two-thirds), over 45 years of age, white, separated, widowed or divorced, live alone, and are either unemployed or retired (2,5). Psychiatric diagnoses tend to differ by age; Suicides younger than 30 years had more substance use disorders and antisocial personality, and suicides older than 30 years suffered more affective disorders (Table 2) (6).

Studies of hospital or clinic populations (8-11) have indicated that most suicides have an affective disorder, schizophrenia, or alcoholism. Although schizophrenia tends to be responsible for more suicides in clinical settings than in the general population (reflecting an overrepresentation of schizophrenia in these settings), it is not a major contributor to suicide in the general population.

Table 1 Psychiatric Diagnoses in Three Selected Studies of Suicides in the General Populatio

	Robins et al. (7)	Barraclough et al. (2)	Rich et al. (6)	
			<30 years	>30 year
Sample Size	134	100	133	150
Depression (%)	47	80	35	52
Alcohol abuse/dependence (%)	25	31	54	55
Drug abuse/dependence (%)	1	4	66	26
Schizophrenia (%)	2	3	5	2
Organic disorders (%)	4	1		7
Personality disorders (%)			10	1
Other disorders (%)	19	1		
Not mentally ill (%)	6	7	4	5

Table 2 Risk Factors for Suicide in General versus Clinical Populations

Risk factor	General	Clinical
Age	Older	Younger
Sex	Male	Female
Marital status	Single, widowed, divorced	Single, widowed, divorced
Diagnosis	Depression, alcoholism	Depression, schizophrenia
Living situation	Lives alone	Lives alone
Employment	Unemployed	Unemployed

Other differences between clinical and general population suicides have been found. Suicides in clinical samples tend to show a more equal sex distribution, although men still predominate (9-11), and tend to be young and have greater relative risk for suicide than the aged (10,11). In fact, as psychiatric patients age, observed rates of suicide approach expected rates within the general population; thus, there is a systematic decrease in the suicide rate as psychiatric patients age (10). Among similarities in a clinical sample, suicides were likely to be unmarried, unemployed, living alone, and depressed, regardless of diagnosis (9). In clinic populations, suicide is greatest around the time of hospital discharge or in the immediate follow-up period. For example, in a study of 5412 hospitalized patients, 68 persons committed suicide during the follow-up; 38% of suicides occurred in first 6 months, 57% within the first year, and 79% by 2 years (10).

SUICIDE ATTEMPTERS VERSUS SUICIDE COMPLETERS

Suicide attempters and suicide completers represent discrete, but overlapping populations (12,13). Nonetheless, up to one-third of patients who commit suicide have a history of suicide attempts (2,7), and an estimated 1% of suicide attempters will complete suicide annually, up to a total of 10% (14). Differences between suicide completers and suicide attempters involve both demographics and clinical characteristics. In a general population sample, men are twice as likely as women to commit suicide; suicides can occur at any age over 14 years, and nearly all completers are mentally ill at the time of their suicide (2,3,7). Suicide completers generally plan their act, use an effective means (e.g., firearms, hanging), and carry out the suicide in private or make provisions to avoid interruption (15). Completers are serious about ending their lives. In contrast, suicide attempters are three times more likely to be female and are usually younger than 35 years (16,17). They often act impulsively, make provisions for rescue, and use ineffective or slowly effective means (e.g., drug overdoses) (16,17).

Suicide attempters and suicide completers also differ diagnostically. Somewhat fewer of those who attempt than those who complete suicide are psychiatrically ill. Although suicide completers are likely to suffer from depression, alcoholism, or both, attempters diagnoses may include depression (often a secondary depression), alcohol or drug abuse, and also diagnoses that are uncommon among successful suicides, such as somatization disorder (Briquet's syndrome) and antisocial personality (19). Furthermore, it has been suggested that between 5 and 20% of those who attempt suicide have no diagnosable mental illness, as opposed to the estimated 3-12% of those who complete suicide who are not considered to be mentally ill (20,21).

Suicide attempters can be further subdivided into those whose attempts are serious and those for whom they are not. Serious attempts result in medically or surgically serious conditions (e.g., a penetrating gunshot wound) or are judged serious on psychological grounds (e.g., a depressed person who had carefully planned a suicide and carried out the attempt in private). However, most suicide attempts are neither medically nor psychologically serious. Serious attempts generally are associated with an affective disorder, higher scores on depression scales, and greater seriousness of intent (22,23). Patients who make serious attempts tend to be older, are more often men, and use more lethal means. Indeed, these patients resemble those who complete suicides, rather than attempted suicides, and more subsequently commit suicide than those whose attempts are rated as less serious (24).

DEPRESSION AND SUICIDE

Affective disorders are the largest single diagnostic group among those who commit suicide. Evidence for the importance of affective disorder in suicide comes mainly from two sources. First, follow-up studies of patients with affective disorder show that suicide is the ultimate outcome for a significant proportion of patients. Guze and Robins estimated that 15% of all persons with major affective disorders ultimately commit suicide (25). This finding means that patients with affective disorders are at about 30 times the risk of suicide as persons in the general population. Miles (26) reviewed 30 follow-up studies of patients with depressive illness and reached the same conclusion, regardless of classification as endogenous or neurotic depression. These estimates gain further support from Helgason (27) who followed a cohort of 5400 Icelanders through 60 years and determined that 103 (or about 2%) developed an affective disorder, and that 18 (or 17%) died by committing suicide.

The second source of evidence supporting the important link between suicide and affective disorder originates in the follow-up studies of suicide victims (2-7). An important observation from these studies is that suicide in affectively ill persons invariably occurs during an episode of depression; thus, suicide rarely, if ever, occurs in a person with a history of affective disorder who is not experiencing a depressive episode. Of the 1037 suicide reported in these six studies, not one was manic at the time of death. Thus, the manic phase of a bipolar illness does not appear to be associated with a substantial suicide risk.

THE DEPRESSED SUICIDE

Clinical Features

Among samples of depressed patients who have committed suicide, relatively few risk factors are consistently identified across studies (Table 3). In fact, Barraclough and Pallis (28) have shown that there are more clinical similarities between depressed suicides and living depressives than there are differences. They compared 64 depressed suicides with a random sample of 128 endogenous depressives matched for age and sex and drawn from the same population as the suicides. The rank order of the frequency of ten leading depressive symptoms was the same for both groups, although their severity was often rated higher in the suicide completers. The two groups differed significantly on only three clinical items: suicides manifested more persistent insomnia, more self-neglect, and more memory impairment. Again, the depressed suicides were more often men, were older if women, had made more attempts at suicide than controls (41% versus 4%), and were more likely to be unmarried and to live alone (28).

Table 3 Clinical Risk Factors for Suicide in the Depressed Suicidal Patient

Factors that correlate	Factors that do not correlate
Hopelessness	Male sex (?)
Living alone	Marital status (?)
Family history of suicide	Older age (?)
Recent discharge	Unemployment (?)
Early parental loss	History of past suicide attempts (?)
Recent change in dwelling	Physical illness
Foreign-born	Life stresses
Mood cycling	Interpersonal conflicts
Agitation	Depressive subtypes
Insomnia, self-neglect, memory impairment	Psychotic features
Anhedonia	
Low CSF 5-HIAA	

Among studies that used control groups, suicide completers were more severely depressed, but less hypochondriacal than controls (29); they were rated as more agitated (30); and, for some, the act was associated with a recent change in dwelling (31). No differences in marital status, amount of physical illness, number of life stresses, or interpersonal conflicts were found, but there was a significant difference in living situations: twice as many victims as controls lived alone (32). Roy (33) compared neurotic depressives who had committed suicide with diagnostically matched living controls on various items and found that more of the suicides were foreign-born, unmarried, and living alone. They also had more previous hospitalizations than controls and had been reported as more depressed and suicidal during their last admission. Roy later (34) compared manic-depressives (unipolar and bipolar) who had committed suicide with diagnostically matched living controls. More of these suicides had early parental loss, a history of suicide attempts, and were living alone. Fawcett et al. (35) presented follow-up data from the Collaborative Depression Study. Among a sample of 954 affectively disordered patients, 25 committed suicide. Compared with the living depressed patients, suicides had experienced more hopelessness, loss of pleasure or interest, and mood cycling during the index episode. However, diagnostic subtype, marital status, suicidal ideation at intake, past suicide attempts, and medical severity of suicide attempts did not correlate with suicide.

Reconciliation of these findings is difficult because they differ in methods, location, and time frame. There are no clinical symptoms that clearly distinguish the potential suicides, but many studies agree that suicides are more likely to live alone. Whether this situation predisposes to suicide or merely reflects a consequence of depression is unknown.

Family History

There is some evidence that a family history of suicide increases the risk for suicide in depressed patients. Data from the Danish adoption study (36) showed a higher incidence of suicide in biological relatives of adoptees who suffered from depression than in their adopted relatives or in the biological or adopted relatives of nondepressed adoptee controls. Egeland and Sussex (37) reported on suicide in the Amish, for whom, despite pacifist ways, strong family ties, and an absence of alcohol abuse, 26 suicides were reported, 92% having had an affective disorder. The suicides clustered in four pedigrees loaded with generations of either bipolar or unipolar affective disorder.

Follow-up

The initial 2 or 3 years of follow-up appear to be the period of greatest risk for suicide in the depressed patient. In a 30- to 40-year outcome study, Tsuang

(38) found that increased risk for suicide was largely limited to the first decade following the initial hospital admission. In the Collaborative Depressive Study (35), nearly one-third of 25 suicides occurred within the first 6 months and one-half within the first year after intake. Similar statistics were found in a study by Black et al. (39) of unipolar and bipolar depressives. Nearly 42% of 36 suicides during follow-up occurred within 6 months of hospital discharge, 58% by 1 year, and 70% by 2 years.

Communication of Intent

Many depressed patients who commit suicide communicate their intent to others. Barraclough et al. (2) reported that 30% of depressives had given warning. Robins et al. (7) found that of 60 manic-depressives, 68% had communicated suicidal ideas, most frequently through a direct and specific statement of their intent to commit suicide. Moreover, these investigators found that communications were diverse, repeated, and expressed to different persons.

Depressive Subtypes

It is uncertain whether or not depressive subtype is associated with suicide, for the data has often been contradictory. Two retrospective studies (40,41) showed that bipolar depressives have lower suicide rates than unipolar patients, but three other studies (38,42,43) failed to show any differences. Two studies in clinic populations (44,45), showed bipolar patients at higher risk for suicide than unipolar, but Martin et al. (11) did not. Moreover, Dunner et al. (45) reported that within the bipolar group, bipolar II patients had a greater risk for suicide than bipolar I. Black et al. (46) demonstrated that among former inpatients with unipolar and bipolar depression, suicide rates were similar. The lower rate of suicide reported in bipolar depression in some studies was hypothesized (46) as being due to the low risk of suicide in mania. Thus, in short-term follow-up studies, patients with bipolar disorders appear to have lower risk for suicide.

Martin et al. (11) concluded from study data of a psychiatric clinical population, that secondary depressives were at greater risk for suicide than primary depressives. They postulated that primary depressives may respond better to somatic treatment, and that their finding may represent a benefit of modern treatment era. However, Black et al. (46) found no difference in suicide rates between primary and secondary depressives. If differences in suicide do exist in depressive subtypes, they are probably minor and unimportant.

Psychosis and Suicide

Psychosis apparently does not predispose to suicide in patients with affective disorders (39,48,49). These findings, however, may not hold true for hospitalized patients, as Roose et al. (50) found that hospitalized psychotic depressives had a suicide risk 7.5 times higher than that of nonpsychotic patients.

BIOLOGICAL FACTORS IN SUICIDE

Monoamines and Their Metabolites

Aggression, suicidal attempts, and suicide, all have been linked to abnormal levels of monoamine and monoamine metabolites in the brain and cerebrospinal fluid (CSF). Specifically, both serotonin, and its metabolite 5-hydroxyindoleacetic acid (5-HIAA) have been correlated with suicidal behavior. Asberg et al. (51) reported that 40% of a group of depressives with low CSF 5-HIAA levels had attempted suicide compared with 15% of a group with normal 5-HIAA levels. They also found that suicide attempts in the low 5-HIAA group were more serious, whereas attempts in the normal 5-HIAA group were confined to drug overdoses. The association between CSF 5-HIAA and suicidal behavior in depressives was subsequently confirmed (52-56), but Secunda et al. (57) found no association. In a related study (58), among treatment-resistant patients with unipolar and bipolar disorders, suicidal unipolar patients tended to have lower CSF 5-HIAA than did the nonsuicidal, but no association was found between suicidality and 5-HIAA level in bipolars. This agrees with the findings of Berrettini et al. (59), who failed to find this association in a sample of bipolars. Thus, the biological correlates of suicidal behavior may differ between unipolar and bipolar patients.

Because suicide attempters do not have a one-to-one relationship with suicide completers, it is unclear whether the association between 5-HIAA and suicidal behavior can be generalized to include subsequent suicide. Asberg et al. (60) reported data from a follow-up study in which 21% of 34 patients, admitted to a psychiatric clinic after a suicide attempt, who had CSF 5-HIAA levels below 90 nm/L later committed suicide; only 2% of 42 patients, admitted to a psychiatric clinic after a suicide attempt, who had CSF levels of 5-HIAA above 90 nm/L committed suicide, which suggests that measurements of CSF 5-HIAA may be of value, but this finding clearly needs replication.

Postmortem studies of monoamines and their metabolites in brains of suicide victims have been more problematic. These reports have mostly investigated unselected suicides, probably half of whom had depression. Differences in concentration of serotonin or 5-HIAA are the most consistently reported findings. In general, decreases have been found in the brain stem (raphe nuclei) and in other subcortical nuclei (i.e., the hypothalamus). Two studies (61,62) found lower levels of serotonin or 5-HIAA in depressed suicide victims than in controls or nondepressed victims. However, not all the reports show abnormalities. Cochran et al. (63) found no differences in levels of serotonin in several brain regions. However, because of several difficult methodologic problems, such as time and mode of death, previous drug treatment, decay of the amines or their metabolites, and the subsequent autopsy itself, the findings are inconclusive.

Binding Studies

The binding of specific drugs to brain tissue in suicides has also been investigated. The most intensively studied ligand has been [^{3}H]imipramine. Two groups (64,65), found lower imipramine-binding levels in the brains of suicides than in those of controls, but another (66) reported increased binding. The data are inconclusive on the binding properties of other ligands.

Hormonal Abnormalities

Abnormalities of the hypothalamic-pituitary-adrenal (HPA) axis are found in a high proportion of patients with a melancholic subtype of major depression. An early study (67), reported that patients who progressed to serious suicide attempts or to complete suicide had an unusually high excretion of cortisol metabolites before the event. These findings were later replicated (68), and it was suggested that the measurement of cortisol might be useful in identifying persons at risk for suicide. A prospective study (69), demonstrated a relationship between high cortisol concentrations in blood and subsequent suicide. Introduction of the dexamethasone suppression test (DST) has renewed interest in a possible association between suicide and cortisol. Carroll et al. (70) found abnormal DSTs results more often in suicidal than in nonsuicidal patients, and of 243 depressed inpatients tested by DST (71), all four who subsequently committed suicide were nonsuppressors. Among 49 depressed patients, significantly more of those who had been admitted after suicide attempts were DST nonsuppressors, as were five patients who eventually committed suicide (72). More recently, Roy et al. (73) found that both low levels of the catecholamine metabolite, homovanillic acid (HVA), in the CSF and DST nonsuppression correlated with suicidal behavior in 27 depressed patients; three of four patients who committed suicide within a year of the study had both low CSF HVA levels and DST nonsuppression. However, three other studies (52,74,75), have failed to find an association between suicide and an abnormal DST.

Blunted thyrotropin (TSH) response after injection of thyrotropin-releasing hormone (TRH) also has been linked to suicidal behavior. For example, Linkowski et al. (76) found a reduced TSH response to TRH in patients with a history of violent suicidal attempts compared with those who had a history of nonviolet attempts or those with no history of suicidal attempts. During a

5-year follow-up, four patients committed suicide, three by violent means and one by overdose, and all four had blunted TSH response to TRH. A second study by these investigators (77) was confirmatory, although in a group of six patients Banki and Arato (78) found no relationship between TSH response and suicide. Although these correlations are interesting, we are not yet able to utilize laboratory tests effectively in assessing suicidality. The association of biological factors and suicide has recently been reviewed (79).

ASSESSMENT OF THE DEPRESSED SUICIDAL PATIENT

The assessment of suicide risk begins with its recognition. Barraclough et al. (2) reported that 53% of 64 depressives made an unequivocal threat of suicide in the month before death. Furthermore, over 60% of depressives contacted their general practitioner in the month before their death. Other investigators have also reported that a high proportion of depressed suicide attempters had seen their physicians just before the act. These figures suggest that with most suicidal depressives there are ample opportunities for intervention, provided that the clues of an impending suicide are recognized.

The accurate assessment of suicide risk must include a thorough psychiatric history, family history, and mental status examination. The clinician should be alert to the possibility of suicide in any depressed patient. In these patients, the assessment will focus on the vegetative signs and cognitive symptoms of depression, death wishes, suicidal ideation, and suicidal plans. Most suicidal patients are willing to discuss their thoughts with a physician if asked (80). Unfortunately, it is clear that many clinicians do not ask patients about suicide. Two separate studies showed that only one physician in six reported an awareness of a patient's suicidal thoughts (7,81). There is no substance to the belief that asking a patient about suicide will give the patient ideas that he or she had not already had. Suicidal thoughts are common in depression; most depressed patients have had these thoughts and may be relieved to talk about them. Patients are often fearful or even feel guilty about having these thoughts. Giving the patient an opportunity to discuss them may provide some relief. Specific questions that may be asked of the patient include:

Are you having any thoughts of harming yourself?
Are you having thoughts about killing yourself?
Have you developed a plan for committing suicide? If so, what is your plan?

The psychiatrist should also assess the patient's history of suicidality.

Have you ever had thoughts of killing yourself?
Have you ever attempted suicide?
If so, could you tell me about the attempt(s)?

The issue of suicide should be approached in a slow and deliberate manner after having developed some rapport and trust with the patient.

Because the condition of depressed patients may fluctuate, vague suicidal thoughts may change into a formulated plan. Therefore, clinicians must reassess suicide risk at each contact with the patient. Patients who have developed well-thought-out plans and have the means to carry them out require surveillance on a psychiatric unit. Most patients will probably agree to a voluntary hospitalization. However, if voluntary admission is not possible, a court order for hospitalization should be sought on an emergency basis. Hospitalization is the only way a physician may reasonably assure the safety of the patient, although suicides in the hospital are not infrequent events. In fact, Robins (15) reported that 27% of 134 suicides had occurred in the hospital.

MANAGEMENT OF THE SUICIDAL PATIENT

Once in the hospital, treatment of the suicidal patient will most likely depend on the diagnosis. Antidepressant medication will be the treatment of choice for most depressed patients, although lithium carbonate or neuroleptic agents may be appropriate adjunctive medications for bipolar and psychotically depressed patients, respectively. Electroconvulsive therapy (ECT) is often recommended for the suicidally depressed patient, especially for those who may not live until an antidepressant begins to work. This, however, is probably not a valid concern if the patient is in the hospital under constant supervision (82). Electroconvulsive therapy may be the treatment of choice for severely retarded or catatonic depressed patients who are not eating or are not taking fluids, conditions that may be life-threatening (83).

Table 4 Recommendations for the Management of the Depressed Suicidal Patient

1. Hospitalization
    - Locked unit
    - Suicide/elopement precautions
    - Close supervision by nursing staff
    - Removal of sharps, belts, etc.
    - Seclusion, restraints
2. Treatment of depression
    - Antidepressants
    - Electroconvulsive therapy
3. Close follow-up postdischarge
    - Prophylactic medication
    - Psychotherapeutic support

If a choice is made to treat on an outpatient basis, close supervision will be necessary. This will include frequent assessments of depression and suicidality, supportive psychotherapy, and frequent prescriptions for small amounts of medication, to avoid the problem of having a large number of pills on hand for an impulsive suicide attempt. Family members may be helpful in monitoring the medication. Regardless, some patients will maintain stores of pills in preparation for a future attempt, but there is little one can do to avoid this problem. Finally, the family should be told to remove all firearms from the home.

The Postdischarge Period

The psychiatrist should continue to follow the depressed patient closely after hospital discharge. Risk for suicide remains high during the first 1-2 years after hospital discharge, particularly during the first few months (10). The physician must be alert to signs of depressive relapse, or to the emergence of a new episode of depression, and adjust treatment accordingly. Follow-up is the cornerstone of suicide prevention. Some patients will require weekly visits, whereas other may be seen only monthly. A tapering schedule of visits may be useful. For example, a clinician may start by seeing the patient weekly for the first month after hospital discharge, then every 2 weeks for 2 months, followed by monthly thereafter for the duration of follow-up. Medication should be continued on a prophylactic basis; both antidepressant medication and lithium carbonate are useful in the unipolar depressive and lithium carbonate in the bipolar patient (84).

Psychotherapeutic support is essential, to improve medication compliance, provide hope, and help restore morale. The psychotherapy should be supportive (85), and the goals of psychotherapy in the suicidal depressed patient should include educating the patient about the time-limited nature of depression and suicidal thoughts, and emphasizing the clinicians' familiarity with the syndrome and its treatment (85). A duration of prophylactic medication of 16-20 weeks has been advocated (86), but many clinicians will be more comfortable with 6 months to a year of prophylaxis (87).

THE PREDICTION AND PREVENTION OF SUICIDE

Prediction

Is it actually possible to predict suicide? Any answer to this question must address two issues: (1) statistical prediction and (2) clinical prediction. Statistical prediction, or the identification of persons at high risk in a given population, is probably not possible. Progress has been made, however, in identifying large groups with greater than average risk (e.g., men, persons over

45 years of age), although these groups are too general to be of practical use. The knowledge that suicide rarely occurs in the absence of a major mental illness further narrows the field. Most persons with mental disorders, however, are not at risk for suicide. These demographic and diagnostic clues are inadequate in isolating potential suicides.

Two prospective studies of high-risk populations have looked at statistical prediction. One (88), taking a psychosocial perspective, looked at how well various models (e.g., "males under 40," "stable with forced change") could be used to predict suicide. The models showed a better than baseline correlation with suicide, but apply to only a small proportion of the suicide population. None of the characteristics identified by discriminant function analysis occurred with a frequency as great as 14% of the original sample. In a subsequent study (89), a scale was developed for estimating risk of suicide within 2 years, based on the original data set of depressed or suicidal inpatients. Although this scale provided valid estimates of population rates for deciles of estimated risk (e.g., first decile "very low risk," tenth decile "very high risk"), it is not useful for prediction of suicide in individual cases. Pokorny (8) used a historic-psychological model to identify characteristics that set apart suicide completers. A high-risk group could be identified, but no predictor variable was unique to the group. A computer program that used the predictor having the greatest discriminating value correctly predicted the 67 suicides that occurred among the 4800 subjects; however, when base rates of suicide were not taken into account, it successfully predicted 35 suicides, but it also predicted suicide for 1206 survivors. When base rates were used, the program failed to identify a single suicide correctly. Thus, statistical modeling of clinical, demographic, and social data appears unsuccessful as a mean of identifying potential suicides.

Conversely, clinical prediction involves small steps, taken with individual patients, that are guided by knowledge of both the phenomenology of suicide and of the individual patient (90). This knowledge takes into account both the inconstancy of the suicidal urge, which may wax and wane, and the state-dependent nature of suicide (i.e., the knowledge that suicide rarely occurs in the affectively ill patient in the absence of depression). Pokorny (8) notes that, under these conditions, psychiatrists appear to know which patients are highly suicidal: "The clinical work is in an entirely different time frame, dealing in minutes, hours, or days. It is commonly recognized that a 'suicidal crisis' will pass . . . so that after a few days the risk has abated and it may be safe for the patient to be discharged." Such a time frame—the clinical time frame, which is omitted from statistical prediction—is probably not researchable. Psychiatrists will never know with certainty that they have prevented a suicide. Therefore, the goal must focus on relieving the despair that forms the basis for most suicides; this may be within reach.

Prevention

Other than treatment of the individual case, general measures to prevent suicides have included suicide prevention centers. These centers, originally established in the late 1950s in both the United States and Great Britain, found early support. Bagley (91) reported evidence of a decline in suicide rates in cities in which branches of a suicide prevention organization, the Samaritans, had been established, and an increase in rates in matched cities that did not have Samaritan branches. A subsequent replication of this study (92), in which the control cities were better matched than those in Bagley's, failed to support the earlier finding, as did three subsequent investigations of suicide prevention centers in the United States (93-95).

Although these centers may not affect general suicide rates, there is some evidence that they may lower rates among young women. Miller et al. (96) found no difference in overall suicide rates between counties in which crisis intervention centers were established between 1968 and 1973 and those lacking these centers, but did find that suicide rates for young white females (i.e., under 24 years) were lower in the counties with crisis intervention centers. They suggest that more than 600 lives might be saved annually if such centers were available throughout the United States. Although it is still not clear whether or not suicide prevention centers actually prevent suicide, these centers appear to perform a useful role by providing a listening post for many lonely, depressed, and unstable persons.

Whether or not specific somatic treatments for depression, including ECT and antidepressants, prevent suicides has also been questioned. Early studies found fewer deaths, including suicides, in ECT-treated patients than in untreated controls (97-99). Electroconvulsive therapy appeared to reduce death rates in depressives at 1- and 3-year follow-up, compared with patients receiving inadequate or no treatment (100), and schizoaffective patients with a lifetime history of ECT had lower death rates than patients who had never received ECT (101). However, neither of these latter two studies showed that ECT reduced suicide rates specifically, and four other studies have not found that ECT reduces suicide rates (82,102-104).

No systematic data are available on the question of whether or not medication has altered suicide rates. Barraclough (105) hypothesized, however, that as lithium is effective in recurrent affective disorder, it might be expected to lower suicide rates. From a study of 64 persons who committed suicide, he concluded that there would have been a 21% reduction in suicides had lithium been used. Two studies (106,107) from lithium clinic samples found that patterns of mortality did not differ from patterns observed in other studies of manic-depressive illness, casting doubt on Barraclough's conclusion.

Do these discouraging findings mean that the clinician can do little for the individual patient to prevent suicide? This pessimistic data should be put into perspective. As Murphy (108) has wisely observed, ". . . a saved life is a statistical non-event" (p. 573). Research methods may not be sensitive enough to measure the effect of treatments in preventing suicide in individual patients: suicide rates might be much higher if depressed patients were not treated, and evidence suggests that comprehensive community-based psychiatric care may, in fact, reduce suicide rates. Walk (109) compared suicide rates of all patients in contact with a psychiatrist during a 5-year period both before and after the introduction of a well-organized psychiatric service organization in Chichester, England. He found a significant decrease in the suicide rates of elderly psychiatric patients. Because the older, depressed patients had benefitted the most and had the greatest increase in level of care, there is a likelihood that the services were responsible for the drop in suicide rates. Thus, although specific somatic treatments and suicide prevention centers may not lower general suicide rates, a comprehensive mental health care system, providing evaluation, treatment, and careful follow-up, might offer the best hope for suicide prevention.

REFERENCES

1. Weed, J. A. (1985). Suicide in the United States 1958-1982. In *Mental Health, United States,* Washington, D.C., NIMH.
2. Barraclough, B., Bunch, J., Nelson, B., and Sainsbury, P. (1974). A hundred cases of suicide: Clinical aspects. *Br. J. Psychiatry 125*:355-373.
3. Beskow, J. (1979). Suicide and mental disorder in Swedish men. *Acta Psychiatr. Scand. Suppl. 277*:1-138.
4. Dorpat, L. and Ripley, H. S. (1960). The study of suicide in the Seattle area. *Compr. Psychiatry 1*:349-359.
5. Chynoweth, R., Tonge, J. I., and Armstrong, J. (1980). Suicide in Brisbane. A retrospective psychosocial study. *Aust. N. Z. J. Psychiatry 14*:37-45.
6. Rich, C. L., Young, D., and Fowler, R. C. (1986). San Diego suicide study I. Young vs. old subjects. *Arch. Gen. Psychiatry 43*:577-582.
7. Robins, E., Murphy, G. E., Wilkinson, R. H., Gassner, S., and Kayes, J. (1959). Some clinical considerations in the prevention of suicide based on a study of 134 successful suicides. *Am. J. Public Health 49*:888-899.
8. Pokorny, A. D. (1983). Prediction of suicide in psychiatric patients. *Arch. Gen. Psychiatry 40*:249-257.
9. Roy, A. (1982). Risk factors for suicide in psychiatric patients. *Arch. Gen. Psychiatry 39*:1089-1095.
10. Black, D. W., Warrack, G., and Winokur, G. (1985). The Iowa Record Linkage Study I. Suicide and accidental death among psychiatric patients. *Arch. Gen. Psychiatry 42*:71-75.
11. Martin, R. L., Cloninger, C. R., Guze, S. B., and Clayton, P. J. (1985). Mortality in a follow-up of 500 psychiatric outpatients II: Cause-specific mortality. *Arch. Gen. Psychiatry 42*:58-66.

12. Avery, D. and Winokur, G. (1978). Suicide, attempted suicide, and relapse rates in depression occurrence after ECT and antidepressant therapy. *Arch. Gen. Psychiatry 35*:749-753.
13. Tefft, B. M., Patterson, A. M., and Babigian, H. M. (1977). Patterns of death among suicide attempters, psychiatric population, and a general population. *Arch. Gen. Psychiatry 34*:1155-1161.
14. Ettlinger, R. (1975). Evaluation of suicide prevention after attempted suicide. *Acta Psychiatr. Scand. Suppl. 260*:1-135.
15. Robins, E. (1981). *The Final Months: A Study of 134 Persons Who Committed Suicide.* New York, Oxford University Press.
16. Clendenin, W. W. and Murphy, G. E. (1971). Wrist cutting. New epidemiologic findings. *Arch. Gen. Psychiatry 25*:415-469.
17. Bancroft, J. H. J., Skrimshire, A. M., and Simkin, S. (1976). The reasons people give for taking overdoses. *Br. J. Psychiatry 128*:538-548.
18. Kreitman, N. (1977). *Parasuicide.* New York, John Wiley & Sons.
19. Woodruff, R. A., Clayton, P. J., and Guze, S. B. (1972). Suicide attempts and psychiatric diagnosis. *Dis. Nerv. Syst. 33*:617-621.
20. Dahlgren, K. G. (1945). *On Suicide and Attempted Suicide. A Psychiatrical and Statistical Investigation.* Lund, P.H. Lindstedts, University Bokhandl.
21. Murphy, G. E. and Wetzel, R. D. (1982). Family history of suicidal behavior among suicide attempters. *J. Nerv. Ment. Dis. 170*:86-90.
22. Pallis, D. J. and Sainsbury, P. (1976). The value of assessing intent in attempted suicide. *Psychol. Med. 6*:487-492.
23. Schmidt, E. H., O'Neil, P., and Robins, E. (1954). Evaluation of suicide attempts as a guide to therapy: Clinical and follow-up study of 109 patients. *JAMA 155*:549-557.
24. Rosen, D. H. (1970). The serious suicide attempt: Epidemiological and follow-up study of 886 patients. *Am. J. Psychiatry 127*:764-770.
25. Guze, S. B. and Robins, E. (1970). Suicide in primary affective disorders. *Br. J. Psychiatry 117*:437-438.
26. Miles, C. P. (1977). Conditions predisposing to suicide: A review. *J. Nerv. Ment. Dis. 164*:231-246.
27. Helgason, T. (1964). The epidemiology of mental disorder in Iceland. *Acta Psychiatr. Scand. Suppl. 173*:1-258.
28. Barraclough, B. M. and Pallis, D. (1975). Depression followed by suicide—a comparison of depressed suicides with living depressives. *Psychol. Med. 5*:55-61.
29. McDowell, A. W. T., Brooke, E. M., Freeman-Browne, D. L., and Robin, A. A. (1968). Subsequent suicide in depressed inpatients. *Br. J. Psychiatry 114*:749-754.
30. Farberow, N. L. and McEvoy, T. C. (1966). Suicide among patients with diagnosis of anxiety reaction or depressive reaction in general medicinal and surgical hospitals. *J. Abnorm. Psychol. 71*:287-299.
31. Sainsbury, P. (1973). Suicide: Opinion and facts. *Proc. R. Soc. Med. 66*:579-587.
32. Murphy, G. E. and Robins, E. (1967). Social factors in suicide. *JAMA 199*:81-86.

33. Roy, A. (1983). Suicide in depressives. *Compr. Psychiatry 24*:487-491.
34. Roy, A. (1984). Suicide in recurrent affective disorder patients. *Can. J. Psychiatry 29*:319-321.
35. Fawcett, J., Scheftner, W., Clark, D., Hedeker, D., Gibbons, R., and Coryell, W. (1987). Clinical predictors of suicide in patients with major affective disorders: A controlled prospective study. *Am. J. Psychiatry 144*:35-40.
36. Kety, S. (1979). Disorders of the human brain. *Sci. Am. 241*:202-214.
37. Egeland, J. A. and Sussex, J. N. (1985). Suicide and family loading for affective disorder. *JAMA 254*:915-918.
38. Tsuang, M. T. (1978). Suicide in schizophrenic, manics, depressives, and surgical controls. *Arch. Gen. Psychiatry 35*:153-155.
39. Black, D. W., Winokur, G., and Nasrallah, A. (1988). The effect of psychosis on suicide risk in 1593 patients with unipolar and bipolar affective disorders. *Am. J. Psychiatry 145*:849-852.
40. Angst, J., Felder, W., and Frey, R. (1979). The course of unipolar and bipolar affective disorders. In *Origin, Prevention and Treatment of Affective Disorder.* Edited by M. Schou and E. Stromgren. London, Academic Press, pp. 215-226.
41. McGlashan, T. H. (1984). Chestnut Lodge follow-up study III. Long-term outcome of schizophrenia and affective disorders. *Arch. Gen. Psychiatry 41*:586-601.
42. Perris, C. and D'Elia, G. (1966). The study of bipolar (manic-depressive) and unipolar recurrent depressive psychoses X. Mortality, suicide, and life cycles. *Acta Psychiatr. Scand. Suppl. 194*:172-183.
43. Week, E. A. and Vaeth, M. (1986). Excess mortality of bipolar and unipolar manic depressive patients. *J. Affect. Disord. 11*:227-234.
44. Morrison, J. R. (1982). Suicide in the psychiatric practice population. *J. Clin. Psychiatry 43*:348-352.
45. Dunner, D. L., Gershon, E. S., and Goodwin, F. K. (1976). Heritable factors in the severity of affective illness. *Biol. Psychiatry 11*:31-41.
46. Black, D. W., Winokur, G., and Nasrallah, A. (1987). Suicide and subtypes of major affective disorder—comparison with general population suicide mortality. *Arch. Gen. Psychiatry 44*:878-888.
47. Martin, R. L., Cloninger, C. R., Guze, S. B., and Clayton, P. J. (1985). Mortality in a follow-up of 500 psychiatric outpatients. I. Total mortality. *Arch. Gen. Psychiatry 42*:47-54.
48. Wolfersdorf, M., Keller, F., Steiner, B., et al. (1987). Delusional depression in suicide. *Acta Psychiatr. Scand. 76*:359-363.
49. Coryell, W. and Tsuang, M. T. (1982). Primary unipolar depression: The prognostic importance of delusions. *Arch. Gen. Psychiatry 39*:1181-1184.
50. Roose, S. P., Glassman, A. H., Walsh, B. T., Woodring, S., and Vital-Herne, J. (1983). Depression, delusions, and suicide. *Am. J. Psychiatry 140*:1159-1162.
51. Asberg, M., Traskman-Bendz, L., and Thoren, P. (1976). 5-HIAA in the cerebrospinal fluid—a biochemical suicide predictor? *Arch. Gen. Psychiatry 33*:1193-1197.
52. Agren, H. (1980). Symptom patterns in unipolar and bipolar depression correlating with monoamine metabolites in the cerebrospinal fluid. II. Suicide. *Psychiatric Res. 3*:225-236.

53. Traskman, L., Asberg, M., Bertilsson, L., and Sjostrand, L. (1981). Monoamine metabolites in CSF and suicidal behavior. *Arch. Gen. Psychiatry 38*:631-636.
54. Montgomery, S. A. and Montgomery, D. (1982). Pharmacological prevention of suicidal behavior. *J. Affect. Disord. 4*:291-298.
55. Palanappian, V., Ramachandran, V., and Somasundaram, O. (1983). Suicidal ideation and biogenic amines in depression. *Indian J. Psychiatry 25*:286-292.
56. Banki, C. M., Arato, M., Papp, Z., and Curcz, M. (1984). Biochemical markers in suicidal patients. Investigations with cerebrospinal fluid, amine metabolites, and neuroendocrine tests. *J. Affect. Disord. 6*:341-350.
57. Secunda, S. K., Cross, C. K., Koslow, S., Katz, M. M., Kocsis, J., Maas, J. W., and Landis, H. (1985). Biochemistry and suicidal behavior in depressed patients. *Biol. Psychiatry 21*:756-767.
58. Roy-Byrne, P., Post, R. M., Rubinow, D. R., Linnoila, M., Savard, R., and Davis, D. (1983). CSF 5-HIAA and personal and family history of suicide in affectively ill patients: A negative study. *Psychiatr. Res. 10*:263-274.
59. Berrettini, W., Nurnberger, J., Narrow, W., Simmons-Alling, S., and Gershon, E. (1986). Cerebrospinal fluid studies of bipolar patients with and without a history of suicide attempts. *Ann. N.Y. Acad. Sci. 487*:197-201.
60. Asberg, M., Nordstrum, P., and Traskman-Bendz, L. (1986). Biological factors in psychiatry. In *Suicide*. Edited by A. Roy. Baltimore, Williams & Wilkins, pp. 47-71.
61. Shaw, D. N., Camps, F. E., and Eccleston, E. G. (1967). 5-Hydroxytryptamine in the hind brain of depressive suicides. *Br. J. Psychiatry 113*:1407-1411.
62. Bourne, H. R., Bunney, W. E., Jr., Colburn, R. W., Davis, J. M., Davis, J. N., Shaw, D. M., and Coppen, A. J. (1968). Noradrenaline, 5-hydroxytryptamine and 5-hydroxyindoleacetic acid in hindbrains of suicidal patients. *Lancet 2*:805-808.
63. Cochran, E., Robins, E., and Grote, S. (1976). Regional serotonin levels in brain: A comparison of depressive suicides and alcoholic suicides with controls. *Biol. Psychiatry 11*:283-294.
64. Stanley, M., Virgilio, J., and Gershon, S. (1982). Tritiated imipramine binding sites are decreased in the frontal cortex of suicides. *Science 216*:1337-1339.
65. Paul, S. M., Rehavi, M., Skolnick, P., and Goodwin, H. (1984). High affinity binding antidepressants to biogenic transport sites in human brain and platelets studies in depression. In *Neurobiology of Mood Disorders*. Edited by R. M. Post and J. C. Ballenger. Baltimore, Williams & Wilkins, pp. 845-953.
66. Myerson, L. R., Wennogle, L. P., Abel, M. S., Coupet, J., Lippin, A., Rauh, C. E., and Beer, B. (1982). Human brain receptor alterations in suicide victims. *Pharmacol. Biochem. Behav. 17*:159-163.
67. Bunney, W. E. and Fawcett, J. A. (1965). Possibility of a biochemical test for suicide potential. *Arch. Gen. Psychiatry 13*:232-239.
68. Bunney, W. E., Fawcett, J. A., Davis, J. M., and Gifford, S. (1969). Further evaluation of urinary 17-hydroxycortocosteroid in the suicidal patients. *Arch. Gen. Psychiatry 21*:138-150.
69. Krieger, G. (1974). The plasma level of cortisol as a predictor of suicide. *Dis. Nerv. Syst. 35*:237-240.

70. Carroll, B. J., Greden, T. F., and Feinberg, M. (1981). Suicide, neuroendocrine dysfunction and CSF 5-HIAA concentrations in depression. *Adv. Biosci. 31*: 307-313.
71. Coryell, W. and Schlesser, M. A. (1981). Suicide and the dexamethasone suppression test in unipolar depression. *Am. J. Psychiatry 138*:1120-1121.
72. Targum, S. D., Rosen, L., and Capodanno, A. E. (1983). The dexamethasone suppression test in suicidal patients with unipolar depression. *Am. J. Psychiatry 140*:877-879.
73. Roy, A., Agren, H., Pickar, D., Linnoila, M., Doran, A. R., Cutler, N. R., and Paul, S. M. (1986). Reduced CSF concentrations of homovanillic acid, homovanillic acid to 5-hydroxyindolacetic acid ratios in depressed patients: Relationship to suicidal behaviors and dexamethasone nonsuppression. *Am. J. Psychiatry 143*:1539-1545.
74. Van Waltere, J. P., Charles, G., and Wilmotte, J. (1983). Test de function a la dexamethasone et suicide. *Acta Psychiatr. Scand. 83*:569-578.
75. Kocsis, J. H., Kennedy, S., Brown, R. P., Mann, J. J., and Mason, B. (1986). Neuroendocrine studies in depression: Relationship to suicidal behavior. *Ann. N.Y. Acad. Sci. 487*:256-262.
76. Linkowski, P., Van Wetterer, J.-P., Kerkhofs, M., Brauman, H., and Mendlewicz, J. (1983). Thyrotropin response to thyrostimulin in affectively ill women in relationship to suicidal behavior. *Br. J. Psychiatry 143*:401-405.
77. Linkowski, P., Van Welterer, J.-P., Gregoire, F., Kerkofs, M., Brauman, H., Mendlewicz, J. (1984). Violent suicidal behavior and the thyrotropin-releasing hormone-thyroid stimulation hormone test: A clinical outcome study. *Neuropsychobiology 12*:19-22.
78. Banki, C. M. and Arato, M. (1983). Amino metabolites and neuroendocrine responses related to depression and suicide. *J. Affect. Disord. 5*:223-232.
79. Stanley, M. and Mann, J. J. (1988). Biologic factors associated with suicide. In *Review of Psychiatry*. Edited by A. J. Francis and R. E. Hales. Washington, D.C., American Psychiatric Association Press, pp. 334-352.
80. DeLong, W. B. and Robins, E. (1961). The communication of suicidal intent prior to psychiatric hospitalization. *Am. J. Psychiatry 117*:695-705.
81. Murphy, G. E. (1975). The physicians responsibility for suicide. II. Errors in omission. *Ann. Intern. Med. 82*:305-309.
82. Black, D. W., Winokur, G., Mohondoss, E., Woolson, R. F., and Nasrallah, A. (1989). Does treatment influence mortality in depressives? A follow-up of 1076 patients with major affective disorders. *Ann. Clin. Psychiatry 1*:165-173.
83. Crowe, R. R. (1982). Electroconvulsive therapy—a current perspective. *N. Engl. J. Med. 311*:163-167.
84. Prien, R. F., Kupfer, D. J., Mansky, P. A., Small, J. G., Tuason, V. B., Voss, C. B., and Johnsen, W. F. (1984). Drug therapy in the prevention of recurrences in unipolar and bipolar affective disorders. *Arch. Gen. Psychiatry 41*:1096-1104.
85. Winokur, G., Clayton, P., and Reich, T. (1969). *Manic-Depressive Illness*. St. Louis, C.V. Mosby.
86. Prien, R. F. and Kupfer, D. J. (1986). Continuation drug therapy for major depressive episode: How long should it be maintained? *Am. J. Psychiatry 143*:18-23.

87. Abou-Saleh, M. T. (1987). How long should drug therapy for depression be maintained [Letter]? *Am. J. Psychiatry 144*:1247-1248.
88. Motto, J. A. (1979). The psychopathology of suicide in a clinical model approach. *Am. J. Psychiatry 136*:516-520.
89. Motto, J. A., Heilbron, D. C., and Juster, R. P. (1985). Development of a clinical instrument to estimate suicide risk. *Am. J. Psychiatry 142*:680-686.
90. Murphy, G. E. (1983). On suicide prediction and prevention. *Arch. Gen. Psychiatry 40*:343-344.
91. Bagley, C. (1968). The evaluation of a suicide prevention scheme by an ecological method. *Soc. Sci. Med. 2*:1-14.
92. Jennings, C., Barraclough, B., and Moss, J. R. (1978). Have the Samaritans lowered the suicide rate? A controlled study. *Psychol. Med. 8*:413-422.
93. Weiner, I. W. (1969). The effectiveness of a suicide prevention program. *Ment. Hyg. 53*:357-363.
94. Lester, D. (1974). Effect of suicide prevention centers on suicide rates. *U.S. Health Serv. Ref. 89*:37-39.
95. Bridges, T. P., Potkin, S. G., Zung, W. W. K., and Soldo, B. J. (1977). Suicide prevention centers: Ecological study of effectiveness. *J. Nerv. Ment. Dis. 164*:18-24.
96. Miller, H. L., Cooms, D. W., Leeper, J. D., and Barton, S. M. (1984). An analysis of the effects of suicide prevention facilities on suicide rates in the United States. *Am. J. Public Health 74*:340-343.
97. Huston, P. E. and Locher, L. M. (1948). Involutional melancholia. Course when untreated and treated with electric shock. *Arch. Neurol. Psychiatry 59*:385-394.
98. Huston, P. E. and Locher, L. M. (1948). Manic depressive psychoses. Course when untreated and when treated with electric shock. *Arch. Neurol. Psychiatry 60*:37-48.
99. Ziskind, F., Somerfield-Ziskind, E., and Ziskind, L. (1945). Metrazol and electric convulsive therapy of the affective psychoses. *Arch. Neurol. Psychiatry 53*:212-217.
100. Avery, D. and Winokur, G. (1976). Mortality in depressed patients treated with electroconvulsive therapy and antidepressives. *Arch. Gen. Psychiatry 33*: 1029-1037.
101. Tsuang, M. T., Dempsey, G. M., and Fleming, J. A. (1979). Can ECT prevent premature death in suicide and schizoaffective patients? *J. Affect. Disord. 1*:167-171.
102. Eastwood, M. R. and Peacocke, J. (1976). Seasonal patterns of suicide, depression, and electroconvulsive therapy. *Br. J. Psychiatry 129*:472-475.
103. Babigian, H. M. and Guttmacher, C. B. (1984). Epidemiological considerations in electroconvulsive therapy. *Arch. Gen. Psychiatry 41*:246-253.
104. Milstein, V., Small, J. G., Small, I. F., and Green, G. E. (1986). Does electroconvulsive therapy prevent suicide? *Convuls. Ther. 2*:3-6.
105. Barraclough, B. (1972). Suicide prevention, recurrent affective disorder, and lithium. *Br. J. Psychiatry 121*:391-392.
106. Glen, A. I. M., Dodd, M., Hulme, E. B., and Kreitman, N. (1979). Mortality on lithium. *Neuropsychobiology 5*:167-173.

107. Norton, B. and Whalley, L. J. (1984). Mortality of a lithium treated population. *Br. J. Psychiatry 145*:277-282.
108. Murphy, G. E. (1986). Suicide and attempted suicide. In *Medical Aspects of Psychiatry*. Edited by G. Winokur and P. Clayton, Philadelphia, W.B. Saunders, pp. 562-580.
109. Walk, D. (1967). Suicide and community care. *Br. J. Psychiatry 113*:1381-1391.

Index

About the Editor

Jay D. Amsterdam is Director of the Depression Research Unit at the Hospital of the University of Pennsylvania and Associate Professor of Psychiatry at the University of Pennsylvania School of Medicine, Philadelphia. The author of numerous publications, he is a member of the International Society of Psychoneuroendocrinology, Society of Biological Psychiatry, American Federation for Clinical Research, and a Fellow of the American Psychiatric Association. Dr. Amsterdam received his B.A. degree (1970) from Syracuse University, Syracuse, New York, and M.D. degree (1974) from Jefferson Medical College, Philadelphia, Pennsylvania.